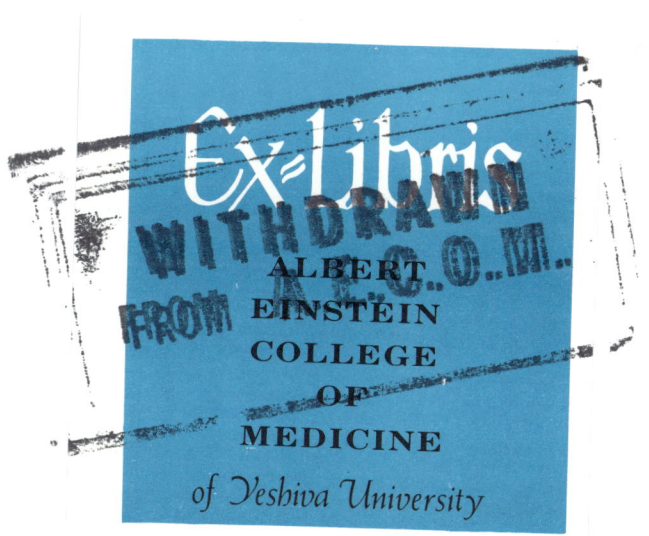

As computerisation in the medical environment has increased, so the advantages of storage and computer analysis of data from various monitoring and measuring equipment have become well recognised. Most medical monitoring and measuring equipment now supports an RS-232 serial interface and therefore allows data to be accessed directly by computer as well as enabling the computer to have control in its turn over the monitoring equipment. This book describes the techniques used for interfacing a PC to a range of medical equipment used internationally in the areas of anaesthesia, intensive care, surgery, respiratory medicine and physiology.

Part I addresses the serial interface, including the RS-232 Standard, transmission of data, and an introduction to serial-interface programming using Microsoft QuickBASIC. Part II looks at electrical safety, the use of Kermit and data analysis. Part III considers the practical aspects of interfacing a PC to a wide range of medical equipment and includes example programs.

This essential practical information constitutes a valuable resource for a very broad audience of PC and measurement equipment users in the medical field.

Interfacing the IBM-PC to medical equipment

INTERFACING THE IBM-PC TO MEDICAL EQUIPMENT:
the art of serial communication

R. W. D. NICKALLS
R. RAMASUBRAMANIAN

With invited contributions by

R. J. HALL
F. JAHAN
J. P. McCARTHY

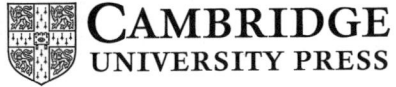

Published by the Press Syndicate of the University of Cambridge
The Pitt Building, Trumpington Street, Cambridge CB2 1RP
40 West 20th Street, New York, NY 10011-4211, USA
10 Stamford Road, Oakleigh, Melbourne 3166, Australia

© Cambridge University Press 1995

First published 1995

Printed in Great Britain at the University Press, Cambridge

A catalogue record of this book is available from the British Library

Library of Congress cataloguing in publication data

Nickalls, R. W. D.
Interfacing the IBM-PC to medical equipment: the art of serial
communication / R.W.D. Nickalls, R. Ramasubramanian; with invited
contributions by R.J. Hall, F. Jahan, J.P. McCarthy.
p. cm.
Includes bibliographical references.
ISBN 0 521 46280 0
1. Medical instruments and apparatus – Data processing.
2. Interface circuits.   3. IBM Personal Computer.   4. Computerized
instruments.   5. Patient monitoring – Data processing.
I. Ramasubramanian, R.   II. Title.
R858.N53 1995
681'.285'4616–dc20   94-19246 CIP

ISBN 0 521 46280 0 hardback

TAG

Contents

List of Contributors		*page* xii
Preface		xiii
Conventions		xvii
Disclaimer		xix
PART I	**THE SERIAL INTERFACE**	**1**
1	**The RS-232 Standard**	**3**
	1.1 Introduction	3
	1.2 Circuits	5
	1.3 Voltages	9
	1.4 Connectors	9
	1.5 Problems with RS-232	10
2	**Transmission of data**	**12**
	2.1 Introduction	12
	2.2 Asynchronous transmission	13
	2.3 Timing of data-line sampling	16
3	**Flow control**	**18**
	3.1 Introduction	18
	3.2 Hardware handshaking	18
	3.3 Software handshaking	19
	3.4 The checksum	21

Contents

4 The PC serial interface — 25
  4.1 Introduction — 25
  4.2 The UART — 25
  4.3 UART addresses — 30
  4.4 UART registers — 32
  4.5 Handling of serial I/O — 41

5 Serial interface programming in QuickBASIC — 44
  5.1 Introduction — 44
  5.2 Opening a serial port — 45
  5.3 Outputting data to a peripheral device — 50
  5.4 Inputting data from the serial port — 51
  5.5 Opening a data-file — 56
  5.6 Reading hidden control characters — 57
  5.7 Accessing data using `ON COM` — 60
  5.8 Accessing a reply code — 63
  5.9 Emptying the Receive buffer — 64
  5.10 Reading a data-file — 65
  5.11 Use of the `LTRIM$` function — 66
  5.12 Time delays — 67
  5.13 Trapping errors — 68
  5.14 Trapping keys — 70
  5.15 The checksum — 71
  5.16 Controlling the output control lines — 72
  5.17 Monitoring the input control lines — 78

PART II MISCELLANEOUS TOPICS — 81

6 Kermit — 83
  6.1 Introduction — 83
  6.2 Setting up Kermit — 83
  6.3 Running Kermit — 85
  6.4 Problems with Kermit — 87

7 Electrical safety and the PC — 88
  7.1 Introduction — 88
  7.2 General aspects of electrical safety — 90
  7.3 Safety of Medical Electrical Equipment — 91
  7.4 General precautions when using PCs — 95

Contents

8	**Data analysis**	**98**
	8.1 General aspects	98
	8.2 Software tools	100
	8.3 Analysis of pulse oximetry data	102
PART III	**THE EQUIPMENT**	**109**
9	**The Ohmeda 3700 and 3740 pulse oximeters**	**111**
	9.1 Introduction	111
	9.2 Serial port	113
	9.3 Auto-output mode	115
	9.4 Control mode	117
	9.5 Trend mode (manual operation)	118
	9.6 Trend mode (initiated by computer)	121
	9.7 Waveform mode	124
	9.8 Slave mode	127
10	**The Nellcor N-200E pulse oximeter**	**129**
	10.1 Introduction	129
	10.2 Serial port	131
	10.3 Beat-to-beat mode	134
	10.4 Computer mode	136
	10.5 Conversation mode	141
	10.6 Accessing stored data	144
11	**The Novametrix 515A pulse oximeter**	**154**
	11.1 Introduction	154
	11.2 Serial port	156
	11.3 Accessing real-time data	158
12	**The Minolta Pulsox-7 pulse oximeter**	**160**
	12.1 Introduction	160
	12.2 Serial port	161
	12.3 Real-time data	162
	12.4 Trend data	164
13	**The Datex Cardiocap™ II and Capnomac Ultima™ series of monitors**	**176**
	13.1 Introduction	176
	13.2 Serial/analog port	179
	13.3 Data format	182

	13.4 Status codes	197
	13.5 Example program	200
14	**The Graseby 3400 syringe pump**	**211**
	14.1 Introduction	211
	14.2 Serial port	214
	14.3 Commands and replies	216
	14.4 Example interactive program	221
	14.5 Programming a continuous infusion	224
15	**The Ohmeda 9000 syringe pump**	**241**
	15.1 Introduction	241
	15.2 Serial port	244
	15.3 Commands and replies	246
	15.4 The checksum	248
	15.5 Data-logging	251
	15.6 Local mode	256
	15.7 Remote mode	257
	15.8 Interactive program for Local/Remote mode	258
	15.9 Programming a continuous infusion	264
16	**The Vitalograph Compact II spirometer**	**272**
	16.1 Introduction	272
	16.2 Serial port	273
	16.3 Communication Modes	275
	16.4 Data format	276
	16.5 Serial Mode 1 (printout without graphs)	280
	16.6 Serial Modes 3, 4, 5 (results and flow data)	283
17	**The Ohmeda 7800 ventilator**	**295**
	17.1 Introduction	295
	17.2 Serial port	296
	17.3 Communication modes	297
	17.4 Commands and replies	298
	17.5 Data formats	300
	17.6 The checksum	304
	17.7 Example interactive program	306
18	**The Dräger Evita intensive care ventilator**	**313**
	18.1 Introduction	313
	18.2 Serial port	314

18.3 Command format 316
18.4 Reply format 317
18.5 Interactive program for accessing telegrams 324
18.6 Program to access the Measured data telegram 329

PART IV APPENDICES 339

Appendix 1 **ASCII control and graphic characters** 341

Appendix 2 **Serial port connector pin-outs** 348

Appendix 3 **Key codes** 350

Appendix 4 **The null modem** 354

Appendix 5 **Program for a device simulator** 358

Appendix 6 **QuickBASIC 4.5 OPEN and OPEN COM statements** 360

Appendix 7 **Plotting data using GNUPLOT** 369

Appendix 8 **Binary and hexadecimal notation** 373

Appendix 9 **Glossary of terms and abbreviations** 375

References 385

Index 395

Contributors

R. J. Hall B.Tech.Eng.
Department of Medical Physics, Nottingham City Hospital NHS Trust, Nottingham, UK.

F. Jahan BSc, MSc.
Department of Medical Physics, Nottingham City Hospital NHS Trust, Nottingham, UK.
email: *100321.600@compuserve.com*

J. P. McCarthy BSc, MSc, C.Eng, MIEE, FIPSM.
Head of Bioengineering Services, University Hospital of Wales and Cardiff Royal Group of Hospitals, Cardiff, UK.
email: *wmpjpm@cardiff.ac.uk*

R. W. D. Nickalls BSc, PhD, MBBS, FRCA.
Senior Lecturer and Consultant, Department of Anaesthesia, University Hospital, Queen's Medical Centre, Nottingham, UK.
email: *dick.nickalls@nottingham.ac.uk*
       100115.1010@compuserve.com

R. Ramasubramanian MBBS, FRCA.
Department of Anaesthesia, Burton Hospitals NHS Trust, Burton-on-Trent, UK.
email: *100016.3245@compuserve.com*

Preface

Most of the monitoring equipment used in hospital medicine has a serial interface, and data can therefore be accessed directly by a PC, processed, and stored on disk. Conversely, many items of medical equipment can also be controlled directly by a PC via the serial interface.

The range of such equipment is growing each year, and currently includes pulse oximeters, non-invasive blood pressure machines, syringe drivers, infusion pumps, spirometers, intravascular oxygen monitors, ventilators, and the comprehensive anaesthesia monitors.

Although most of these devices are extensively used in the fields of anaesthesia, intensive care, and respiratory medicine, there is an increasing use of many of them in other fields. For example, pulse oximeters are now widely used to monitor patients on both medical and surgical wards; they are also beginning to appear in dental clinics. In addition, non-invasive blood pressure monitors and spirometers are appearing increasingly in general practitioner clinics.

However, serial interfacing to such equipment tends to be little used and poorly documented. Furthermore, information regarding the serial interface is widely dispersed throughout a myriad texts and articles.

This book therefore represents an attempt to bring together both the details of serial communication as they relate to an IBM-compatible PC, and the problems associated with interfacing specific items of equipment. Part I addresses the serial interface, including the RS-232 Standard, transmission of data, and an introduction to serial-interface programming using Microsoft QuickBASIC™. Part II addresses a number of related topics, namely electrical safety, analysis of data, and the use of Kermit. Part III considers the practical aspects of interfacing an IBM-compatible PC to a range of equipment found principally in the domains of medicine and physiology, and includes example programs for collecting data and, in some cases, for controlling the equipment directly. The Appendices include a glossary, as well as sections on binary and hexadecimal notation, the ASCII code, pin-outs of serial connectors, programming information, key codes, the null modem, and a note on using the freeware package GNUPLOT.

The programs

All programming examples have been written in QuickBASIC 4.5 since not only is it the most popular compiled BASIC, but it is also particularly well suited for measurement and control applications involving the serial interface. In addition, since QuickBASIC is very similar to the interpreted QBASIC which comes as standard with MS-DOS 5.0 or greater, most of the example programs will also run using QBASIC. Furthermore, a QuickBASIC program can be easily modified for use with Visual Basic.

Although an elementary grounding in BASIC programming will be an advantage when reading this book, prior experience with QuickBASIC or QBASIC is not strictly necessary. However, newcomers to programming will need to have a QuickBASIC manual to hand.

All the example programs have been written with the beginner in mind and are fairly simple; they are not meant to be comprehensive *'all singing, all dancing'* programs. They are simply meant to illustrate one way of either accessing data, or controlling a device, and the reader is expected to modify and expand the programs as necessary to suit his/her particular requirement. For example, while an item of equipment may output several groups of data, the example program may well only demonstrate how to access one particular group of data. Each of the example programs is preceded by a series of 'program points' which we hope are useful.

ASCII font for TeX *and* LaTeX

The manuscript was typeset on a 386-PC using Eberhard Mattes' EmTeX implementation of LaTeX. However, since we were unable to find a TeX font which contained all the symbols commonly used to represent the ASCII control characters (☺ ♪ ‡ etc.; see Appendix 1), we were therefore driven to make our own font.

In due course a font compatible with PostScript printers was eventually made, consisting of the 128 standard ASCII characters *including* the usual symbols for all the control characters. Finally, the font was uploaded to the TeX CTAN archive (**ftp.tex.ac.uk**) as a package called ASCII (see the directory **/pub/archive/fonts/ascii**) which includes the font in various sizes, together with a LaTeX style option called ASCII.STY (Ramasubramanian, Nickalls & Reed, 1993, 1994).

Acknowledgments

First and foremost RWDN would like to thank Elisabeth, Frances and Oliver, for their patience and support throughout the evolution of this book. Special thanks are due to Robert Hall, Faisal Jahan, and Justin McCarthy for becoming involved and contributing Chapters 7 and 16. We also thank all the staff at Cambridge University Press who were involved in the publishing process, and the many people from industry who helped with technical information.

We also thank the British Standards Institution, the American National Standards Institute, and Microsoft Corporation, for allowing us to reproduce material from their publications regarding electrical standards, ASCII, and QuickBASIC 4.5 respectively. We also thank D.J. Sapsford, I.D. Somerville and J.G. Jones for allowing us to reproduce one of their compressed spectral array graphs; Bob Winter for suggesting we include a chapter on Kermit; Novametrix Medical Systems Inc. for supplying the photograph used in Chapter 11; and the Department of Medical Photography (City Hospital, Nottingham) for supplying all the other photographs.

Brand names and product names mentioned in the book are trademarks or registered trademarks of their respective holders.

Subsequent editions

It is envisaged that subsequent editions of this book will incorporate new items of equipment as they become available.

R.W.D. Nickalls
R. Ramasubramanian

June 1994

Conventions

Throughout this book the term PC is used to mean either an IBM-PC or an IBM-compatible PC.

Notation

- All numerals are decimal unless qualified by the suffix b (binary) or h (hexadecimal). Occasionally, in order to avoid confusion, a decimal number may have the suffix d.
- Tall anglebrackets ⟨ ⟩ are used to indicate either ASCII control characters or fields.
  The codes used for representing ASCII control characters are those shown in Appendix 1. For example, the Carriage Return and Start of Header control characters are represented as ⟨CR⟩ and ⟨SOH⟩ respectively.
  A field may be part of a received string of data or part of a string to be sent to a peripheral device, and may represent a number or text or an alphanumeric code. In the following example, ⟨command-code⟩ is a variable field which is included in a command string to be transmitted to a peripheral device.

  ⟨ESC⟩VT⟨command-code⟩⟨CR⟩

  Where a field consists of a specific number of *digits*, the size of the field is often indicated by the appropriate number of n's, e.g. nnnn. However, where a field consists of a specific number of *characters* (i.e. either letters or digits) then this is indicated by the appropriate number of x's, e.g. Cxx.
- Shallow anglebrackets <> are used to indicate a key to be pressed. For example, the key 'Q' is represented as <Q>.

- Throughout this book a 'space' character which is transmitted in a string is represented by the symbol ␣. For example, a device may output a string of 3-digit data fields which are separated by a space; this would be represented as follows.

nnn␣nnn␣nnn␣

- The symbol ^ is used for Ctrl. For example, Ctrl-Q is written as ^Q.

Programs

- All programs are written in Microsoft QuickBASIC 4.5, and are printed using a **bold face typewriter** font, with QuickBASIC 'key words' being printed in uppercase letters, as follows.

```
buffer$ = INPUT$(LOC(1), #1)
```

- Note that QuickBASIC programs consist of a 'main module' and a variable number of 'subroutines' (often known as subprograms) which are called using the CALL statement.
- In program listings some lines are necessarily longer than the page width, in which case they are continued on the next line. However, where this occurs it may not be immediately obvious to those readers not familiar with QuickBASIC. In view of this, the following convention is adopted throughout the book.

Where program lines are *not* normally indented (i.e. in the main module) then line continuations are printed flush with the right margin as follows.

```
OPEN "COM1:1200,E,7,2,CS,DS,CD" FOR RANDOM ACCESS
                                     READ WRITE AS #1
```

Where program lines *are* normally indented (i.e. in subroutines) then line continuations are printed to start flush with the left margin as follows.

```
        CALL emptybuffer
        IF s$ = CHR$(6) THEN message$ = "identification
data telegram"
        IF s$ = CHR$(5) THEN message$ = "measured data
telegram"
```

Disclaimer

The authors and the publisher make no warranties, express or implied, that the programs contained in this volume are free of error, or are consistent with any particular standard of merchantability, or that they will meet your requirements for any particular application. They should not be relied on for solving a problem whose incorrect solution could result in injury to a person or loss of property. If you do use the programs in such a manner, it is at your own risk. The authors and publisher disclaim all liability for direct or consequential damages resulting from your use of the programs.

PART I
THE SERIAL INTERFACE

(1) The RS-232 Standard

(2) Transmission of data

(3) Flow control

(4) The PC serial interface

(5) Serial interface programming in QuickBASIC

1
The RS-232 Standard

1.1 Introduction

The RS-232 serial interface is a so-called low-performance character interface, which converts digital information from the parallel format used within computers and peripherals to the serial format used when sending data from one device to another. It is intended for linking devices which handle data in units of characters, and was originally used to connect computer terminals to modems.

The Standard for the serial interface was established in 1960 by the Electronic Industries Association,† and published as their Recommended Standard 232, hence RS-232. However, in 1986 the prefix RS was superseded by the prefix EIA. This was purely to make clear the origin of their documents, there being no *technical* significance to the change. In 1988 the Telecommunications Industry Association (TIA) was formed by the merger of the US Telephone Suppliers Association and EIA/ITG, and subsequent documents are therefore prefixed by EIA/TIA.

Where an EIA Standard has been approved as an American National Standard this fact is indicated by the prefix ANSI, for example ANSI/EIA-232-D-87, where the last two digits indicate the year of approval as an ANSI Standard.

Over the years the RS-232 Standard has undergone a number of revisions; the third revision in 1969 being known as RS-232-C. This was revised in 1987 and called EIA-232-D. The most recent document at the time of writing is that of the fifth revision in July 1991, known as EIA/TIA-232-E (ANSI/EIA/TIA-232-E-91). However, in spite of the various names and revisions, the interface is still generally known as

---

† Electronic Industries Association, 2001 Pennsylvania Avenue, NW Washington, DC 20006, USA. Tel: +1–202–457–4942. Fax: +1–202–457–4985.

'RS-232', and for convenience will be referred to as such throughout this book.

Useful overviews of the RS-232 Standard are those by Maine (1986), Friend *et al.* (1988), Hughes (1989), and Honig & Hoover (1990). Details of all EIA standards can be found in the annual catalogue of a firm called Global Engineering Documents,† which is the primary distributor for all EIA standards and publications. Some of the documents which relate to the serial interface and connectors are as follows.

- EIA/TIA-232-E (ANSI/EIA/TIA-232-E-91).
  Interface between data terminal equipment and data circuit-terminating equipment employing serial binary data interchange. Electrical Industry Association, July 10th 1991.
- EIA/TIA-530.
  High speed 25-position interface for data terminal equipment and data circuit-terminating equipment. Electrical Industry Association, March 1987.
- Industrial Electronics Bulletin No. 12.
  Application notes on interconnection between interface circuits using EIA-449 and EIA-232-D. Electrical Industry Association, 1987.
- EIA/TIA-363.
  Standard for specifying signal quality for transmitting and receiving data-processing terminal equipment using serial data transmission at the interface with non-synchronous communication equipment. Electrical Industry Association.
- EIA/TIA-404.
  Standard for start-stop signal quality for non-synchronous data communication equipment. Electrical Industry Association.
- CCITT, Blue Book, Fascicle VIII.1, Recommendation V.24.
  List of definitions for interchange circuits between data terminal equipment (DTE) and data circuit-terminating equipment (DCE).
- ISO 2110.
  25-pole DTE/DCE interface connector and contact number assignments. International Standards Organisation.
- EIA/TIA-574.
  9-position non-synchronous interface between data terminal equipment and data circuit-terminating equipment employing serial binary data interchange. Electrical Industry Association.

† Global Engineering Documents, 1990 M Street N.W., Washington, DC 20036, USA. Tel: +1-202-429-2860. Fax: +1-202-331-0960.

The RS-232 Standard

The EIA/TIA-232-E revision is a 36-page document which includes a number of modifications to circuit definitions, a specification for an alternative 26-pin interface connector (EIA/TIA-232-E ALT A), a list of 'Recommendations and explanatory notes', and a Glossary. Four aspects of the communications interface are addressed, as follows.

- Functional characteristics of the three circuit groups (data, control, timing).
- Electrical and grounding characteristics of the signals.
- Mechanical characteristics of connectors and cables.
- Standard interfaces for selected communication system configurations.

1.2 Circuits

The RS-232 Standard allocates specific serial communications circuits to specific pins of 25/26-pin connectors, as shown in Table 1.1. Since the pin number of the various circuits varies with the connector (9, 15, and 25/26 pins), the standard three-letter function codes are always used when referring to the RS-232 circuits in order to avoid confusion.

The EIA-232-D revision gave two of the circuits new names (see Honig & Hoover, 1990). Thus the circuit previously known as Data Terminal Ready (DTR) was renamed DTE Ready. Similarly, Data Set Ready (DSR) was renamed DCE Ready. However, since virtually all books on the subject still use the old RS-232-C names, the function codes DTR and DSR will continue to be used throughout this book.

Note that in practice only 9 of the circuits shown in Table 1.1 are generally used by the PC's serial interface, hence the widespread use of the 9-pin interface connector. These circuits (Table 1.2) together with their direction (input or output) are shown in Figure 1.1.

The serial interface circuits running between the computer and the peripheral device can be classified into four groups as follows.

- Ground
- Data
- Control
- Timing

These will now be described in some detail with the exception of the timing circuits, since these are not used in the asynchronous form of data transmission employed by IBM compatible PCs.

Table 1.1. *EIA/TIA-232-E pin assignments for 25/26-pin connectors.*

Pin No.	Code	Descriptive name
1		Shield
2	TxD	Transmits data
3	RxD	Receives data
4	RTS	Request to send/ready for receiving
5	CTS	Clear to send
6	DSR	Data set ready (DCE ready)
7	GND	Signal ground
8	DCD	Data carrier detect (received line signal detector)
9		RESERVED FOR TESTING
10		RESERVED FOR TESTING
11		UNASSIGNED
12		Secondary received line signal detector
13		Secondary clear to send
14		Secondary transmitted data
15		Transmitter signal element timing—DCE source
16		Secondary received data
17		Receiver signal element timing
18		Local loopback
19		Secondary request to send
20	DTR	Data terminal ready (DTE ready)
21		Remote loopback/signal quality detector
22	RI	Ring indicator
23		Data signal rate selector
24		Transmitter signal element timing—DTE source
25		Test mode
26		Alt A connector only—not connected

Table 1.2. *Pin assignments for 9-pin serial port connectors.*

Pin No.	Code	Descriptive name
1	DCD	Data carrier detect
2	RxD	Receives data
3	TxD	Transmits data
4	DTR	Data terminal ready
5	GND	Signal ground
6	DSR	Data set ready
7	RTS	Request to send
8	CTS	Clear to send
9	RI	Ring indicator

1.2.1 Ground circuits

Two ground circuits exist, namely

- Shield (chassis ground)
- Signal ground (GND)

The shield pin, when available,† should be connected to the equipment chassis. Where a shielded cable is used, then the shield should be connected to the shield pin at one end only.‡ *Never* connect the shield at both ends of the cable (Friend *et al.*, 1988). Note that the protective ground is not used with 9-pin connectors.

Signal ground (GND) is the reference for all cables and must, therefore, be connected at both ends.

1.2.2 Data circuits

Two wires are assigned to carry data, one for each direction. The 25-pin connectors have the computer receiving data on pin-3 (Receives data; RxD), and transmitting data on pin-2 (Transmits data; TxD). Note that this order is reversed when using 9-pin connectors (see Tables 1.1 and 1.2).

When interfacing computers to other equipment, therefore, it is important to check that the pin receiving data at the computer (RxD) is connected to the pin used for transmitting data from the peripheral device (TxD), and vice versa.

1.2.3 Control circuits

Six control circuits are used by microcomputers, and are commonly known as 'handshaking' lines. The control circuits are used to enable the computer and the other device to communicate to each other such things as whether they are switched on or not, or whether they are ready to receive data or not. This is achieved very simply by setting the respective control line voltage either HIGH (positive) or LOW (negative).

For example, when a printer using hardware handshaking runs out of paper, it will set one of its control lines either HIGH or LOW depending on the particular code used. This voltage change will be sensed by the

---

† A pin is allocated for the shield only on 25-pin connectors, and on the new alternative (Alt A) 26-pin connector described in EIA/TIA-232-E.

‡ EIA/TIA-232-E indicates that *Normally the DCE should make no connection to the interface connector contact number 1.*

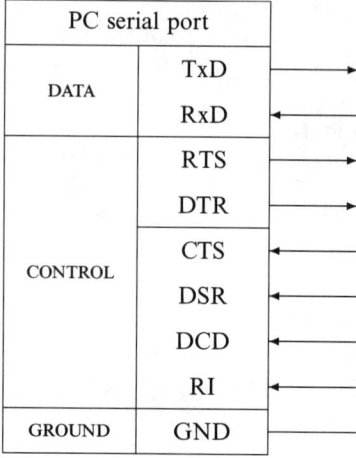

Fig. 1.1. Schematic diagram showing the 9 circuits used by the PC's serial port. Note that the PC has 4 *input* control lines, but only 2 *output* control lines.

computer and interpreted as a signal to stop sending data. When the paper tray has been reloaded the printer resets the control line, and the computer will resume sending data.

The six control circuits, together with their short codes, are as follows.

- Request to Send (RTS)
- Clear to Send (CTS)
- Data Set Ready (DSR)
- Data Carrier Detect (DCD)
- Data Terminal Ready (DTR)
- Ring Indicator (RI)

The curious names of the control circuits arise from the fact that the circuits were originally designed for connecting equipment to modems. Both the names and the number of circuits therefore reflect the fairly complex control-line signalling which modems use when synchronising the flow of data traffic in the two data lines RxD and TxD.

It is important to appreciate the *direction* of signalling in the various control lines—see Figure 1.1. The PC has two output control circuits (RTS, DTR) which it can use to communicate with the peripheral device. These two output control circuits are controlled by the computer's Modem Control Register (see Chapter 4). Conversely, the PC receives incoming control signals from the peripheral device via the remaining four control circuits (CTS, DSR, DCD, RI). The status of these four input control circuits is monitored by the computer's Modem Status Register (see Chapter 4).

1.3 Voltages

The RS-232 Standard specifies certain conditions as follows.

- Positive voltages should be in the range +3 to +15 volts; negative voltages should be in the range −3 to −15 volts.
- The interface should tolerate without damage up to ±25 volts at the input.
- It should be possible to short across any two lines without damage.

The transmission line voltages produced by RS-232 line-driver chips are usually within the range ±9 to ±15 volts depending on the particular line-driver chip used. The range of transmission line voltages is, therefore, considerably greater than that of the TTL (transistor-transistor logic) circuits used within the PC (0–5 volts). The reason for this difference is historical, since RS-232 predates modern chip technology.

The interpretation of the RS-232 transmission voltages is initially somewhat confusing, since those on the two *data* lines (TxD, RxD) are inverted relative to the TTL voltages used within the devices, while those on the six *control* lines (RTS, CTS, etc) are not inverted.

Thus a positive control line voltage is counted as HIGH (ON, TRUE, RAISED, ASSERTED), and a negative one as LOW (OFF, FALSE, LOWERED). However, for the data lines, logic 1 (Marking) is transmitted as a negative voltage, and logic 0 (Spacing) as a positive voltage.† The idle, or inactive, line state which exists on the data lines between data transmissions is a negative voltage.

1.4 Connectors

Although an interface connector was not defined in the original RS-232 Standard, the 25-pin D-shell connector has been generally adopted, and was incorporated into the EIA-232-D revision (Honig & Hoover, 1990). The mechanical aspects of the connector are detailed in the document EIA/TIA-530. The convention is that computers have male connectors and peripherals have female connectors, although not all manufacturers adhere to this.

† The terms Marking, Spacing are often contracted to Mark, Space.

A new aspect of the EIA/TIA-232-E revision is the inclusion of a specification for a smaller Alternative 26-pin D-shell interface connector (EIA/TIA-232-E Alt A). The 26-pin Alt A connector is about half the size of the usual 25-pin connector. Note that the Alt A connector has the *same* pin-outs as the 25-pin connector, with the addition of pin-26 which is unallocated.

Since IBM's implementation of RS-232 makes use of only nine channels, many devices and computers have adopted the 9-pin D-shell connector. However, a large number of peripheral devices still use either a 15 or 25-pin D-shell connector, and utilise either unassigned channels or those nominally reserved for testing, in order to transmit a number of useful signals. These are commonly additional power lines (either AC or DC or both), analog signals, or extra signal ground (GND) lines.

The D-shell connectors are sometimes named according to a 'DXn' convention, where D codes for the shape of the shell, X codes for the size, and n gives the number of pins (Honig & Hoover, 1990). Consequently, the 25-pin and 9-pin serial port connectors are occasionally referred to as DB25 and DE9 respectively.

1.5 Problems with RS-232

Although the RS-232 interface is widely used and works well, there are limitations, particularly with regard to the maximum bit rate (20 K bits/sec), transmission distance, and the use of a common signal ground (see Friend *et al.*, 1988). As a result of these and other problems, a number of different interface standards have been developed which are capable of much greater bit rates, e.g. RS-423 (100 K bits/sec), RS-422 (10 M bits/sec).

Of these newer interface standards, only the RS-423 interface (logic 1 +3.6 to +6 volts; logic 0 −3.6 to −6 volts) is compatible with RS-232. Note that since RS-232 signals are considerably greater than those for RS-423 circuits, any connection between the two circuits should use an appropriate attenuator circuit (see Maine, 1986).

A comparison of the electronic specifications of the various EIA standards (RS-232, RS-423, RS-422, RS-485) is given in the RS Data Sheet 6985.†

---

† RS Components Ltd., Birchington Road, Weldon, Corby, Northamptonshire, NN17 9RS, UK.

1.5.1 Distance

The RS-232 Standard specifies maximum limits for the duration of the transition time from HIGH to LOW, and vice versa. For example, for data circuits the transition time must be less than 4% of the bit period. This therefore restricts the amount of stray capacitance allowed in a cable since the transition time is a function of capacitance. In addition, the Standard also specifies that the total cable capacitance should be less than 2500 picofarads (pF). Since the capacitance of cables used in data communications is in the range 40–200 pF/m† the maximum length can theoretically be as great as 62 m depending on the particular cable. In practice, such long lengths are not recommended since the likelihood of noise being picked up and causing data corruption increases with length. However, since the bit period is inversely related to the bit rate, even greater lengths (e.g. 1000 feet) can work satisfactorily providing slow bit rates are used (Campbell, 1989a).

1.5.2 Ground

Because the RS-232 interface is technically an 'unbalanced' system (i.e. all the control and data signals are referenced to a common signal ground), there is the possibility that transmission errors may arise if there is a significant difference in ground potential between the two ends of the cable. This is another reason for keeping the interface cable relatively short since the further the peripheral device is from the PC, the greater the likelihood that their GND pins will be at significantly different potentials (Friend *et al.*, 1988).

† The flat Speedbloc ribbon cable commonly used for serial interfacing has a nominal capacitance of 49 pF/m (RS Catalogue).

2
Transmission of data

2.1 Introduction

All data which passes between the PC and a peripheral device is transmitted along one of the two data-lines, namely the Transmit (TxD) and Receive (RxD) lines. The data itself consists of a stream of characters (e.g. letters, numbers, symbols), and in view of this the RS-232 interface is known as a character interface.

Each character is coded as a unique sequence of either seven or eight logic states, consisting of combinations of logic 1 (negative) or logic 0 (positive). The individual 1's and 0's which collectively represent a character are known as **bits**, and a group of eight bits is known as a **byte**.

The most widely used character code is the ASCII code (American Standard Code for Information Interchange).† The 'standard' ASCII code is a 7-bit code (see Appendix 1), which represents a fixed set of 128 control and graphic characters ($128 = 2^7$). However, by using 8 bits the code is extended to include an additional 128 characters and symbols making a total of 256 ($256 = 2^8$). The additional 128 characters is known as the 'extended' ASCII code.

7-bit formats are commonly used by peripheral devices which are able to output data directly to a computer; familiar examples being some of the automatic blood pressure machines and pulse oximeters. For such devices the 7-bit ASCII code is often quite adequate, since they usually use only a limited number of characters for transmitting alpha-numeric data.

Other character codes do exist but are not widely used, namely the 5-bit Baudot code (used in old telex machines), the 5-bit Murray code, and the 8-bit EBCDIC code (Extended Binary-Coded-Data Interchange Code) (Maine, 1986).

† American National Standard X3.4 (1986). Available from American National Standards Institute, 11 West 42nd Street, New York, N.Y. 10036, USA.

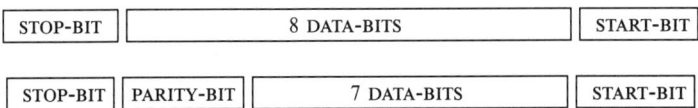

Fig. 2.1. Character-frames for 7 and 8-bit codes.

During transmission, the PC sends bits one at a time along the Transmit data line (TxD). However, since the bits are coded as a voltage—either positive (logic 0) or negative (logic 1)†—a system of synchronisation is required to enable the receiver to know when to sample the voltages, and so determine the nature of the bits (logic 1 or 0). To this end, a number of techniques for serial synchronisation exist, namely **synchronous**, **enchronous**, **isochronous**, and **asynchronous** (Cripps, 1989). In the synchronous form, both the sending and receiving devices have their resident clocks synchronised using an extra cable running in parallel, which allows the receiving device to identify bits according to their timing.

Since distance communication has to be achieved using only a single wire (allowing telephone lines to be used), an asynchronous form of serial interfacing was developed which allows data to be transmitted intermittently, without the need for an extra synchronisation cable.

2.2 Asynchronous transmission

Asynchronous transmission is the method used by all IBM compatible PCs for serial interfacing. It is achieved by embedding the data-bits within a so-called **frame** of extra control bits which indicate the beginning (**start-bit**) and end (**stop-bit**) of the data-bits (see Dettmann, 1989). This sequence of bits, including the start and stop-bits, is known as a **character-frame**.

The great advantage of this system is that it keeps the timing *within* a character-frame correctly synchronised using only the resident timing clock, while allowing the interval *between* character-frames to be quite variable.

The total number of bits in a character-frame is usually 10.‡ Providing all the codes which need to be transmitted are included within the standard 128 character ASCII code, then only seven data-bits are required. In this case the redundant eighth bit can then be used for checking

† See Section 1.3.
‡ If two stop-bits are used then the character-frame will consist of 11 bits.

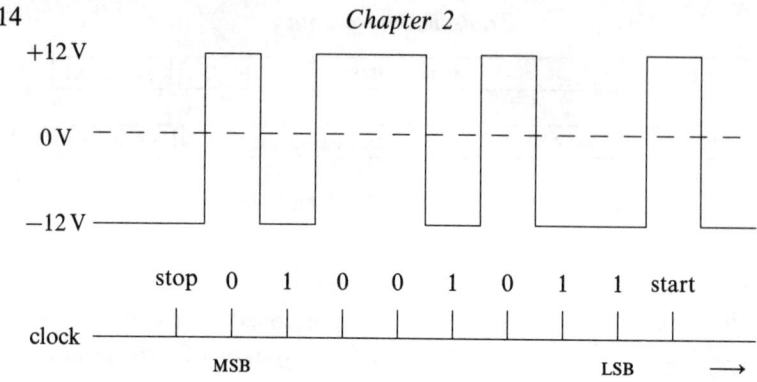

Fig. 2.2. Character-frame representing the letter K.

purposes, whereupon it is termed a **parity-bit** (see Section 2.2.3). The structure of a typical character-frame when using 7-bit and 8-bit codes is shown in Figure 2.1.

Asynchronous transmission is, therefore, a relatively inefficient system since only 7 or 8 bits in each frame represent data. However, this slight disadvantage is more than offset by the fact that such a system allows data to be transmitted intermittently since, providing both the transmitter and receiver process bits at the same frequency (**bit rate**), the receiver can read the data-bits accurately by first detecting the start-bit.

The data-bits are always transmitted in reverse order, with the least significant bit (LSB) being sent first, and the most significant bit (MSB) being sent last. The reason for this is that some character codes use less than 8 data-bits, and therefore bit-7 is not always a data-bit, but bit-0 is *always* the first data-bit (Microsoft, 1990b).

The transmission speed is expressed as bits-per-second (bps); typical bit rates being 2400, 4800, 9600 bps. The term **baud** (after Jean Maurice Emile Baudot, 1845–1903) is also commonly referred to in this context, although strictly it refers to modulation rate (Banks, 1990).† However, for systems transmitting one bit at a time bps and baud are identical (Honig & Hoover, 1990).

An example of how a character is transmitted via one of the RS-232 data lines (RxD, TxD) is shown in Figure 2.2, which illustrates a data-frame representing the character K (01001011b; 75d; 4Bh) travelling

---

† See also the articles in the CompuServe communications forum IBMCOM, e.g. baud.thd, baudrt.thd, bit-ba.txt, bitsbaud.txt.

Table 2.1. *Parity options.*

Odd	Parity-bit makes the total odd
Even	Parity-bit makes the total even
Mark	Parity-bit is always set to 1
Space	Parity-bit is always set to 0
None	No parity-bit used

from left to right, consisting of 8 data-bits, 1 start-bit, and 1 stop-bit. Note that the inactive state for a data line is a negative voltage.

2.2.1 Start-bit

In asynchronous transmission a start-bit is always sent immediately before the data-bits which code for the character being transmitted.

2.2.2 Data-bits

These are the bits representing the character being sent. If the standard ASCII character set is being used (128 characters), then only 7 data-bits are required, in which case the eighth bit is used as a parity-bit. The extended ASCII character set uses 256 characters, and therefore requires 8 data-bits.

2.2.3 Parity-bit

Parity is a simple error-checking system used for determining whether a character has been received correctly, and can only be used with a 7-bit character code. Parity is implemented by adding-up the data-bits set to 1, and then setting a parity-bit (either 1 or 0) depending on the parity system being used. For example, with Even parity, the parity-bit is calculated to make the total even. When an 8-bit code is used, there is no parity-bit, and the parity option None is used. The parity options are shown in Table 2.1.

2.2.4 Stop-bit

In asynchronous transmission, a stop-bit (or bits) is sent following the parity-bit (if used) (a) to give the receiver time to process the data-bits,

Table 2.2. *Protocol options.*

Bit rate	110, 150, 300, 600, 1200, 1800, 2400, 4800, 9600, 19200
Data-bits	5, 6, 7, 8
Parity	Even, Odd, None, Mark, Space
Stop-bits	1, 1.5, 2

and (b) to return the data line to the inactive negative voltage state (see Figure 2.2).

It is usual to use only one stop-bit. However, two stop-bits are sometimes used. For example, the Dräger Evita ventilator described in Chapter 18 uses two stop-bits and can accommodate bit rates as low as 50 bps. Systems using only five data-bits use 1.5 stop-bits (Waite *et al.*, 1990).

2.2.5 *Communications protocol*

The particular bit rate and configuration of bits within a character-frame is generally known as the **protocol**. While a range of protocols can often be used, the protocol must of course be the same for both the computer and the peripheral device.

In practice, a suitable protocol is first selected from the options available for the computer and the peripheral device. This is then set on the peripheral device, and also specified in the computer program which will control the computer's serial interface.† The usual protocol options are shown in Table 2.2.

2.3 Timing of data-line sampling

Accurate sampling of incoming data voltages is achieved by having the receive clock running considerably faster than the bit rate, usually at 16 times the bit rate (Friend *et al.*, 1988). Such a fast rate allows the onset of the start-bit to be detected within a small fraction of the normal bit period. Once the voltage transition from negative (logic 1) to positive (logic 0) which marks the beginning of the start-bit is detected, the receiver counts 8 cycles, which takes it very close to the middle of the start-bit, and checks to see if the voltage is still positive. If it is not, then the transition is assumed to be due to noise, and the receiver waits for

† See the OPEN COM statement in Chapter 5 and Appendix 6.

another start-bit. If the voltage is still positive, then the receiver assumes that a true start-bit has been detected, and it starts measuring the line voltage on every subsequent 16th cycle, i.e. close to the middle of each bit period. After counting the correct number of bits the receiver finally checks that the stop-bit has the correct voltage; any problem here signals a **framing** error.

The receiver resets its counter with each voltage transition, and so eliminates errors which might otherwise arise if the timing clocks in the computer and peripheral device differed significantly in rate (Cripps, 1989). Furthermore, the fact that the start-bit (positive) and stop-bit (negative) have opposite polarity means that there will always be at least one voltage transition for each character, which means that the two resident clocks can theoretically differ by up to 5% without giving rise to a framing error.

3
Flow control

3.1 Introduction

A number of techniques exist for controlling the flow of data via the serial port (Cullimore, 1987; Friend *et al.*, 1988; Campbell, 1989b). Such control is termed **handshaking**, and can be achieved either by setting positive (HIGH) or negative (LOW) voltages on the control lines (**hardware handshaking**), or by sending certain control characters or escape sequences via the data lines (**software handshaking**).†

Checking for data corruption during transfer is commonly achieved using some form of **checksum** or **cyclic redundancy check**.

3.2 Hardware handshaking

This form of handshaking refers to the method by which the computer and peripheral device signal to one another using the serial port control lines. These lines are often known as handshaking lines and are used in a variety of ways.

One of the roles of the handshaking lines is to *control* data outflow. For example, many peripheral devices will not output data unless one of their input control lines (often CTS) is held HIGH by the computer, which must therefore use one of its two output control lines (either RTS or DTR) to do this. Usually the computer maintains the control line HIGH until all the data has been downloaded.

Sometimes, however, the data from a peripheral device can only be accessed by the computer repeatedly toggling one of the control lines LOW and then HIGH. For example, the Minolta Pulsox-7 pulse oximeter (see Chapter 12) only transmits three bytes of Trend data in response

† See Chapter 1 for details of the control lines.

to each transition of its CTS from LOW to HIGH. Although complicated, such a system can be useful if a lot of data processing has to be done *en route*, since it allows the computer to access the data when it is ready.

Hardware handshaking is often used to indicate an alarm state. For example, the Nellcor N-200E pulse oximeter sets its pin-9 (RI) HIGH whenever any of its alarms are activated. The computer can therefore be made aware of the alarms by having this pin connected to one of the computer's spare input control lines, and then monitoring the line by inspecting the computer's Modem Status Register (see Chapter 4).

Because most devices set at least one of the output control lines HIGH when powered up and running, the PC can determine whether or not communications can proceed by monitoring the appropriate line. In addition, some devices use one of their output control lines to indicate when they are ready to receive commands. For example, the Graseby 3400 syringe pump (see Chapter 14) sets its RTS HIGH when it is powered up, and sets its DSR HIGH when the pump is able to receive and process commands from the PC.

3.3 Software handshaking

Software handshaking is achieved by transmitting certain control characters and/or escape sequences via the data lines. In this case only three lines are needed for communications, namely transmit (TxD), receive (RxD), and signal ground (GND).

Two well established software control systems are in common use, namely the character protocol XON/XOFF, and the automatic repeat request (ARQ) protocol ETX/ACK which incorporates error-checking codes (e.g. checksum). In practice, however, there is no standardisation in this area with respect to medical equipment, and the particular codes and formats vary considerably, with many devices using either a variation of one of the standard protocols, or their own non-standard software codes.

3.3.1 Escape sequence

The ⟨ESC⟩ control character (ASCII 27) is one of the three 'code extension' control characters (see Appendix 1), and is used to indicate that the consecutive sequence of characters following the escape character (i.e. the escape sequence) is to be considered as a special code or instruction.

Table 3.1. *Transmission control characters.*

Char	Dec	Hex	DOS		Meaning
SOH	1	01h	^A	☺	start of heading
STX	2	02h	^B	☻	start of text
ETX	3	03h	^C	♥	end of text
EOT	4	04h	^D	♦	end of transmission
ENQ	5	05h	^E	♣	enquiry
ACK	6	06h	^F	♠	acknowledge
DLE	16	10h	^P	►	data link escape
NAK	21	15h	^U	§	negative acknowledge
SYN	22	16h	^V	▬	synchronous idle
ETB	23	17h	^W	‡	end transmission block

3.3.2 XON/XOFF

This system uses the two device control characters ⟨DC1⟩ and ⟨DC3⟩ known as Device Control 1 and Device Control 3 respectively. They are also commonly known as XON and XOFF respectively (see Appendix 1).

Sending XOFF tells the peripheral device to stop sending data, while sending XON tells the device to resume data transmission (Cullimore, 1987). For example, where this system is used with a printer, the printer will send XOFF to the PC when its input buffer is approximately 80% full, and send XON when the buffer size has fallen to about 20% full (Friend et al., 1988).

Neither QuickBASIC nor Microsoft BASIC supports the XON/XOFF protocol (Microsoft, 1991a). However, the program QBserial 2.0, which is available from the CompuServe QuickBASIC forum and runs using QuickBASIC 4.5, contains serial I/O routines which do support XON/XOFF handshaking.

3.3.3 ARQ protocols

There are a number of file transfer systems based on an automatic repeat request (ARQ) protocol, which uses four of the transmission control characters, namely ⟨STX⟩, ⟨ETX⟩, ⟨ACK⟩, and ⟨NAK⟩ (see Table 3.1), to facilitate accurate data transfer (Cullimore, 1987; Campbell, 1989b; Jackson, 1992).

The principle underlying the ARQ protocol is that the data to be transmitted is split up into a number of relatively small data-blocks, each of which is then transmitted within a so-called **data-packet**. Each

Flow control

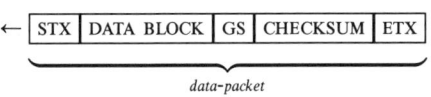

Fig. 3.1. The structure of a data-packet. In this example the group separator ⟨GS⟩ is used to separate the checksum from the data. The arrow indicates that the control character ⟨STX⟩ is transmitted first.

data-packet consists of a **data-block** and **checksum** (used for checking purposes; see Section 3.4), bracketed by the control characters ⟨STX⟩ and ⟨ETX⟩ as shown in Figure 3.1. The group separator ⟨GS⟩ is sometimes used to separate the checksum from the data.†

After sending each data-packet, the transmitting device waits for the control character ⟨ACK⟩ before sending the next data-packet. If the receiving device finds that the data-block does not tally with the checksum it sends back the control character ⟨NAK⟩, whereupon the transmitting device sends the data-packet again. If the received data-block agrees with the relevant checksum then the reply is ⟨ACK⟩, whereupon the transmitting device then sends the next data-packet.

Both the error-checking techniques and the size of the data-block used vary considerably. For example, XMODEM transmits data in 128-byte blocks and uses an 8-bit checksum; XMODEM-1K allows the use of 1028-byte data-blocks; XMODEM/CRC uses a 16-bit cyclic redundancy check (CRC) error code with each block (Gofton, 1986); and ZMODEM allows the option of using a 32-bit CRC code (Jackson, 1992).

3.4 The checksum

A checksum is an error-checking device used when sending data, and is a numeric value derived from the characters making up the data. Providing the received checksum agrees with that derived from the received data, it is assumed that the received data is correct.

Unfortunately the usual terminology is somewhat ambiguous, with two quite different checksums being referred to as the 'checksum'. When the term **checksum** is unqualified, it is taken to mean the remainder left over after dividing the sum of the ASCII decimal codes of all the relevant characters by some arbitrary value (commonly either 128 or 256). To avoid confusion, this book will refer to this particular checksum as a

† The four ASCII information separators ⟨FS⟩, ⟨GS⟩, ⟨RS⟩, ⟨US⟩ are described in Appendix 1.

$\leftarrow \underbrace{\langle\text{STX}\rangle\langle\text{data}\rangle\langle\text{CR}\rangle\langle\text{LF}\rangle}_{checksum}\langle\Sigma\text{-checksum}\rangle\langle\text{ETX}\rangle$

Fig. 3.2. Format of a Nellcor N-200E pulse oximeter data-packet, showing that the Nellcor checksum is calculated from the data *and* the $\langle\text{CR}\rangle\langle\text{LF}\rangle$ pair.

Σ-checksum.† However, a variation is the **two's complement checksum** which, when added to the character sum and then divided, gives a remainder of zero. This book will refer to this particular checksum as a TC-checksum. Both checksums are described in detail below.

Note that the particular characters on which the checksum is calculated vary considerably from one device to another, and it is therefore important to determine exactly which characters in the transmitted string are included in the checksum. Furthermore the form the checksum takes also varies, being either the equivalent ASCII character, the decimal value, or the hexadecimal value. For example, the Nellcor N-200E pulse oximeter (see Chapter 10) which transmits data using the format shown in Figure 3.2, uses a Σ-checksum (transmitted as the equivalent ASCII character) which includes all data characters *and* both the $\langle\text{CR}\rangle\langle\text{LF}\rangle$ control characters but *not* the $\langle\text{STX}\rangle$ or $\langle\text{ETX}\rangle$ control characters.

3.4.1 Σ-checksum

Typically the Σ-checksum is an 8-bit value, and therefore represents the lowest 8 bits of the sum of the character codes; i.e. the remainder left over after dividing the sum by 256. Since the lowest 8 bits represent a number in the range 0–255, an 8-bit Σ-checksum is also referred to as a *modulo*256 Σ-checksum. A 7-bit Σ-checksum is also commonly used, and is the remainder after dividing by 128; i.e. it is a *modulo*128 Σ-checksum. Thus, if the sum was 130 then the remainder after dividing by 128 would be expressed as $(130) modulo 128 = 2$.

As an example, consider the Graseby 3400 syringe pump (see Chapter 14) which uses a two-character 8-bit hexadecimal Σ-checksum (e.g. A3). Suppose it is necessary to determine the checksum required when sending the command 'STOP'. The command format for this device requires that the command is enclosed in anglebrackets <> which are also included in the checksum as follows.

† The prefix Σ (sigma) is chosen here in view of its use in mathematics to signify a summation.

$\underbrace{\text{<STOP>}}_{checksum}$ ⟨hex Σ-checksum⟩⟨CR⟩⟨LF⟩

The 8-bit Σ-checksum is derived as follows; note that the sum of the ASCII codes of the 6 characters <STOP> is 448.

$$\begin{aligned}\text{8-bit Σ-checksum} &= (\text{<STOP>}) modulo 256 \\ &= (60 + 83 + 84 + 79 + 80 + 62) modulo 256 \\ &= (448) modulo 256 \\ &= 192 \\ &= \text{C0h}\end{aligned}$$

In this case the hexadecimal Σ-checksum is C0, which is two hexadecimal characters and therefore satisfies the Graseby 3400 command format. The full command string to be sent to the pump is therefore as follows.

<STOP>⟨C0⟩⟨CR⟩⟨LF⟩

However, if the Σ-checksum is less than 16 (decimal), then its hexadecimal equivalent is only a single character. In this case, therefore, the hexadecimal Σ-checksum would have to be prefixed with a zero in order to make it two characters, and so satisfy the Graseby command format. For example, if the hexadecimal Σ-checksum was B (11 decimal), it would have to be transmitted as the two characters 0B.

A QuickBASIC function for calculating an 8-bit Σ-checksum and converting it to a two-character hexadecimal checksum is given in Chapter 5. This function is also used in the example interactive program for the Graseby 3400 syringe pump (see Chapter 14).

3.4.2 Two's complement checksum (TC-checksum)

The TC-checksum is a numeric value such that when it is included in the character sum and then divided, the remainder is zero. For a 7-bit TC-checksum this is equivalent to the following equation, where 'data' represents the sum of the relevant data characters, and $(data) modulo 128$ means the remainder after dividing the data sum by 128.

$$\text{TC-checksum} = 128 - (data) modulo 128$$

The 7-bit TC-checksum is used by a number of medical devices; two such devices being the Ohmeda 7800 ventilator (see Chapter 17) and the Ohmeda 9000 syringe pump (see Chapter 15).

For example, when the Ohmeda 7800 ventilator's TC-checksum is enabled the affirmative reply string in response to a command is as follows.

:VTYC⟨CR⟩

In this case the reply to be sent to the computer is actually the string :VTY, following which the ventilator adds the TC-checksum which in this case is the character C (ASCII 67). Here the TC-checksum relates to the string :VTY and is calculated as follows.

$$
\begin{aligned}
\text{TC-checksum} &= 128 - (\text{:VTY}) modulo 128 \\
&= 128 - (58 + 86 + 84 + 89) modulo 128 \\
&= 128 - (317) modulo 128 \\
&= 128 - 61 \\
&= 67 \\
&= C
\end{aligned}
$$

Two's complement is related to **one's complement**, which is equivalent to the logic operation NOT; the relationship is as follows.

$$\text{two's complement} = \text{one's complement} + 1$$

In order to illustrate this, the previous example worked out using the binary notation would be as follows.

$$
\begin{aligned}
100111101 &= \text{:VTY} = 58 + 86 + 84 + 89 = 317 \\
011000010 &= \text{one's complement} (= \text{NOT } 317) \\
011000011 &= \text{two's complement} (= \text{one's complement} + 1) \\
11000011 &= \text{7-bit two's complement checksum} (= \text{lowest 7 bits}) \\
&= 67 \\
&= C
\end{aligned}
$$

A QuickBASIC function to calculate a two's complement checksum is given in Chapter 5. This function is used in the example interactive program given in Chapter 15 on the Ohmeda 9000 syringe pump.

3.4.3 *Cyclic redundancy check (CRC)*

This is a powerful error-checking technique involving *modulo 2* arithmetic, and is generally used for checking file transfers (Campbell, 1989b; Gofton, 1986; Goodwin, 1992; Halsal, 1992). CRC is not used by any devices described in this book.

4
The PC serial interface

4.1 Introduction

Most PCs have at least one serial communication port which, from a programming point of view, is known as a COM port since COM is the term that the operating systems MS-DOS and OS/2 use to identify the serial interface. Thus COM1 and COM2 refer to serial ports 1 and 2 respectively.

MS-DOS versions prior to 3.3 supported only 2 serial ports (COM1 & COM2). MS-DOS 3.3 extended this to the use of 4 serial ports. The OS/2 operating system allows the use of up to 8 serial ports (Honig & Hoover, 1990).

4.2 The UART

IBM compatible PCs receive and transmit bits in and out of the serial port using a chip known as the UART (Universal Asynchronous Receiver/Transmitter), which is based on the Intel 8250 Asynchronous Communications Controller (Dettmann, 1989; Aitken, 1992; Van Gilluwe, 1994). A number of devices are available for performing serial I/O (see Vears, 1990), and these are variously named according to their abilities, as shown in Table 4.1.

The 8250 UART was used in the original XT specification. This has since been superseded in the AT and PS/2 machines by the faster backward-compatible UARTs 16450 and 16550 respectively (Margolis, 1989, 1990; Phoenix, 1991; O'Brien, 1992).

However both the 16450 and the 8250 have only a 1-byte data-holding register for input and output, and consequently tend to lose data with very fast bit rates. This is because data may arrive faster than it can be processed, with the effect that new data overwrites the old data in

Table 4.1. *Serial I/O devices.*

UART	Universal Asynchronous Receiver/Transmitter
USART	Universal Synchronous/Asynchronous Receiver/Transmitter
DART	Dual Asynchronous Receiver/Transmitter
ACIA	Asynchronous Communications Receiver/Transmitter
SIA	Serial Input/Output controller

the Receive data register. In order to accommodate faster bit rates and multi-tasking environments, the UART therefore required a significant data buffer of its own. This problem led to the development of the 16550 UART, which had a 16-byte cache FIFO (first-in-first-out) data buffer associated with each of the Receive and Transmit registers (Prosise, 1989; Collin, 1992; Goodwin, 1992; O'Brien, 1992; Oliver, 1993).

While both the 16550 and the later 16550A had problems associated with the FIFO buffer, these were corrected in the later AF, C, and CF versions (Van Gilluwe, 1994). The AFN upgrade (16550AFN) features FIFO queues, DMA† transfer, and speeds up to 250,000 bps (see Eggebrecht, 1990; Genois, 1992; Dvorak & Anis, 1992; Oliver, 1993).

Another UART which is sometimes used is the Intel 82510. While this is also 8250 compatible with FIFO options, it has many additional modes and registers and consequently is significantly more complicated to program (Van Gilluwe, 1994).

4.2.1 Registers

The UART coordinates and controls a number of activities which can be categorised as (a) transmitting data, (b) receiving data, (c) control, (d) status, and (e) timing (Duncan, 1988). Each of these activities is associated with one or more 1-byte UART **registers** (see Table 4.2), which can be accessed by the programmer in order to control and monitor the serial interface.

While most UART registers have both Read and Write access, some allow only one or the other. For example, the Interrupt Identification Register (IIR) is a read-only register. Similarly, reading from the **base address** reads only the Received Data Register (RDR), while writing a byte to the base address writes it only to the Transmitter Holding Register (THR).

† Direct memory access.

Table 4.2. *UART registers.*

Function	Name	Read/Write
Transmit	Transmitter holding register	W
Receive	Received data register	R
Control	Interrupt enable register	R/W
	Interrupt identification register	R
	Line control register	R/W
	Modem control register	R/W
	Modem status register	R
	FIFO control register (16550 UART)	W
Status	Line status register	R
Timing	Baud rate divisor latch register : high byte	R/W
	Baud rate divisor latch register : low byte	R/W

Each serial port has an additional register (the scratch register) which is not used in serial interfacing, making a total of 11 UART registers. However, the UART has only 3 **register-select lines** with which it can access only 8 register addresses. In order to be able to access 11 registers, bit-7 of the Line Control Register (known as the Divisor Latch Access Bit; DLAB) is therefore used as a fourth register-select line (Campbell, 1989b). The use of the DLAB is shown in Table 4.5.

The more recent UARTs have an additional write-only register known as the FIFO Control Register, which allows software control of its additional facilities (Margolis, 1989; Goodwin, 1992; O'Brien, 1992; Van Gilluwe, 1994).

While full details of all UART registers are given in the data sheets supplied by the manufacturers, an excellent overview of UART registers including various undocumented aspects and 'bugs' is given by Van Gilluwe (1994).

4.2.2 Control of RS-232 lines

In general, the UART chip is able to handle two RS-232 outputs (RTS, DTR), and four RS-232 inputs (CTS, DSR, RI, DCD). The voltage on the PC's output control lines (RTS, DTR) is controlled using software by writing either a 1 or 0 to the appropriate bit of the Modem Control Register (MCR) for the COM port in question (see Figure 4.1). Details

Table 4.3. *Baud rate divisors.*

Bit rate	Master clock frequency	Reference clock frequency	Baud rate divisor		
			Dec	High byte	Low byte
300	4800 Hz	1.8432 MHz	384	01h	80h
1200	19200 Hz	1.8432 MHz	96	00h	60h
2400	38400 Hz	1.8432 MHz	48	00h	30h
4800	76800 Hz	1.8432 MHz	24	00h	18h
9600	153600 Hz	1.8432 MHz	12	00h	0Ch

of how to do this using QuickBASIC without altering any of the other bits in the register are given in Chapter 5.

4.2.3 Timing

The UART derives both the Receive and Transmit bit rate from the **Master clock**, which itself is derived from a **Reference clock** which is either generated by the UART itself (using a crystal oscillator) or supplied from an external source (Campbell, 1989b). The frequencies commonly used for the Reference clock are either 1.8432 MHz or 3.072 MHz. Although the Transmit and Receive bit rates are usually the same, the UART has the facility to make these different if necessary, since some modems transmit and receive at different rates.

The Master clock frequency is derived by sequential division from the Reference clock, and is considerably greater than the bit rate (usually 16 times greater), since this allows the middle of each bit period to be located with greater precision (see Section 2.3). The bit rate is then derived by dividing the Master clock frequency by 16.

The Master clock frequency is derived by dividing the Reference clock frequency by a 16-bit integer (**baud rate divisor**) which is held as two 8-bit bytes (high and low bytes) occupying the two baud rate divisor latch registers having offset 0 (low byte) and offset 1 (high byte). For example, in order to generate a bit rate of 1200 bps from a 1.8432 MHz Reference clock, a baud rate divisor of 0060h (= 96) would generate a Master clock frequency of 19200 Hz, which would then be divided by 16 to give a bit rate of 1200 (19200 = 16 × 1200). For this particular baud rate divisor (0060h), the high byte is 00h and the low byte is 60h. A table giving bit rates and the corresponding baud rate divisors for the main crystal frequency of 1.8432 MHz is given in Table 4.3. Comprehensive

Table 4.4. *NS8250 protocol options.*

Bit rate	110 – 9600 bps (XT)
	110 – 19200 bps (AT and EISA)
Data bits	5, 6, 7, 8
Parity	Even, Odd, None, Mark, Space
Stop bits	1, 1.5, 2

tables are given for various crystal frequencies in the data-sheets for the National Semiconductor UARTs NS16450 (1.8432, 3.072, 8.0 MHz), and NS16550AF (1.8432, 3.072, 18.432 MHz).

4.2.4 Protocol

The 16550 and 16450 UARTs are both fully downward compatible with the 8250, which handles data with the specifications shown in Table 4.4.

4.2.5 Programming

For general aspects of the interface and serial interface programming for PCs see Schwaderer (1986), Gofton (1986), Campbell (1989b), Schildt (1989), Dettmann (1989), Waite *et al.* (1990), Eggebrecht (1990), Brown & Kyle (1991), Tischer (1991), Goodwin (1992), Monk (1992), and Van Gilluwe (1994). For programming serial communications for Windows see Monk (1992), and Appleman (1993).

A number of useful freeware utilities are available for documenting the serial port(s), and for interacting with the UART and its various registers. Good sources for such programs are the IBMCOM forum in CompuServe, and the Public Domain Software Archive at Lancaster, UK (**pd-software.lancaster.ac.uk**). Some examples of the available utilities are as follows.

- CHK_UART.COM   See Genois (1992) for details of this program.
- 16550DET.COM   This program determines the variety of UART used by a PC. It is described by Oliver (1993). Both the hexadecimal code and the assembler code are given.
- O'Brien (1992) describes an interactive program which accesses and displays UART registers.
- INIT14.COM   This is a TSR program† written by Nance (1992), and

† Terminate and stay resident.

offers service subroutines for initialising COM1 and COM2, reading and writing characters to the ports, functions for purging the buffer, as well as many other things.

- LITES.COM   This program by Prosise (1989) helps diagnose I/O problems, and displays in real-time the status of the six serial port control lines.
- An assembly language interrupt handler is described by Margolis (1990). The code shows how to discriminate between all four types of UART interrupt, and is available for downloading.
- An RS-232 serial monitor is described by Livingstone & Livingstone (1993).
- A wide range of diagnostic utilities relating to the serial port are supplied on the disk which accompanies the recent book by Van Gilluwe (1994).

The practicalities of connections and accessing data are considered by Thompson & Kuckles (1989), Baran (1991), Bedford (1991, 1992a), Carr (1991), Perry (1993). The null modem is considered in Appendix 4.

4.3 UART addresses

The addresses of the various UART registers are defined in terms of an **offset** from the COM port's **base address** (offset 0); these are summarised in Table 4.5.

The address of a particular UART register is at a given offset from the base address of that particular COM port. For example, consider the Line Control Register (LCR) for COM2. The base address for COM2 is 02F8h, and the offset for its LCR is 3. This means that the address of the LCR for COM2 is 02F8h + 3 = 02FBh.

The UART register addresses are known as **port** addresses, and are read from and written to using different programming commands to those used for the ordinary *memory* addresses. Thus QuickBASIC uses the command INP for reading a port register, and OUT for writing to a port register. The equivalent commands for accessing the ordinary memory addresses are PEEK and POKE respectively. Details regarding the QuickBASIC syntax for read/write operations are given in Chapter 5.

Note that the UART base addresses for COM3 and COM4 are not standardised; thus Windows 3.0 and 3.1 use different addresses (Livingstone & Livingstone, 1993) as shown in Table 4.6.

Table 4.5. *UART register addresses.*

COM1	COM2	Offset	DLAB	Code	Register
03F8h	02F8h	0	0	THR	Transmitting holding reg.
03F8h	02F8h	0	0	RDR	Receiver data register
03F8h	02F8h	0	1	BRDL	Baud rate divisor, low byte
03F9h	02F9h	1	1	BRDH	Baud rate divisor, high byte
03F9h	02F9h	1	0	IER	Interrupt enable register
03FAh	02FAh	2	–	IIR	Interrupt identification reg.
03FAh	02FAh	2	–	FCR	FIFO control register
03FBh	02FBh	3	–	LCR	Line control register
03FCh	02FCh	4	–	MCR	Modem control register
03FDh	02FDh	5	–	LSR	Line status register
03FEh	02FEh	6	–	MSR	Modem status register
03FFh	02FFh	7	–		Scratch register

Table 4.6. *UART COM port base addresses.*

Port	Usual address	Windows 3.0	Windows 3.1
COM1	03F8h	03F8h	03F8h
COM2	02F8h	02F8h	02F8h
COM3	03E8h	02E8h	03E8h
COM4	02E8h	02E0h	02E8h

4.3.1 Numerical registers (THR, RDR, BRDL, BRDH)

Four of the UART registers hold 1-byte numbers, which are either proper numbers in their own right (THR, RDR), or are the high byte (BRDH) and low byte (BRDL) of a 16-bit proper number known as the Baud Rate Divisor (BRD).

4.3.2 Bit-mapped registers (IER, IIR, LCR, MCR, LSR, MSR)

Six of the UART registers are said to be 'bit-mapped' or 'bit-encoded', indicating that the 8 bits making up the byte in these particular registers do not code for a real number; instead, each bit codes separately for some particular function.

For example, consider bit-4 of the Modem Status Register (MSR) which codes for whether the handshaking line CTS is set HIGH or not. When CTS is HIGH (positive voltage) then bit-4 of MSR is set to 1 (see Figure 4.3).

4.4 UART registers

The UART registers are particularly important when it comes to programming the serial port, and these will now be dealt with in some detail (see also Gofton, 1986; Campbell, 1989b; Dettmann, 1989; Margolis, 1989, 1990; Waite *et al.*, 1990; Phoenix, 1991; Tischer, 1991; Goodwin, 1992; Monk, 1992; O'Brien, 1992; Nance, 1992; Appleman, 1993; Van Gilluwe, 1994). The method of reading from and writing to the various registers is described in Chapter 5.

Since the development of UARTs is a fast moving and complicated field, this Section will deal primarily with the earlier 8250/16450 UARTs, and indicate the areas where the more recent 82510 and 16550 series of UARTs differ. In practice, the main difference is that the 16550 and later series of UARTs have an additional register (FIFO Control Register). There are also a number of changes to the following registers.

- Interrupt Identification Register
- Interrupt Enable Register
- Line Status Register
- Modem Control Register

4.4.1 Transmitter Holding Register (THR)
[write only] [COM1 = 03F8h] [COM2 = 02F8h] [DLAB = 0]

This register holds the data byte which is about to be sent. Data can only be written to this register when bit-5 of the Line Status Register is set to 1, which indicates that the THR is currently empty (see Figure 4.4).

4.4.2 Received Data Register (RDR)
[read only] [COM1 = 03F8h] [COM2 = 02F8h] [DLAB = 0]

This register holds the last incoming data byte, and can be read when bit-0 of the Line Status Register is set to 1, which indicates that a byte has been received from the serial port (see Figure 4.4).

4.4.3 Modem Control Register (MCR)
[read/write] [COM1 = 03FCh] [COM2 = 02FCh]

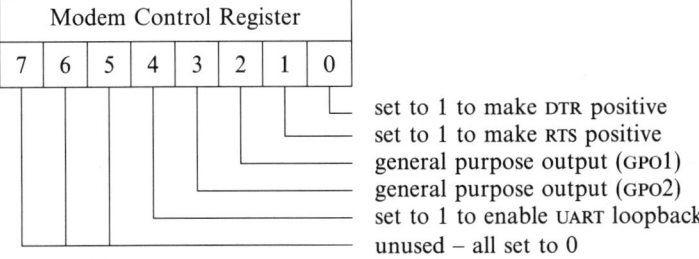

Fig. 4.1. Modem Control Register.

This register controls the state of the two output control lines RTS and DTR, and therefore allows the programmer to control these two lines by writing to this address. The bit assignments of this register are shown in Figure 4.1.

One of the functions controlled by this register is the UART **loopback** facility (bit-4), which can be useful when testing programs which read from and write to the serial port. Setting bit-4 to 1 directs the output of the transmitter shift-register into the receiver shift-register input of the same COM port. For further details regarding the loopback facility see Campbell (1989b), Van Gilluwe (1994).

Bit-2 controls a general purpose output line (GPO1) which can be used to reset an internal modem. Bit-3 controls another general purpose output line (GPO2) which is used in conjunction with enabling interrupts; this bit must be set to 1 in order to enable interrupts set by the Interrupt Enable Register (see Figure 4.6). Note that serial port interrupts also require the relevant IRQ bit to be set in the Interrupt Mask Register (21h) of the 8259 Peripheral Interrupt Controller (Goodwin, 1992). COM2 and COM4 are serviced by IRQ3 (bit-3); COM1 and COM3 are serviced by IRQ4 (bit-4).

16C1450/16C1550/82510 UARTs

See Van Gilluwe (1994) for details of differences associated with these UARTs.

4.4.4 Line Control Register (LCR)
[read/write] [COM1 = 03FBh] [COM2 = 02FBh]

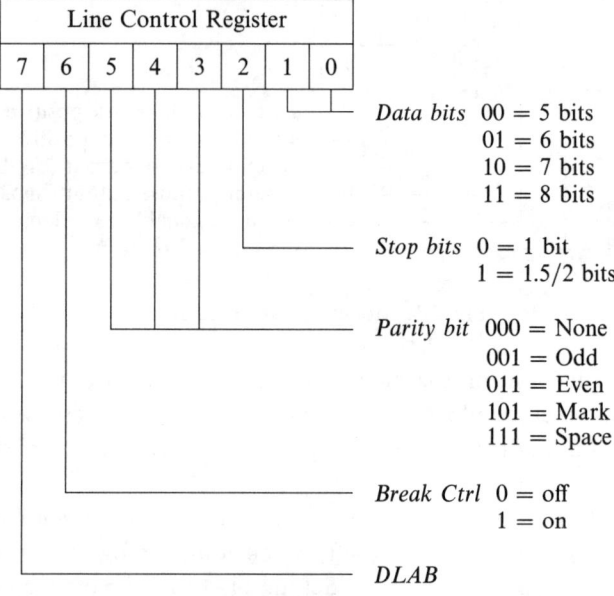

Fig. 4.2. Line Control Register.

This register holds the protocol used for serial communications and is shown in Figure 4.2. Bit-7 (the Divisor Latch Access Bit; DLAB) controls access to the various 'doubled-up' registers. For example, when bit-7 is set to 1 then the UART registers 0 (THR/RDR) and 1 (IIR) become BRDL (low byte) and BRDH (high byte) respectively (see Table 4.5) allowing the baud rate divisor to be set.

Bit-6 of the LCR is used to force what is known as a **hardware break** signal (see Section 4.5.4), which is used to signal that a communication problem exists (Schwaderer, 1986). Setting bit-6 to 1 forces the Transmit data line (TxD) to a positive voltage (known as the Space state), and the line will then remain in this state until bit-6 is set to zero.

Note that if the protocol requires 5 data bits to be used, then the 1.5 stop bits which are always used in this case are set by configuring bit-2 to 1.

4.4.5 Modem Status Register (MSR)

[read only] [COM1 = 03FEh] [COM2 = 02FEh]

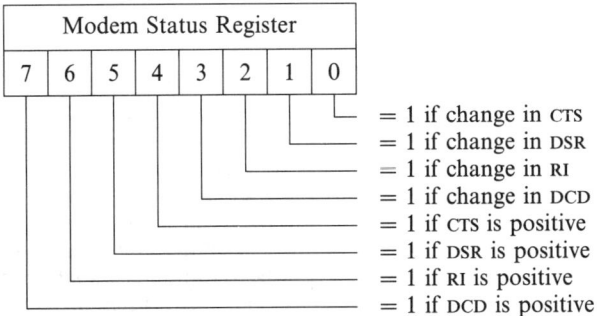

Fig. 4.3. Modem Status Register.

This register indicates the status (HIGH or LOW) of the four RS-232 input lines CTS, DSR, DCD and RI. The bit assignments of this register are shown in Figure 4.3.

Note that if one of the PC's input control lines is not connected to anything (i.e. on open circuit), then its status will be recorded as a 0 in the relevant bit of the Modem Control Register. Thus a zero bit could indicate either that the line is being held LOW (i.e. is connected to a negative voltage),† or that the line is just not connected to anything externally.‡

The Modem Status Register also indicates any *change* in the status of the four input control lines, as these bits (0–3) are set to 1 if the line status has changed since the register was last read.

Note that bit-2 (RI) is **edge-sensitive** in that it detects the trailing edge, i.e. it only detects a change from HIGH to LOW (Campbell, 1989b; Phoenix, 1991).

---

† Note that for control lines, LOW = negative voltage.
‡ The pins of the serial port are held LOW internally by an appropriate resistor, so that the voltage does not 'float' when the pin is not connected to anything—i.e. on open circuit.

4.4.6 Line Status Register (LSR)

[read only] [COM1 = 03FDh] [COM2 = 02FDh]

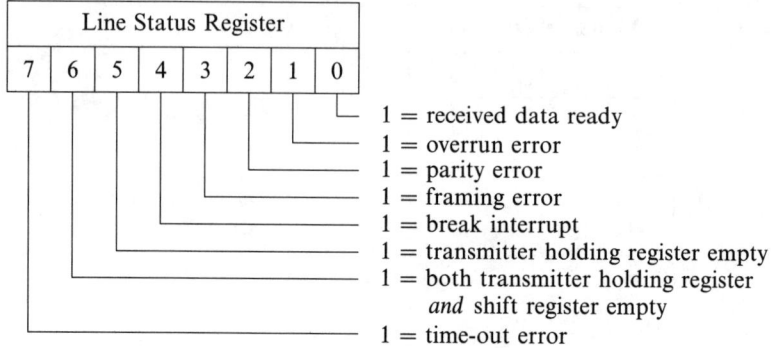

Fig. 4.4. Line Status Register.

This register indicates the status of the Receive and Transmit registers, as well as identifying serial communication errors. The bit assignments of this register are shown in Figure 4.4.

A bit is set to 1 when the respective event occurs. For example, bit-7 is set to 1 if a time-out error occurs (Phoenix, 1991). Note that each time the register is read, the bits are automatically reset to 0.

Bit-6 is used to indicate when *all* the data has been transmitted, since both the Transmitter Shift Register and Holding Register will be empty when the last data character has been transmitted.

16550 UART

Bit-7 is set to 1 when the FIFO mode is enabled; see Van Gilluwe (1994) for details.

4.4.7 Interrupt Identification Register (IIR)
[read only] [COM1 = 03FAh] [COM2 = 02FAh]

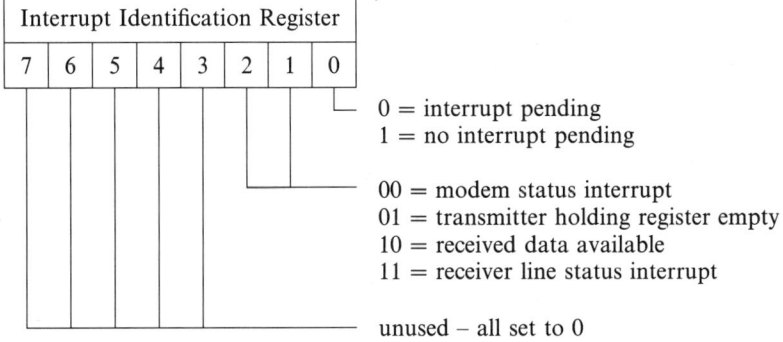

Fig. 4.5. Interrupt Identification Register.

This register gives information regarding pending interrupts. For example, if there are no interrupts pending, then bit-0 is set to 1. If an interrupt is pending (waiting to be serviced by the microprocessor) then this is indicated by bits 1 and 2 as shown in Figure 4.5.

Bit-1 and bit-2 are set in response to a status change in any of the PC's four input control lines CTS, DSR, RI, DCD. Which particular control line is involved will be indicated by the Modem Status Register.

If an interrupt arises from an error at the Receive data register, then the particular error (overrun, framing, BREAK etc.) is indicated by the Line Status Register. See also Margolis (1990) and Alford (1992).

16550 UART

Port 2 of the 16550 UART accesses two separate registers, of which the Interrupt Identification Register is the Read-only register.† There are differences in the use of bits 3, 6, 7.

Bit-3 is associated with a character time-out. Bits 6 and 7 are variously set to 1 when FIFO is enabled, depending on the particular UART of this series (see Van Gilluwe (1994) for details).

---

† The other register is the FIFO Control Register, which is the corresponding Write-only register.

4.4.8 Interrupt Enable Register (IER)

[read/write] [COM1 = 03F9h] [COM2 = 02F9h] [DLAB = 0]

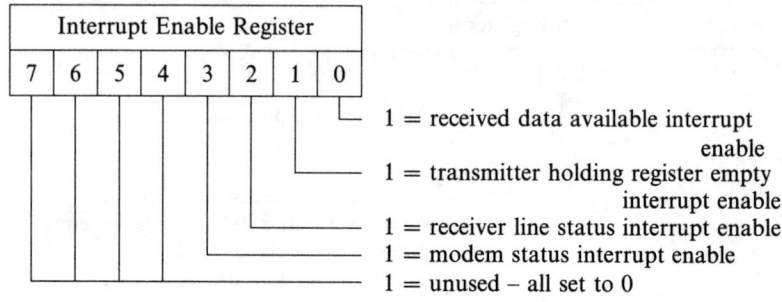

Fig. 4.6. Interrupt Enable Register.

This register controls which events cause interrupts. Setting a bit to 1 will enable the respective interrupt. The bit assignments of this register are shown in Figure 4.6.

Note that after enabling an interrupt in this register, it is also necessary to set bit-3 (GPO2) in the Modem Control Register as well as bits in other registers (Goodwin, 1992). See also Margolis (1990) and Alford (1992).

16550/82510 UARTs

There are differences in the use of bits 0, 4, 5 (see Van Gilluwe (1994) for details).

4.4.9 FIFO Control Register (FCR)

[write only] [COM1 = 03FAh] [COM2 = 02FAh]

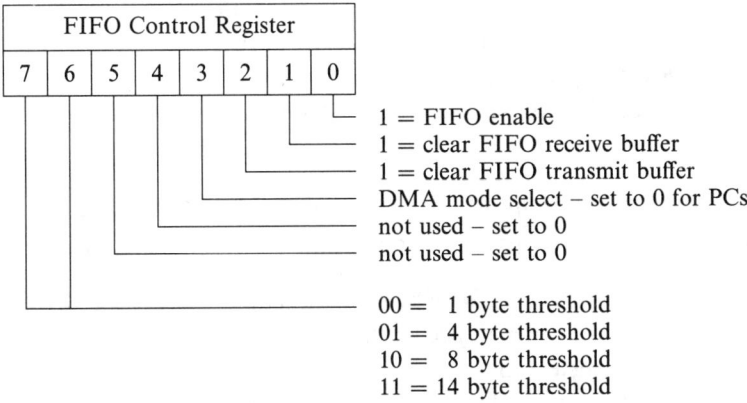

Fig. 4.7. FIFO Control Register.

This register controls the FIFO buffer facility of the 16550 UART In addition to enabling and clearing the buffers, this register allows the threshold at which the Receive buffer full interrupt is set to be varied between 1, 4, 8, and 14 bytes. The bit assignments of this register are shown in Figure 4.7. See also Margolis (1989), Goodwin (1992) and Van Gilluwe (1994).

16552 dual UART

This dual UART has an additional register (Alternate Function Register) which controls one of the general purpose output lines† (see Van Gilluwe (1994) for details).

---

† See Section 4.4.3.

4.4.10 Baud Rate LSB Divisor Latch Register (BRDL)
[read/write] [COM1 = 03F8h] [COM2 = 02F8h] [DLAB = 1]

This register allows the *low* byte of the baud rate divisor to be set (see Figure 4.8). In order to access this register, the DLAB (bit-7 of the Line Control Register) must be first set to 1. After the BRDL register has been accessed, the DLAB must be returned to 0 in order to allow continued access to the Receive and Transmit data registers.

4.4.11 Baud Rate MSB Divisor Latch Register (BRDH)
[read/write] [COM1 = 03F9h] [COM2 = 02F9h] [DLAB = 1]

This register allows the *high* byte of the baud rate divisor to be set (see Figure 4.8). In order to access this register, the DLAB (bit-7 of the Line Control Register) must be first set to 1. After the BRDH register has been accessed, the DLAB must be returned to 0 in order to allow continued access to the Interrupt Enable Register.

Baud Rate Divisor															
15	14	13	12	11	10	9	8	7	6	5	4	3	2	1	0
high byte register (BDRH)								low byte register (BDRL)							

Fig. 4.8. Baud Rate Divisor Registers.

4.5 Handling of serial I/O

For a computer and peripheral device to communicate effectively via the serial interface they have to be able to do the following.

- Indicate that they are switched on and powered up.
- Indicate that they want to send data.
- Indicate that they are ready to receive data.
- Indicate that they want the other device to temporarily stop sending data.
- Indicate that they are experiencing a communication problem, and that the other device should stop sending data altogether.

In practice these aspects of serial communication are most easily controlled using a general programming language, for example QuickBASIC 4.5 which is described in Chapter 5.

4.5.1 On/off status

The on/off status of the PC's serial port is generally indicated by the status of its DTR line. If it is necessary for the peripheral device to know whether the PC's serial port is 'open' and therefore available for communication, the peripheral device can monitor the PC's DTR line using one of its own input control lines.

Consequently when a serial port is opened the program automatically sets the PC's DTR line HIGH (positive) indicating that the serial port is now active and ready for communication.

4.5.2 Outputting data

The usual convention is that a device intending to transmit data first holds its RTS line HIGH, in order to indicate that it wishes to transmit, and then waits for the other device to signal that it is ready to receive by setting its own RTS line HIGH. In view of this, the peripheral device's RTS line is generally wired to the PC's CTS pin. If the PC detects that the peripheral device is holding the PC's CTS HIGH, the PC interprets this as indicating that it is Clear To Send the data (hence, CTS).

In practice, the PC checks the status of its own CTS before outputting each byte. If during data transmission the peripheral device suddenly holds the PC's CTS LOW, the PC will stop transmitting and wait until its CTS is held HIGH again by the peripheral device.

If the PC's CTS is not reset HIGH within a specified time then a time-out error will occur, resulting in bit-7 of the Line Status Register being set to 1 (see Figure 4.4). Note that when using QuickBASIC, if a CTS time-out parameter is not specified† *and* the PC's CTS continues to be held LOW then data transmission will cease indefinitely.

Often a PC is connected to a device which is not using hardware handshaking, in which case it is necessary to make the PC transmit data *without* first checking the status of its CTS line.‡

4.5.3 Receiving data

During the input of each byte, the PC checks the status of its DSR, since the PC requires its DSR pin to be held HIGH in order to enable it to read the incoming byte.

If the PC's DSR is suddenly held LOW then the PC waits for its DSR to be set HIGH before reading in any more of the incoming data. If the PC's DSR is not reset HIGH within a specified period then a time-out occurs, and bit-7 of the Line Status Register is set to 1 (see Figure 4.4).

Often a PC is connected to a device which is not using hardware handshaking, in which case it is useful to be able to have the PC able to receive data without first checking the status of its DSR line.§

4.5.4 The hardware BREAK signal

This is a signal which can be sent by the PC to indicate to the peripheral device that it is experiencing a problem receiving data. However, since the PC has only two output control lines (RTS, DTR) and these are already allocated, the PC has only the data transmit line (TxD) left to use.

The hardware BREAK signal is defined as setting a positive voltage (logic 0)¶ on the data line (TxD) for *longer* than the time to transmit a single character (Phoenix, 1991). The duration ought to be at least two full character frames at the current baud rate (Van Gilluwe, 1994).

The BREAK signal is controlled by bit-6 of the PC's Line Control Register (see Figure 4.2). Setting bit-6 to 1 results in the TxD line being forced positive (logic 0), where it will stay until the bit is reset to 0.

† See Chapter 5 for details.
‡ QuickBASIC uses the CS parameter in the OPEN COM statement.
§ QuickBASIC uses the DS parameter in the OPEN COM statement.
¶ See Sections 1.3, 2.2 and Figure 2.2.

Details of how to set bits in a register are given in Chapter 5. See also Microsoft (1989c, 1990b).

If the PC receives a BREAK signal (i.e. on its RxD line) QuickBASIC 4.5 issues a 'device I/O error' (error 57), and the program stops. However data already sent to the PC's transmit buffer will continue to be transmitted. Note that in this event QuickBASIC 4.5 does not reset RTS and DTR to LOW, and the program will have to be run again unless provision is made for trapping this event as described earlier.

5
Serial interface programming in QuickBASIC

5.1 Introduction

QuickBASIC is an excellent programming language for serial interfacing. Not only is it easy to use and widely available, but it is particularly well suited for measurement and control applications, owing to the fact that the serial port is so easily programmed using this language (Penfold, 1992; Appleby, 1992; Smith, 1993). QuickBASIC's main advantage over QBASIC is that it is a compilable BASIC, and therefore free-standing executable (.EXE) programs can be formed. In addition QuickBASIC allows string lengths up to 32,767 bytes, and assembly language routines can be used more easily with it (Wyatt, 1990). However, although all the programs in this book are written in QuickBASIC 4.5, they will also run under QBASIC which now comes as standard with MS-DOS.

Serial I/O using QuickBASIC is not generally well documented; indeed the topic is omitted in most books on QuickBASIC. Useful texts in this regard have been Aitken (1992), Microsoft (1988, 1989a–h, 1990a–i, 1991a–f, 1992a–d), Gofton (1986), Nameroff (1989), Schwaderer (1986), Waite *et al.* (1990). Note that Microsoft maintains an extensive library of documents on QuickBASIC, and these can be downloaded from CompuServe's Microsoft KnowledgeBase forum (GO MSKB). The Microsoft documents relevant to serial interfacing are listed in the references at the end of this book under Microsoft. A valuable listing of reported problems associated with compiled BASICs including QuickBASIC 4.5, entitled QUIRKS.TXT, is also maintained (see Novisoff, 1991).

5.1.1 Program structure

In order to access data from a peripheral device, the program usually has to perform most if not all of the following key routines.

- Open communications via the serial port(s) using an appropriate protocol.
- Set output control lines (RTS, DTR) either HIGH or LOW as necessary.
- Determine the status of input control lines (CTS, DSR, DCD, RI).
- Send appropriate control characters to the peripheral device to enable data to be output from the device.
- Read input data from the buffer and print the data to the screen.
- Save the data on a disk, adding the date and time of sampling if these parameters are not included in the data.
- Re-format the data, if necessary, in an appropriate form to facilitate further processing by another program or software package.

In practice, it is often convenient to allocate many of these components of the program to separate subroutines or functions which can then be called as required. It is also useful to include in the program some menu-driven subroutines which (a) allow the peripheral device's various output modes to be selected, and (b) allow recently collected data to be printed to the screen.

5.2 Opening a serial port

Unsupported, QuickBASIC 4.5 can handle two serial ports; namely those designated as COM1 and COM2 (Microsoft, 1990f, 1992a, 1992c). QuickBASIC can be made to access as many as four serial ports, by making use of certain DOS services (see Microsoft, 1991d).

If it is necessary to have two serial ports operating simultaneously, i.e. having both COM1 and COM2 open at the same time, then QuickBASIC will service COM2 first (Microsoft, 1990a).

5.2.1 The OPEN COM statement

Communication via one of the serial ports is established using the OPEN COM statement. Since this is such a key statement with respect to serial interfacing, the relevant material from Microsoft (1988) is reproduced in Appendix 6.

The OPEN COM statement is a single-line statement which sets the following parameters.

Table 5.1. *Protocol parameters for QuickBASIC 4.5.*

Bit rate	75, 110, 150, 300, 600, 1200, 1800 2400, 4800, 9600, 19200
Parity	Even, Odd, None, Mark, Space
Data bits	5, 6, 7, 8
Stop bits	1, 2

- The serial port to be used (COM1 or COM2).
- The protocol.
- The optional control-line parameters to be used.
- The size of the Receive and Transmit buffers.
- The direction of data flow (input, output, or both).
- The file number used to refer to the port (#1, #2, etc.).

For example, the following OPEN COM statement opens serial port 2 (COM2) for receiving data (INPUT) as file number one (#1) without using CTS or DSR handshaking; sets a 5 second time-out limit for opening the port (OP5000); increases the Receive buffer to 2000 bytes (RB2000); and uses the following protocol: bit rate 1200, 1 stop-bit, 8 data-bits, no parity-bit.

OPEN "COM2:1200,N,8,1,CS,DS,OP5000,RB2000" FOR INPUT AS #1

The various parameters for the OPEN COM statement are now described in detail (see also Appendix 6).

5.2.2 *The protocol parameters*

The first four parameters following the colon (:) in the OPEN COM statement (see above) are reserved for the **protocol** parameters which are shown in Table 5.1. The four protocol parameters must be in the strict order bit rate (baud), parity, data-bits, stop-bits.

5.2.3 *The optional parameters*

The optional parameters are detailed below (Microsoft, 1988, 1989a, 1990a, 1991d; Nameroff, 1989; Waite *et al.*, 1990). Note that where a control line option takes a parameter (e.g. DSn, CSn, CDn), if the parameter is zero (e.g. CS0) then the relevant time-out is disabled. If the parameter is omitted the default is zero. Thus both CS and CS0 will disable the CTS time-out. See Appendix 6 for further details.

- **OPn** This option gives the total time in ms to wait for the OPEN COM statement to be executed before giving rise to a time-out, e.g. OP5000 (waits 5 seconds).
- **DSn** This option gives the time in ms to wait for DSR to go HIGH before giving rise to a time-out, e.g. DS5000 (waits 5 seconds). This is because the PC requires its DSR to be HIGH in order to be able to read an input byte, unless the DS option is used to disable DSR checking. If the DS option is omitted the default time is 1 second. DSR is also involved in the execution of the OPEN COM statement. Thus if neither the DS nor the DS0 option is used, then QuickBASIC will not execute the OPEN COM statement unless the PC's DSR is *already* being held HIGH. Using either the DS or DS0 option will disable the DSR time-out, and therefore allow communications to proceed without checking the status of the computer's DSR.
- **RS** This option stops the PC from automatically setting its RTS line HIGH on opening the serial port. Consequently when this option is used the PC does not check to see whether CTS is HIGH or not prior to outputting data via the serial port, e.g. following a PRINT# or WRITE# statement. Note that RS does not take a parameter. If the RS option is *not* used, then in order for a PRINT# or WRITE# statement to be executed successfully either CTS checking must be disabled (use the CS option), or the CTS line must go HIGH within the stated CTS wait time (default is 1 second).
- **CSn** This option gives the time in ms to wait for CTS to go HIGH before giving rise to a time-out, e.g. CS5000 (waits 5 seconds). This is because the PC requires its CTS to be set HIGH in order to output a byte, unless the CS option has been used to disable CTS checking. If the CS option is omitted the default time is 1 second. Both the CS and CS0 options will disable the time-out, and therefore allow communications to proceed without checking the status of CTS (i.e. without the need for CTS to go HIGH). If the RS option is *also* used (i.e. to prevent QuickBASIC setting RTS HIGH on opening the serial port), then CTS checking is automatically disabled, in which case the CSn option is unnecessary.
- **CDn** This option gives the time in ms to wait for DCD to go HIGH before giving rise to a time-out, e.g. CD5000 (waits 5 seconds). The CDn option is generally only used when interfacing to a modem, when it is used to monitor the line status of the modem's Carrier Detect line. If the CD option is omitted the default time is 1 second. Both the CD and CD0 options will disable the time-out, and therefore allow

communications to be opened without checking the status of the PC's DCD.
- **ASC**   This option specifies characters as ASCII, expands tabs (i.e. shows tabs as spaces), forces a carriage return ⟨CR⟩ at the end of each line, and treats Ctrl-Z (^Z) as the End Of File (EOF) marker.
- **LF**   This option puts a linefeed character ⟨LF⟩ after each carriage return character ⟨CR⟩. It is therefore used in conjunction with serial printers.
- **RBn**   This option sets the size (in bytes) of the Receive buffer. The value of **n** must be in the range 0 to 32767. The default buffer size is 512 bytes.
- **TBn**   This option sets the size (in bytes) of the Transmit buffer. The value of **n** must be in the range 0 to 32767. The default size is 512 bytes.
- **PE**   This option enables parity checking during communications, and results in a 'device I/O error' if the two communicating programs have different parities. If the PE option is not used, then parity compatibility is not checked for (see Microsoft, 1990i).

5.2.4 Filename

QuickBASIC treats the serial port as an ordinary data-file, and therefore requires a file number (#1, #2, etc.) to identify it. The file number follows the keyword AS in the OPEN COM statement (e.g. AS #2).

5.2.5 Input/output

When dealing with either Random or Sequential files, then one of the commands RANDOM, INPUT, OUTPUT, or APPEND should follow the keyword FOR in the OPEN COM statement, in order to indicate how the serial port is to be used (e.g. FOR INPUT). The default parameter is RANDOM.

If a serial port is to be opened for either input or output *only*, then the port should be opened using either FOR INPUT or FOR OUTPUT. An example of the syntax is as follows.

OPEN "COM2:4800,E,7,1,CS,DS,OP5000" FOR INPUT AS #1

However, if a serial port has to be opened for both input *and* output traffic (i.e. data is to be flowing in both directions), then the port must be opened FOR RANDOM in conjunction with the ACCESS READ WRITE command, in order to indicate that data will be both written to and read from the same port. An example of the syntax in this case is as follows.

OPEN "COM2:4800 ... " FOR RANDOM ACCESS READ WRITE AS #1

5.2.6 Executing the OPEN COM statement

On entering the QuickBASIC environment, QuickBASIC sets the PC's TxD, RTS and DTR to the negative voltage state. Note that the EIA/TIA-232 Standard requires that the idle state of the data lines (TxD, RxD) is negative (see Chapter 1).

When QuickBASIC executes the OPEN COM statement, it allocates the appropriate size to the Receive and Transmit buffers (default size is 512 bytes), and enables the appropriate serial port interrupts. Following this the DTR line is set HIGH, and then after about 1/4 second pause the RTS line is also set HIGH (unless the RS option has been used—see above). Further details of the sequence adopted by QuickBASIC in opening the port are given in Appendix 6.

Unless either the DS or DS0 option has been used in the OPEN COM statement QuickBASIC now checks to see whether its DSR line is held HIGH by the peripheral device (Appendix 6; Microsoft, 1990f). Providing this condition is satisfied within the time specified by the DSn parameter in the OPEN COM statement, then the serial port will be opened successfully, as indicated by QuickBASIC executing the next statement in the program.†

In practice therefore, it is useful to have a successful opening of the serial port indicated on the screen, for example by placing the following statement immediately after the OPEN COM statement.

PRINT "serial port opened successfully"

5.2.7 Failure to execute the OPEN COM statement

If neither the DS nor the DS0 option is used in the OPEN COM statement *and* the PC's DSR is not held HIGH by the peripheral device within the wait time specified in the OPEN COM statement,‡ then a 'device time-out' error occurs, and QuickBASIC 4.5 terminates the program after first setting both RTS and DTR back to the initial LOW (negative) state.

The error-checking sequence used during the execution of the OPEN COM statement is detailed in Microsoft (1990f).

† i.e. QuickBASIC executes the OPEN COM statement.
‡ Note that if DS is omitted altogether, then the default wait time is 1 second.

5.2.8 Time-out following successful opening of a port

If a time-out occurs at some stage *after* a successful execution of the OPEN COM statement, then QuickBASIC 4.5 does *not* reset the PC's DTR and RTS, in which case the program will have to be run from the beginning using the START command (shift-F5), as QuickBASIC automatically resets the serial port before running a program.

5.3 Outputting data to a peripheral device

Data is output via the serial port using the PRINT# or WRITE# statement. For example, the phrase 'Hello world' would be transmitted to a device via a serial port designated as #3 in the OPEN COM statement by the following line of QuickBASIC.

PRINT #3, "Hello world"

When data is sent to the PC's Transmit buffer, QuickBASIC first checks that the PC's CTS is held HIGH (positive) before transmitting the data, unless instructed to do otherwise by the use of a CSn option in the OPEN COM statement. Note that the amount of room (bytes) left in the Transmit buffer is returned by the LOF(n) function (Microsoft, 1990f).

Thus, in order to output data from a serial port using a PRINT# or WRITE# statement, either CTS checking must be disabled (use either the CS or CS0 option in the OPEN COM statement), or the CTS line must be held HIGH within the wait-time indicated by the CSn option (default is 1 second). The error-checking sequence used while outputting data is detailed in Microsoft (1990f).

5.3.1 The PRINT statement

When sending data or instructions to a peripheral device, the precise format of the information transmitted is often critical. In view of this it is important to understand that the PRINT and the PRINT# statements both automatically add the two control characters ⟨CR⟩⟨LF⟩ on to the end of the characters to be transmitted, *unless* instructed otherwise by using a semicolon on the end of the relevant PRINT or PRINT# statement (Microsoft, 1988).

For example, the statement PRINT #1, "Hello" will actually transmit the characters Hello⟨CR⟩⟨LF⟩ from the serial port designated as #1. If it is important not to send the extra two control characters, then add a semicolon to the end of the PRINT# statement as follows.

```
PRINT #1, "Hello";
```

Although most peripheral devices will accept extra ⟨CR⟩ characters, some will not (e.g. the Graseby 3400 syringe pump—see Chapter 14). It is therefore important to know the *exact* command format used by the peripheral device.

5.3.2 Sending commands and control characters

Commands and control characters are sent to a peripheral device via the serial port by writing them to the computer's Transmit buffer, using either a PRINT# or a WRITE# statement. However, the PRINT# statement is generally the preferred output statement for transmitting commands, since the WRITE# statement adds inverted commas around the string to be sent.

For example, a typical command to be sent to the Ohmeda 9000 syringe pump might be ⟨ESC⟩SP?␣⟨CR⟩.† Since the ASCII code for ⟨ESC⟩ is 27, and that for a space ␣ is 32, then this command would be transmitted via a serial port using the PRINT# and WRITE# statements as follows.

```
PRINT #2, CHR$(27) + "SP?" + CHR$(32)
WRITE #2, CHR$(27) + "SP?" + CHR$(32)
```

When the PRINT# statement is used the pump will receive the command exactly as intended, namely as ⟨ESC⟩SP?␣⟨CR⟩. However, when the WRITE# command is used, the command will arrive at the pump with added inverted commas as "⟨ESC⟩SP?␣"⟨CR⟩. Although some peripheral devices will accept both forms, it is generally safer to use the PRINT# statement.

5.3.3 Sending a hardware BREAK

See section 4.5.4. Programming aspects are detailed in Microsoft (1989c, 1990b).

5.4 Inputting data from the serial port

In order for the PC to be able to read a byte arriving at the serial port either the computer's DSR must be held HIGH, or DSR checking must be disabled using either the DS or DS0 option in the OPEN COM statement.

† Throughout this book the symbol ␣ indicates a space.

The error-checking sequence used while receiving data is detailed in Microsoft (1990f).

Once a character has been read in from the serial port, QuickBASIC then saves the character in a software Receive buffer, the size of which is controlled by the RBn option in the OPEN COM statement.

If data accumulates in QuickBASIC's Receive buffer faster than it is being extracted by the program, then before long the buffer will fill, resulting in a 'communications-buffer overflow' error, and the program will terminate. This can be remedied by trying one of the following options.

- Using some form of handshaking to control the flow of data into the Receive buffer from the peripheral device.
- Increasing the size of the Receive buffer using the RBn option (default size is 512 bytes) in the OPEN COM statement. For example, including RB2000 will increase the size of the Receive buffer to 2000 bytes.
- Using the INPUT$ function to input the data.
- Using some combination of these.

If there are problems handling data from the Receive buffer, it is often useful to check the exact format of the data being received, for example by using the subroutine FULLCODE (see Section 5.6).

5.4.1 *Using the* INPUT$ *function*

Data is best read from the Receive buffer using the INPUT$ function, which places the received data into a string which can then be manipulated by the program.

The INPUT$ function should be used in a loop in conjunction with the LOC function (see Microsoft, 1990a). This method has the advantage that it inputs all the characters which have arrived in the Receive buffer since the last cycle of the loop, and is therefore able to keep up with very high rates of incoming data. The recommended use of the INPUT$ function (Microsoft, 1990a) is illustrated in the following example.

Suppose the data arriving at the Receive buffer consists of a series of data-strings, each of which is terminated by the ⟨CR⟩⟨LF⟩ pair of control characters, whose ASCII values are 13 and 10 respectively (see Appendix 1). The following example QuickBASIC routine, which consists of two 'do-loops', initially inputs data from the Receive buffer into the string a$, and then determines how many characters there are up to and including the next ⟨LF⟩ control character. The outer loop then places this

Serial interface programming in QuickBASIC 53

group of characters into the string data$, and prints it to the screen and to a file designated as #2. The remaining characters of the string a$ are then combined with all the characters which have arrived in the Receive buffer since the last cycle of the inner loop (see Figures 5.1a and 5.1b).

If data stops arriving at the serial port, the number of characters in both the Receive buffer and the string a$ will shrink to zero as the remaining data is printed to the screen and saved in a file, whereupon the program exits the outer loop and continues with the rest of the program. The amount of data in the Receive buffer varies depending on the rate of data input via the serial port *and* on the rate of data transfer into a$.

```
1.  OPEN "COM1: ......." FOR INPUT AS #1
2.  OPEN "b:datafile.dat" FOR OUTPUT AS #2
        ...
        ...
3.  LF$ = CHR$(10)
4.  DO
5.        DO
6.            a$ = a$ + INPUT$(LOC(1), #1)
7.            L% = INSTR(1, a$, LF$)
8.        LOOP UNTIL L% > 0
9.        data$ = MID$(a$, 1, L% - 2)
10.       PRINT "data = "; data$
11.       PRINT #2, "data = "; data$
12.       a$ = RIGHT$(a$, LEN(a$) - L%)
13. LOOP UNTIL LEN(a$) = 0
        ...
        ...
14. CLOSE #1,#2
```

As an example, Figure 5.1a shows the above program operating on the following data arriving at the serial port from a pulse oximeter.

HR072:SAT092⟨CR⟩⟨LF⟩
HR073:SAT093⟨CR⟩⟨LF⟩
HR074:SAT094⟨CR⟩⟨LF⟩
HR075:SAT095⟨CR⟩⟨LF⟩
HR076:SAT096⟨CR⟩⟨LF⟩
HR077:SAT097⟨CR⟩⟨LF⟩
HR078:SAT098⟨CR⟩⟨LF⟩

a$ =
Receive buffer = HR072:SAT092⟨CR⟩⟨LF⟩⟨EOF⟩

```
3.  LF$ = CHR$(10)
4.  DO
5.      DO
6.          a$ = a$ + INPUT$(LOC(1), #1)
7.          L% = INSTR(1, a$, LF$)
```

	LEN(a$)=11	
a$ =	$\overbrace{\text{HR072:SAT09}}$	
	L%=0	
Receive buffer = 2⟨CR⟩⟨LF⟩HR073:SAT093⟨CR⟩⟨LF⟩HR074:⟨EOF⟩		

```
8.      LOOP UNTIL L% > 0
6.          a$ = a$ + INPUT$(LOC(1), #1)
7.          L% = INSTR(1, a$, LF$)
```

	LEN(a$)=39	
a$ =	$\overbrace{\text{HR072:SAT092⟨CR⟩⟨LF⟩}}$ $\overbrace{\text{HR073:SAT093⟨CR⟩⟨LF⟩HR074:SAT09}}$	
	L%=14	RIGHT$(a$, LEN(a$)-L%)
Receive buffer = 4⟨CR⟩⟨LF⟩HR075:SAT095⟨CR⟩⟨LF⟩HR076:SAT096⟨CR⟩ ⟨LF⟩HR077:SAT0⟨EOF⟩		

```
8.      LOOP UNTIL L% > 0
9.      data$ = MID$(a$, 1, L% - 2)
```

data$ = HR072:SAT092

```
10.     PRINT "data = "; data$
11.     PRINT #2, "data = "; data$
12.     a$ = RIGHT$(a$, LEN(a$) - L%)
```

a$ = HR073:SAT093⟨CR⟩⟨LF⟩HR074:SAT09
Receive buffer = 4⟨CR⟩⟨LF⟩HR075:SAT095⟨CR⟩⟨LF⟩HR076:SAT096⟨CR⟩ ⟨LF⟩HR077:SAT097⟨CR⟩⟨LF⟩HR078:S⟨EOF⟩

```
13. LOOP UNTIL LEN(a$) = 0
```

Fig. 5.1 a. Accessing data from the Receive buffer using the INPUT$ function. In this example program data is transferred from the Receive buffer into the string a$, from which the data between ⟨CR⟩⟨LF⟩ pairs is transferred to the string data$ and then printed to the screen and to a file. The boxes indicate the current status of the Receive buffer, a$, and data$. Note that the INSTR function is looking for a ⟨LF⟩ character (ASCII 10), and that it returns a value of 0 until a ⟨LF⟩ appears in the Receive buffer, whereupon it then returns the number of characters up to and including the ⟨LF⟩ character. The line numbers refer to the program on the previous page and to Fig. 5.1 b opposite.

Figure 5.1a is designed to be viewed in conjunction with the notes in Figure 5.1b, and shows how the various lines of the program process the incoming data by manipulating the contents of the QuickBASIC Receive buffer as well as the strings a$ and data$. Note that the line numbers in the above example program and those in Figures 5.1a and 5.1b refer to the same program statements. The end of the Receive buffer is indicated by the ⟨EOF⟩ marker (^Z).

An example of a program which illustrates the use of the INPUT$ function to access real-time data from a pulse oximeter is **ohm374-r.bas**, which is described in Section 9.3.1.

Line 1: Opens the serial port designated COM1 for receiving data.
Line 2: Opens a file (datafile.dat) on a disk in drive B to save the data, and designates the file #2.
Line 3: Renames the ⟨LF⟩ control character (ASCII 10) as LF$ for convenience in order to make the program more readable.
Line 6: Removes all the characters currently in the Receive buffer and adds them to the end of the string a$. Note that the LOC(1) statement returns the number of characters in the Receive buffer up to the ⟨EOF⟩ marker.
Line 7: The INSTR function examines the string a$ character by character, and returns an integer value representing the number of characters in the string a$ up to and including the specified character, which in this example is the ⟨LF⟩ control character. Note that the INSTR function returns a value of zero until the specified character is found, whereupon it returns the number of characters up to and including the specified character.
Line 8: The condition terminating the inner loop is when L% is greater than zero; i.e. when the INSTR function has found the next ⟨LF⟩.
Line 9: Copies the first L% - 2 characters from a$ (i.e. all those up to but not including the first ⟨CR⟩ control character) into a separate string called data$.
Line 10: Prints the data (data$) to the screen.
Line 11: Prints the data (data$) to the file designated as #2; i.e. datafile.dat on the disk in drive B (see line 2).
Line 12: Renames the rest of a$ following the first ⟨LF⟩ control character as a$. This effectively deletes the first part of a$ up to and including the first ⟨LF⟩ control character.
Line 13: This line terminates the loop when there are no characters left in a$; i.e. when the Receive buffer is empty.
Line 14: Closes down file 1 and file 2 before terminating the program. Note that if the statement CLOSE is used without any file numbers then it will close *all* files which are currently open.

Fig. 5.1 b.

5.4.2 Using the INPUT# function

Although use of the INPUT$ function is generally recommended for inputting data, use of the INPUT# function instead is often quite satisfactory providing the required data-strings are terminated by the ⟨CR⟩ control character, since the INPUT# function inputs all data up to the first ⟨CR⟩ (Microsoft, 1990a). However, if the inflow of data is too high for too long the Receive buffer will eventually fill. In this case, simply increasing the size of the Receive buffer may suffice. Alternatively, the INPUT$ function may have to be used, since this can always keep up with the inflow of data.

Note that care is needed when using INPUT# to read in data items from a sequential file—see Microsoft (1992d).

The following example uses the INPUT# function to input data into a string called data$. The routine inputs data via the serial port (COM2 opened as #1), prints the data to the screen, and then saves it in a file (opened as #2) on a disk.

```
OPEN "COM2: ......." FOR INPUT AS #1
OPEN "b:datafile.dat" FOR OUTPUT AS #2
 ...
 ...
DO
    INPUT #1, data$
    PRINT data$
    PRINT #2, data$
LOOP
```

An example of a program which illustrates the use of the INPUT# function to access real-time data from a pulse oximeter is **nel-bk-r.bas**, which is described in Section 10.3.1.

5.5 Opening a data-file

A data-file is accessed using the OPEN statement, which defines the destination drive, direction of data flow, and filename. Details of the OPEN statement are given in Appendix 6. Note that the direction of data flow is relative to the computer's RAM.

For example, the following OPEN statement establishes a file called datafile.dat in drive B to receive data—i.e. the data will be output from the RAM. Note that the file number (#n) must, of course, be different from that of the OPEN COM statement.

```
OPEN "b:datafile.dat" FOR OUTPUT AS #2
```

If the data-string to be saved is oximdata$, then the following statement will save the data-string on the disk. Note the use of #2 to identify the data-file and its location.

```
PRINT #2, oximdata$
```

If the data-string (oximdata$) is being saved to a disk in real time from a pulse oximeter and does not already contain the sampling time, then the current time can be added by the computer using the DATE$ and TIME$ functions, and saved with each data-string as follows.

```
PRINT #2, oximdata$, DATE$, TIME$
```

5.6 Reading hidden control characters

It is often useful to know exactly where all the spaces ⊔ and the ⟨CR⟩ and ⟨LF⟩ control characters are in received data-strings, as well as the location of all the other control characters. An example subroutine (FULLCODE), which looks at each character in a string r$ and reveals all the control characters and spaces, is shown below. All control characters which are not among those listed in the subroutine as their uppercase letter codes (e.g. <LF>) are displayed as their decimal ASCII value (e.g. <28>).

```
SUB fullcode (r$)
    code$ = ""
    FOR j = 1 TO LEN(r$)
        ch$ = MID$(r$, j, 1)
        IF ASC(ch$) < 33 THEN
            char$ = "<" + LTRIM$(STR$(ASC(ch$))) + ">"
            IF ch$ = CHR$(13) THEN char$ = "<CR>"
            IF ch$ = CHR$(10) THEN char$ = "<LF>"
            IF ch$ = CHR$(32) THEN char$ = "<SPACE>"
            IF ch$ = CHR$(27) THEN char$ = "<ESC>"
            IF ch$ = CHR$(7) THEN char$ = "<BEL>"
        ELSE
            char$ = ch$
        END IF
        code$ = code$ + char$
```

```
    NEXT j
    PRINT "fullcode = "; code$
    PRINT #2, "fullcode = "; code$
END SUB
```

This example subroutine (FULLCODE) is probably most useful when inputting data using the INPUT$ function, in order to help determine how best to input data-strings which are bracketed by control characters.

For example, suppose data is to be collected from a new pulse oximeter which outputs data every 2 seconds, and it is not clear from the manual exactly how the data is formatted. In this case the following program will collect all the data into a long string (a$), and then display the complete code when <Q> is pressed by calling the subroutine FULLCODE. It is probably most convenient to use a small LED on the PC's RxD line to indicate the flow of incoming data-strings,† and then press <Q> when a reasonable amount of data has been received. Note that FULLCODE will save the data to a disk (#2) as well as printing it to the screen.

```
OPEN "COM1: ......." FOR INPUT AS #1
OPEN "B:datafile.dat" FOR OUTPUT AS #2
PRINT "port open and waiting for data"
PRINT "press <Q> to view collected data"
DO
    a$ = a$ + INPUT$(LOC(1), #1)
    key$ = INKEY$
    IF UCASE$(key$) = "Q" THEN
        CALL fullcode(a$)
        CLOSE
        END
    END IF
LOOP
END
```

When the program is run, and <Q> pressed after the outputs of a few data-strings from the pulse oximeter, the result might appear as follows.

=Ø67<SPACE><CR><LF>SaO2=Ø94<SPACE>PR=Ø66<SPACE><CR><LF>SaO2=Ø93<SPACE>PR=Ø68<SPACE><CR><LF>SaO2=Ø92<SPACE>PR=Ø69<SPACE><CR><LF>

From this initial trial run using the example subroutine FULLCODE,

† A commercial RS-232 line monitor is very useful in this respect.

Serial interface programming in QuickBASIC

it is immediately clear that the oximetry data consists of a number of similar strings, each starting with SaO2=... and ending with the control characters ⟨CR⟩⟨LF⟩.

Note that in the above example only the *last* part of the first data-string output by the device has been collected, since in this particular example the program was started while the first data-string was being output by the oximeter.

Once the complete data has been made 'visible' using the FULLCODE subroutine, it becomes clear that these oximetry data-strings could be captured either by using the INPUT# statement (because each string ends with ⟨CR⟩—see Section 5.4.2), or by using the more versatile INPUT$ technique, in conjunction with the INSTR statement looking for the ⟨LF⟩ control character. In the latter case, this could be done by using the statement L% = INSTR(1, a$, CHR$(1Ø))—see Section 5.4.1.

Once all the control characters have been made 'visible' it is then relatively easy to write a QuickBASIC program to collect, display, and save the oximetry data. For example, in this particular case the following QuickBASIC code could be used.

```
DO
    DO
        a$ = a$ + INPUT$(LOC(1), #1)
        L% = INSTR(1, a$, CHR$(1Ø))
    LOOP UNTIL L% > Ø
    data$ = LEFT$(a$, 1, L% - 2)
    PRINT data$
    PRINT #2, data$
    a$ = RIGHT$(a$, LEN(a$) - L%)
LOOP UNTIL LEN(a$) = Ø
```

This short program will display and save the previous data as follows.

```
=Ø67
SaO2=Ø94 PR=Ø66
SaO2=Ø93 PR=Ø68
SaO2=Ø92 PR=Ø69
```

It is now clear that part of the first data-string has been missed, which is invariably the case when the peripheral device is already outputting data before the program starts.

Note that in this example the data could just as easily have been collected by having the INSTR function look for the ⟨CR⟩ control character

(ASCII 13) by using L% = INSTR(1, a$, CHR$(13)) instead. However, if this approach is used, whenever the program exits the first loop (i.e. when L% > ∅) the string a$ will now start with the ⟨LF⟩ control character as follows.

⟨LF⟩SaO2=098␣PR=074␣⟨CR⟩⟨LF⟩SaO2= ...

In this case the number of characters to be moved into the string data$ is L%-2 as before, but this time the required characters start with the second character in a$ (namely S) since ⟨LF⟩ is the first character. The string data$ therefore has to be defined as follows.

data$ = MID$(a$, 2, L% - 2)

Thus in order to use the INPUT# statement there must be a ⟨CR⟩ in the string (see Section 5.4.2); in order to use the INPUT$ function a terminal character must be specified in the INSTR statement.

Sometimes however, the output data does not contain a ⟨CR⟩, and at the same time it is not clear what all the characters are in the output data. An example of this problem is when trying to access data which is formatted in such a way as to be understood by a specific printer.

For example, the Novametrix 515A pulse oximeter is able to output Trend data to a Hewlett-Packard ThinkJet printer which automatically prints the data as a graph. Since this particular oximeter does not output Trend data formatted in the usual way for a PC, the only way for a PC to access this data is to capture the Trend data as formatted for the printer, and then to reformat the data.

The problem is that when data is formatted for a printer, numerous extra control characters and 'escape' sequences are added to the data in order to control the printer. Additional spaces ␣ and ⟨NUL⟩ characters are also used. If the Trend data is accessed and displayed using the subroutine FULLCODE described above, it will become clear how to write a program to extract the embedded Trend data. An example of Novametrix 515A Trend data formatted for the Hewlett-Packard ThinkJet printer is shown in Figure 5.2.

5.7 Accessing data using ON COM

Sometimes it is useful for a program to only access the serial port when data arrives, since this frees the program to do other things in the meantime. This is achieved in QuickBASIC by using the ON COM(n) GOSUB

0><0><0><0><0><0><0><0><LF><ESC>0<ESC>2<LF><ESC>U1<0><LF><ESC>E<18><14>NOVAMETRIX
<SPACE>*<SPACE><SPACE><SPACE><SPACE><SPACE><SPACE><SPACE><SPACE><SPACE><SPACE>
<SPACE><SPACE><SPACE><SPACE><SPACE>515A<SPACE>PULSE<LF><LF><ESC>E<18><14>
MEDICAL<SPACE>SYSTEMS<SPACE>INC.<SPACE><SPACE><SPACE><SPACE><SPACE><SPACE><SPACE>
<SPACE><SPACE><SPACE>OXIMETER.<LF><LF><ESC>E<18><14>T-JET<SPACE>DRIVER<SPACE>PRINTED
<SPACE>AT<SPACE>21:48<SPACE>JUL/30/93<LF><LF><ESC>E<18><14>PATIENT<SPACE>NAME<SPACE>
                         <LF><LF><ESC>E<18><14>SENSOR<SPACE>TYPE<SPACE>-------------
<SPACE>FIO2<SPACE>------   <LF><LF><ESC>E<18><14>NOTES<SPACE>-------------------
<LF><LF><ESC>E<18><14>FULL<SPACE>TREND<SPACE>PRINTOUT<SPACE><SPACE><SPACE><SPACE>
<SPACE><SPACE><SPACE><SPACE><SPACE><SPACE><SPACE><SPACE><SPACE><SPACE><SPACE>
<SPACE><SPACE><SPACE><LF><0><0><0><0><0><0><0><0><0><0><0><0><0><0><0><0><0>
<0><0><0><0><0><0><0><0><0><0><0><0><0><0><0><0><0><0><0><0><0><0><0><0><0>
<0><0><0><0><0><0><0><0><0><0><0><0><0><0><0><0><0><0><0><0><0><0><0><0><0>
<0><0><0><0><0><0><0><0><0><0><0><0><0><0><0><0><0><0><0><0><0><0><0><0><0>
<0><0><0><0><0><0><0><0><0><0><0><0><0><0><0><0><0><0><0><0><0><0><0><0><0>
<0><0><0><0><0><0><0><0><0><0><0><0><0><0><0><0><0><0><0><0><0><0><LF><ESC>E
<18><14>COL.<SPACE>A<SPACE>=<SPACE>MUTE<SPACE>STATUS<SPACE>-<SPACE>=<SPACE>AUDIO<SPACE>
MUTE<SPACE>ON<SPACE><LF><LF><ESC>E<18><14>COL.<SPACE>B<SPACE>=<SPACE>EVENT<SPACE>MARKS
<SPACE>-<SPACE>=<SPACE>EVENT<SPACE>MARKED<SPACE><SPACE><LF><ESC>A<8><LF><0><0><0>

Fig. 5.2. Part of the Trend data output from a Novametrix 515A pulse oximeter formatted for the ThinkJet printer. This is the output printed using the subroutine FULLCODE. Control characters are given in anglebrackets. A numeric value in anglebrackets indicates the ASCII value of the control character. See text for details.

statement, which specifies the location of an event-handling subroutine which is used to process the data as and when it arrives at the serial port.

An example program demonstrating the general structure of such a program is shown below. The program just prints consecutive numbers to the screen; however, when data arrives at the serial port it breaks off to collect the data, which it prints to the screen (just to show that the data has been collected) and then prints it to a file (coms.dat). Note that the line label getCOMportdata: must be terminated by a colon.

```
REM program to demonstrate the use of ON COM
REM on-com2.BAS
OPEN "COM1:1200,0,7,1,CS,DS,RB10000" FOR INPUT AS #1
OPEN "c:coms.dat" FOR OUTPUT AS #2
CLS : LOCATE 7
PRINT "communications open OK"
ON COM(1) GOSUB getCOMportdata
COM(1) ON
DO
    REM print consecutive nos to screen
    j = j + 1 : PRINT j
    SLEEP 1
    KEY$ = INKEY$
    IF UCASE$(KEY$) = "Q" THEN
        CLOSE #1, #2
        COM(1) OFF
        END
    END IF
LOOP

getCOMportdata:
a$ = ""
DO
    DO
        a$ = a$ + INPUT$(LOC(1), #1)
        L% = INSTR(1, a$, CHR$(13))
        KEY$ = INKEY$
        IF UCASE$(KEY$) = "Q" THEN
            CLOSE #1, #2
            END
        END IF
```

```
        LOOP UNTIL L% > 0
        data$ = MID$(a$, 1, L% - 2)
        PRINT data$
        PRINT #2, data$
        a$ = RIGHT$(a$, LEN(a$) - L%)
LOOP UNTIL LEN(a$) = 0
COM(1) OFF: COM(1) ON
RETURN
END
```

5.8 Accessing a reply code

Sometimes a reply code is sent back to the PC from a peripheral device in response to a command or 'escape' sequence which has been sent by the PC. However, it is not uncommon to find that some commands which cause a reply to be returned take the peripheral device longer to process than others. For example, it may well take significantly longer to return a long string of data in response to a command from the PC than to return a one or two character reply.

If two commands or codes are sent immediately one after another, then the order in which the replies appear in the PC's Receive buffer may not be as expected, if the time required for the peripheral device to generate the replies is not taken into account.

In general it is best to collect each reply immediately following the requesting command, as shown in the following example which calls the subroutines SEND and GETREPLY to transmit commands and collect replies.

```
CALL send(command1)
CALL getreply
CALL send(command2)
CALL getreply
```

A simple subroutine (SEND) to send a command (z$) is as follows.

```
SUB send(z$)
    PRINT #1, z$
END SUB
```

Note that most peripheral devices require their commands to be formatted in a particular way. For example, the Ohmeda 9000 syringe pump requires its command-codes to be sent in a string having the following format.

⟨ESC⟩SP⟨command-code⟩␣⟨CR⟩

Since the ASCII codes for the characters ⟨ESC⟩ and ␣ are 27 and 32 respectively, these would be transmitted as CHR$(27) and CHR$(32). An example subroutine (SENDCODE) to send the command-code code$ using the Ohmeda format is given below, and would be called using the statement CALL sendcode(code$). The ⟨CR⟩ character is added by the PRINT# statement (see Section 5.3.1).

```
SUB sendcode(z$)
    ohmeda$ = CHR$(27) + "SP" + z$ + CHR$(32)
    PRINT #1, ohmeda$
END SUB
```

If the command-code from the PC generates a reply terminated by ⟨CR⟩, then the following simple subroutine (GETREPLY) could be used to collect the reply from the Receive buffer and print it to the screen.

```
SUB getreply
    a$ = ""
    DO
        DO
            a$ = a$ + INPUT$(LOC(1), #1)
            L% = INSTR(1, a$, CHR$(13))
        LOOP UNTIL L% > 0
        data$ = MID$(a$, 1, L% - 1)
        PRINT data$
    LOOP UNTIL LEN(a$) = 0
END SUB
```

Note that in the above example, the subroutine GETREPLY looks for reply strings terminated by ⟨CR⟩ by using CHR$(13) in the INSTR function, since ⟨CR⟩ is equivalent to ASCII 13.

5.9 Emptying the Receive buffer

A precaution against collecting the wrong reply is to empty the Receive buffer immediately prior to sending a command which generates a reply.

A convenient way of emptying the Receive buffer is to use the following subroutine, which empties the buffer in response to the statement CALL emptybuffer. Note that in this example the subroutine empties the buffer associated with the COM port designated as #1.

```
SUB emptybuffer
    DO WHILE NOT EOF(1)
        buffer$ = INPUT$(LOC(1), #1)
    LOOP
    PRINT "buffer empty"
END SUB
```

The number of characters currently in the Receive buffer (#1) can be determined using the LOC statement as follows (see also Microsoft, 1990f).

```
PRINT "No of characters in buffer = "; LOC(1)
```

5.10 Reading a data-file

It is frequently useful to be able to look at the data as it accumulates in the data-file, while the program is running. Although a QuickBASIC routine can be written to do this, it is usually more convenient to use one of the many sophisticated utilities which are available, e.g. SHOW.COM[†] or VIEW.EXE.[‡]

For example, the file-viewing utility SHOW.COM could be used to view the contents of the file datafile using the command show in conjunction with the SHELL statement as follows.

```
SHELL "show datafile"
```

In order to use this file-viewer to view data which is being collected in datafile configured as #2, include the following lines in the do-loop which collects and saves the data. Pressing <V> then invokes the file-viewer.

```
DO
    ...
    ...
    KEY$ = INKEY$
    IF UCASE$(KEY$) = "V" THEN
        CLOSE #2
```

[†] SHOW.COM is available from Clockwork Software, Bidbury House, Havant, Hampshire, PO9 3JG, UK; Tel: +44–(0)1705–483217; Fax: +44–(0)1705–454233.
[‡] VIEW.EXE is part of the Treacles utilities available from Puppy Power Software, PO Box 54, Whitstable, Kent, CT5 3YW, UK.

```
         SHELL "show datafile"
         OPEN "datafile" FOR APPEND ACCESS READ WRITE AS #2
      END IF
LOOP
```

Once <V> is pressed the program closes the file in order to prevent any data being lost from the buffer when using the SHELL statement (see Microsoft, 1990g). The program then SHELLs out to DOS and invokes SHOW.COM. On quitting the file-viewer, the data-file is re-opened in such a way as to allow more data to be written to the end of the file, and the program continues as before.

5.11 Use of the LTRIM$ function

It is frequently necessary to send an alphanumeric code to a peripheral device. For example, a syringe pump may change its infusion rate to 30 ml/hr in response to the command 'rate30'.

A program to send this command interactively by typing 30 at the keyboard would require the word rate and the number 30 to be combined with no intervening space. However, the space immediately before the number is reserved for the sign, which means that for positive numbers the unused sign space has to be removed before adding it to the other string. The method is to first convert the number to a string using the STR$ function, and then remove the first space using the LTRIM$ function.

An example of the code to do this is as follows. Note that the value 30 has been entered into the variable volume.

```
volume = 30
command$ = "rate" + LTRIM$(STR$(volume))
PRINT #1, command$
```

Another common use for the LTRIM$ function is to print numbers in a fixed width format (fixed frame); for example, printing elapsed time in the format 16:15:23, or printing a variable infusion rate with five digits including one decimal place, e.g. 0032.0 ml/hr.

Since the QuickBASIC TIMER function returns the time since midnight in seconds, the function ELAPSEDTIME$ which is described below might be used to print the elapsed time in the fixed frame format hh:mm:ss as follows.

```
timestart = TIMER
...
```

Serial interface programming in QuickBASIC

```
...
PRINT "elapsed time = ;" elapsedtime$(TIMER - timestart)
...
END

FUNCTION elapsedtime$ (seconds)
    REM prints time as hh:mm:ss (16:15:04)
    min% = INT(seconds / 60) MOD 60
    hour% = INT(seconds / 3600) MOD 24
    sec% = INT(seconds) MOD 60
    hour$ = RIGHT$("0" + LTRIM$(STR$(hour%)), 2)
    min$ = RIGHT$("0" + LTRIM$(STR$(min%)), 2)
    sec$ = RIGHT$("0" + LTRIM$(STR$(sec%)), 2)
    elapsedtime$ = hour$ + ":" + min$ + ":" + sec$
END FUNCTION
```

Note that the above example routine defines the start of the time interval using the `timestart = TIMER` statement, and that spaces are filled with leading zeros.

5.12 Time delays

A simple routine for generating a time delay in a program is as follows.

```
FOR j = 0 TO 2000 : NEXT j
```

However, the *exact* time resulting from this construction depends on the particular microprocessor and clockspeed used by the PC. A more precise time delay is achieved using the SLEEP n command. This is shown in the following example which generates a 5 second delay.

```
SLEEP 5
```

5.12.1 Time-out

The QuickBASIC TIMER function, which returns the number of seconds since the previous midnight, has many uses. A common use is for generating a time-out. This is particularly useful in communications, as it allows the program to either exit or follow some other path if there is a communication failure. A common problem is where the peripheral device fails to reply to some command from the PC.

In the following example, the program exits the do-loop if a reply is not received within 2 seconds. This construction is frequently used in the programs given in Part III of this book, usually in the subroutine GETREPLY.

```
starttime = TIMER
DO
    DO
        a$ = a$ + INPUT$(LOC(1), #1)
        L% = INSTR(1, a$, CHR$(13))
        IF TIMER > starttime + 2 THEN EXIT DO
    LOOP UNTIL L% > 0
    ...
    ...
LOOP UNTIL LEN(a$) = 0
```

Alternatively an error handling subroutine (e.g. ERRORHANDLER) could be called if the time-out is exceeded, using the following line instead.

```
IF TIMER > starttime + 2 THEN CALL errorhandler
```

This construction is used in the subroutine GETREPLY in the program **grasebyb.bas** in Chapter 14.

5.13 Trapping errors

It is useful for a program to branch to a special error-handling routine when a program error occurs. This is achieved in QuickBASIC by using the ON ERROR GOTO statement. Different routines can then be instituted depending on the error code returned by the ERR function. The device causing the error can be established using the ERDEV and ERDEV$ functions. If the error is recoverable, then the program can be made to continue using the RESUME statement, as follows.

```
...
ON ERROR GOTO errortrap
...
...
END

errortrap:
PRINT "error = "; ERR
RESUME
```

Serial interface programming in QuickBASIC 69

5.13.1 Error messages

Extensive lists of QuickBASIC's error codes and messages are given by Microsoft (1988, 1989f, 1990f) and Waite *et al.* (1990). Some of the common errors associated with the serial port are as follows. Note that the error code is a value which is returned when using the ERR function in an error-trapping routine.

Error 24 **Device timeout**
Communication links were not established before the specified or default wait-times.

Error 25 **Device fault**
A device has returned a hardware error. If this message occurs while data are being transmitted to a communications file, it indicates that the signals being tested with the OPEN COM statement were not found in the specified period of time.

Error 52 **Bad file name or number**
A statement of command references a file with a file name or number that is not specified in the OPEN statement, or is out of the range of file numbers specified earlier in the program.

Error 54 **Bad file mode**
Executing an OPEN COM statement using the wrong file mode. For example, trying to write to a file opened FOR INPUT (see Microsoft (1988) for further details).

Error 55 **File already open**
This arises when an OPEN statement is issued for a file that is already open, or a KILL statement is given for a file that is open.

Error 57 **Device I/O error**
This indicates an error caused by overrun, framing, or parity errors, or a break signal.

Error 64 **Bad file name**
An illegal form is used for the file name with LOAD, SAVE, KILL, or OPEN. For example, the file name has too many characters.

Error 68 **Device unavailable**
The device to be accessed is not on line or does not exist. For example, trying to open a serial port which does not exist.

Error 69 **Communication-buffer overflow**
The Receive buffer size was exceeded.

5.14 Trapping keys

Trapping a character key is achieved by using either the character itself or its 'key' code (see Appendix 3). For example, the following QuickBASIC statements will exit the program when <Q> is pressed.

```
DO
    key$ = INKEY$
    IF UCASE$(key$) = "Q" THEN
        CLOSE #1, #2
        END
    END IF
    ...
    ...
LOOP
```

Since Q is a character, the "Q" can be replaced by the ASCII value of the character (i.e. ASCII 81), namely CHR$(81). The conditional line would then read as follows.

```
IF UCASE$(key$) = CHR$(81) THEN ...
```

Similarly, if it was necessary to use the key combination Ctrl-E to quit the program, the above line would be as follows, since the Table of key codes in Appendix 3 shows that QuickBASIC returns the single byte 5 when Ctrl-E is pressed.

```
IF key$ = CHR$(5) THEN ...
```

In order to trap one of the extended keys, i.e. one of the keys associated with a two-byte key code (say, F1; 0, 59), both codes must be used in the correct order as follows.

```
IF key$ = CHR$(0) + CHR$(59) THEN ...
```

An alternative strategy is to handle the trapped key using an ON KEY GOSUB construction. However this technique requires a second key press to exit the INKEY$ loop on returning from the key handler. See Microsoft (1990h) for further details, and for alternative strategies requiring only a single keypress.

5.15 The checksum

Checksums are most easily determined using the QuickBASIC MOD function. For example an 8-bit (*modulo* 256) Σ-checksum† would be determined by the following statements, where sum% is the decimal sum of the characters of the string datastring$.

```
sum% = 0
FOR J = 1 TO LEN(datastring$)
    sum% = sum% + ASC(MID$(datastring$, J, 1))
NEXT J
checksum% = sum% MOD 256
```

Sometimes the checksum is required to be in hexadecimal notation, in which case the above checksum% can be converted using the following statement.

```
checksumhex$ = HEX$(checksum%)
```

Sometimes the command format of a device requires that the checksum is transmitted as a fixed number of characters. In this case a variable number of leading zeros may need to be added depending on the value of the checksum.

For example, since HEX$(11) will return the single character B, if the hexadecimal checksum must be returned as a two-character value, then a single leading zero can be added to give 0B using the following statement, where checksum% is the decimal value of the checksum.

```
checksumhex$ = RIGHT$("0" + HEX$(checksum%), 2)
```

In view of the way checksums are used, it is often more convenient to calculate the checksum using a function rather than a subroutine.

For example, the function CHECKSUMHEX$ (shown below) could be used to transmit both the data (say, data$) and its two-character hexadecimal Σ-checksum via the serial port designated as #1, using the following statement. Note that this particular checksum is used by the Graseby 3400 syringe pump (see Chapter 14).

```
PRINT #1, data$ + checksumhex$(data$)
...
...
FUNCTION checksumhex$ (c$)
    REM generates a two character hex 8-bit checksum
```

† See Chapter 3 for details of the various checksums.

```
    sum% = 0
    FOR J = 1 TO LEN(c$)
        sum% = sum% + ASC(MID$(c$, J, 1))
    NEXT J
    checksum% = sum% MOD 256
    REM add leading zero to give at least two characters
    checksumhex$ = RIGHT$("0" + HEX$(checksum%), 2)
END FUNCTION
```

The following function (TWOSCHECKSUM$) could be used in a similar manner to determine the 7-bit (*modulo* 128) two's complement checksum (TC-checksum†) which is used by the Ohmeda 9000 syringe pump. Note that with this particular syringe pump the command (c$) has to be preceded by ⟨ESC⟩SP, which must also be included in the checksum (see Chapter 15).

```
FUNCTION twochecksum$ (c$)
    REM generates a two's complement 7-bit checksum
    k$ = CHR$(27) + "SP" + c$
    sum% = 0
    FOR J = 1 TO LEN(k$)
        sum% = sum% + ASC(MID$(k$, J, 1))
    NEXT J
    twochecksum$ = CHR$(128 - sum% MOD 128)
END FUNCTION
```

5.16 Controlling the output control lines

Each serial port has two output control lines (RTS and DTR),‡ and sometimes it is necessary to switch one of these control lines HIGH or LOW during the running of the program. This is done by changing the appropriate bit in the UART's Modem Control Register (Microsoft, 1990c, 1992b).

Note that with regard to the control lines, the term HIGH is associated with a positive voltage, and logic 1. Similarly, the term LOW is associated with a negative voltage, and logic 0 (see Chapter 1).

Figure 5.3 shows that bit-0 of the Modem Control Register controls DTR, and bit-1 controls RTS (see also Section 4.4.3). The problem is that the relevant bit or bits must be set either HIGH (1) or LOW (0) without

---
† See Chapter 3 for details.
‡ See Chapter 1 for details of the serial port control lines.

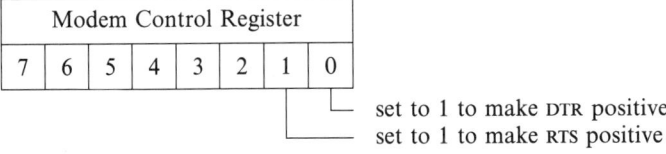

Fig. 5.3. Modem Control Register.

altering any of the other bits in the register. The solution to the problem involves both writing to and reading from port registers, as well as using the logical operators AND, OR, NOT, and Exclusive OR. These are described below.

5.16.1 Reading a register

Serial port registers are read using the INP(address) function. The address value is commonly given in hexadecimal, in which case Quick-BASIC requires that it is prefixed by &H, which indicates that the port address is a hexadecimal (H) long integer (&).

For example, the port address of COM2's Modem Control Register is 02FCh (see Section 4.4.3), and its value would be read into the integer variable mcrcom2% by the following statement.

```
mcrcom2% = INP(&H02FC)
```

Since the decimal equivalent of 02FCh is 764, the statement to read the port address could also be written as follows.

```
mcrcom2% = INP(764)
```

Note that since a port address is an integer, it is always better to use an integer variable for the address (e.g. mcrcom2%),† as integer manipulations are processed considerably faster than those for non-integers (see Microsoft, 1989g).

5.16.2 Writing to a register

Port registers are written to using the OUT statement which takes the two parameters address and value. For example, the value 151 would be

† QuickBASIC uses the suffix % to define an integer variable.

Table 5.2. *Logic table for OR.*

OR		
0 OR 0	=	0
0 OR 1	=	1
1 OR 0	=	1
1 OR 1	=	1

written to the address of the MCR of COM2 (02FCh) by the following statement.

OUT &H02FC, 151

5.16.3 Setting a bit HIGH (1)

The port register is first read using the INP function. Since the bit in question is to be set to 1, the logical operation OR is used to generate a new value, which is then written back to the same register, using the OUT statement.

In practice the value initially read from the port register is ORed with a special binary number known as a 'bit-mask', which has a 1 *only* in the same bit position as that required to be set to 1. Defining the bit-mask in this way has the advantage that the bit-mask for a particular operation can be expressed easily in terms of the bit number. Thus the bit-mask to enable a change to bit-5 will be 2^5 etc. The logic table for the OR operation is shown in Table 5.2.

For example, suppose it is necessary to make the PC's RTS line HIGH (positive). Figure 5.3 shows that RTS is controlled by bit-1 of the Modem Control Register (MCR), which has an offset of 4 from the base address (see Section 4.3). If COM2 is being used (base address 02F8h), then the port address of COM2's MCR will be 02F8h + 4 = 02FCh. Having determined the address of the relevant MCR, the MCR is then read using the INP function for this address. Suppose this returns a decimal value of 133. This has a binary equivalent of 10000101, and since bit-1 (2nd bit from the right) is 0, this indicates that RTS is LOW. If this register value is now ORed with a mask in the bit-1 position, namely 00000010 ($= 2^1$), the result is the binary value 10000111, which is the same as the first number except it now has a 1 in the bit-1 position. This new number is then written back to the same port address using the OUT statement, whereupon the PC sets RTS HIGH (positive).

This particular OR operation is summarised below; the arrows indicate the position of bit-1.

$$\begin{array}{rl} \downarrow & \\ 10000101 \;=\; & \text{initial value of MCR } (= 133) \\ \underline{\text{OR } 00000010} \;=\; & \text{mask for bit-1 } (= 2^1) \\ 10000111 \;=\; & \text{final value of MCR } (= 135) \\ \uparrow & \end{array}$$

The above OR operation is expressed in QuickBASIC as follows.

```
INP(&H02FC) OR 2^1
```

Note that if the original value in the register had a 1 at the bit-1 position (e.g. 10000111), then the OR operation described above would still leave the number having a 1 in the bit-1 position, i.e. the number would be unchanged by this operation. This is because 1 OR 1 = 1.

The complete QuickBASIC statement which sets RTS HIGH, i.e. sets bit-1 of the MCR of COM2 to 1, is therefore as follows.

```
OUT &H02FC, INP(&H02FC) OR 2^1
```

However, when writing a program it is less confusing if the MCR port address is assigned to a meaningful integer variable, say mcrcom2%, in which case the above line of QuickBASIC would be as follows.

```
mcrcom2% = &H02FC
OUT mcrcom2%, INP(mcrcom2%) OR 2^1
```

If more than one bit needs to be set HIGH (1) at the same time, then all the bit positions can be included in the same command. For example, if both DTR (controlled by MCR bit-0) and RTS (controlled by MCR bit-1) need to be set HIGH (1) at the same time, then this can be done using the following statements.

```
mcrcom2% = &H02FC
OUT mcrcom2%, INP(mcrcom2%) OR (2^1 + 2^0)
```

5.16.4 *Setting a bit* LOW *(0)*

The port register is first read using the INP function. Since the bit in question is to be set to 0, the inverse of the bit-mask is first generated using the logical operator NOT. The logical operator AND is then used

Table 5.3. *Logic table for AND and NOT.*

AND	NOT
0 AND 0 = 0	NOT 0 = 1
0 AND 1 = 0	NOT 1 = 0
1 AND 0 = 0	
1 AND 1 = 1	

to generate a new value which is which is then written back to the same register, using the OUT statement. The logic tables of both AND and NOT are shown in Table 5.3.

Suppose it is necessary to set the DTR line LOW (negative). Since DTR is controlled by bit-0 of the MCR (see Figure 5.3) it is necessary to set bit-0 to 1, for which the required bit-mask is therefore 00000001 ($= 2^0$). The inverse of the bit-mask is given by NOT 00000001, which is 11111110. The inverse bit-mask is now ANDed to the initial value of the port register, and the result is then written back into the same register.

For example, if the value in the MCR is 115, which is 01110011 in binary, this indicates that DTR is currently HIGH (positive) since bit-0 is 1. Following the AND operation using the inverse bit-mask the result is 01110010, which is the same as the original value except with bit-0 set to 0 as required. This particular AND operation is summarised below, where the arrows indicate the bit-0 position.

$$
\begin{array}{rcl}
\downarrow & & \\
01110011 & = & \text{initial value of MCR } (= 115) \\
\text{AND } 11111110 & = & \text{NOT } 00000001 \ (= \text{NOT } 2^0) \\
01110010 & = & \text{final value of MCR } (= 114) \\
\uparrow & &
\end{array}
$$

The above AND operation is expressed in QuickBASIC as follows.

```
mcrcom2% = &H02FC
INP(mcrcom2%) AND (NOT 2^0)
```

Note that if the original port address value had a 0 in the bit-0 position (e.g. 01110010), then the AND operation described above would still leave the number having a 0 in the bit-0 position, i.e. the number would be unchanged by the operation. This is because 0 AND 0 = 0.

The QuickBASIC statements which set DTR LOW (negative), i.e. set bit-0 of the MCR of COM2 to 0, are as follows.

Table 5.4. *Logic table for Exclusive OR.*

Exclusive OR
0 EOR 0 = 0
0 EOR 1 = 1
1 EOR 0 = 1
1 EOR 1 = 0

```
mcrcom2% = &H02FC
OUT mcrcom2%, INP(mcrcom2%) AND (NOT 2^0)
```

5.16.5 *Use of the Exclusive OR function (XOR)*

Sometimes it is necessary to *reverse* the state of one or more bits of a register, in which case the Exclusive OR operator is used (Stephenson, 1983). Note that although Exclusive OR is often abbreviated to EOR, QuickBASIC uses the code XOR for this operator. The logic table for Exclusive OR is shown in Table 5.4.

The bit-mask in this case must contain a 1 in only those bit positions where the bit is required to change state. For example, if bits 1 and 4 need to have their status reversed, the bit-mask will therefore be 00010010 (= $2^4 + 2^1$). Following the EOR operation bits 1 and 4 will each have their status reversed, as shown below where the arrows indicate the bit-1 and bit-4 positions.

```
           ↓  ↓
       01100011   =   initial value of the register (= 99)
EOR    00010010   =   mask for bits 1 and 4
       01110001   =   final value of the register (=113)
           ↑  ↑
```

The above EOR operation is expressed in QuickBASIC as follows.

```
finalvalue% = 99 XOR (2^4 + 2^1)
```

5.16.6 *Example subroutines for setting output control lines*

It is very useful to have subroutines which facilitate changing the states of the output control lines (RTS, DTR) from HIGH to LOW and vice versa. For example, the following two subroutines (SETRTS and SETDTR) will set

RTS and DTR HIGH or LOW by using 'high' or 'low' as the second parameter; e.g. by using CALL RTS(com1, high) and CALL DTR(com2, low) etc.

```
SUB setRTS(com$, status$)
    IF com$ = "com1" THEN register% = &H03FC : REM MCR com1
    IF com$ = "com2" THEN register% = &H02FC : REM MCR com2
    IF status$ = "high" THEN
        OUT(register%), INP(register%) OR 2^1
    ELSE
        OUT(register%), INP(register%) AND (NOT 2^1)
    END IF
END SUB


SUB setDTR(com$, status$)
    IF com$ = "com1" THEN register% = &H03FC : REM MCR com1
    IF com$ = "com2" THEN register% = &H02FC : REM MCR com2
    IF status$ = "high" THEN
        OUT(register%), INP(register%) OR 2^0
    ELSE
        OUT(register%), INP(register%) AND (NOT 2^0)
    END IF
END SUB
```

5.17 Monitoring the input control lines

It is often necessary to determine whether one of the computer's four input control lines (CTS, DSR, DCD, RI) is HIGH or LOW during the running of a program. This is done by inspecting the appropriate bit in the UART's Modem Status Register (see Figure 5.4) using the logical operator AND (see also Section 4.4.5).

5.17.1 *Testing for a* LOW *bit (0)*

This is achieved by ANDing the bit-mask with the current MSR value.

For example, suppose it is necessary to determine whether CTS is LOW. Since CTS status is coded by bit-4 of the MSR, the bit-mask for CTS is 2^4. Therefore, if ANDing the value of the Modem Status Register with 2^4 gives a value of zero, then bit-4 of the MSR must also be zero since

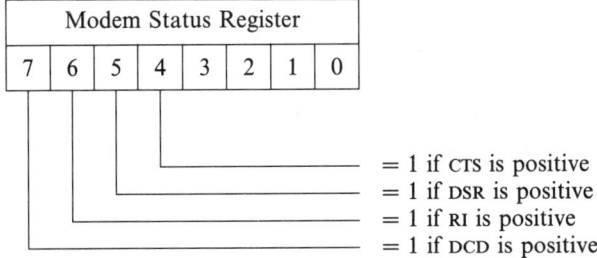

Fig. 5.4. Modem Status Register.

0 AND 1 = 0. This AND operation is shown below, where the arrows indicate the bit-4 position.

$$\begin{array}{rl} \downarrow & \\ 01100011 & = \text{value of MSR } (= 99) \\ \text{AND } 00010000 & = \text{mask for bit-4} \\ 00000000 & = 0 \\ \uparrow & \end{array}$$

The following QuickBASIC statements will therefore indicate whether the CTS of COM2 is LOW (0).

```
msrcom2% = &H02FE
IF (INP(msrcom2%) AND 2^4) = 0 THEN PRINT "CTS = low"
```

Since the sign of 0 is zero, an alternative way of doing this is to use the sign statement (SGN) as follows.

```
IF SGN(INP(msrcom2%) AND 2^4) = 0 THEN PRINT "CTS = low"
```

5.17.2 Testing for a HIGH bit (1)

If ANDing the value of the Modem Status Register with the bit-mask gives the *same* value as the bit-mask, then the bit in question must be 1, since 1 AND 1 = 1.

For example, the following statements can be used to test whether bit-5 of the MSR is a 1; i.e. whether the DSR of COM2 is HIGH.

```
msrcom2% = &H02FE
IF (INP(msrcom2%) AND 2^5) = 2^5 THEN PRINT "DSR = high"
```

This AND operation is summarised below, where the arrows indicate the bit-5 position.

$$\begin{array}{rl} \downarrow & \\ 01110011 & = \text{ value of MSR } (= 115) \\ \text{AND } 00100000 & = \text{ mask for bit-5} \\ 00100000 & = 2^5 \\ \uparrow & \end{array}$$

Since the sign of a positive integer is +1, then an alternative method is to use the sign statement (SGN) as follows.

```
msrcom2% = &H02FE
IF SGN(INP(msrcom2%) AND 2^5) = 1 THEN PRINT "DSR = high"
```

As the value of the MSR cannot be negative, then this will suffice for all occasions.

5.17.3 Example function for testing the status of input control lines

Since the status of an input control line is usually required in order to satisfy a conditional statement (i.e. IF DSR$ = "high" THEN...), it is useful to construct a function to facilitate line status testing.

For example, the following function allows the status of the DSR line of COM2 to be used as follows: IF dsrcom2$ = "low" THEN ...

```
FUNCTION(dsrcom2$)
    msrcom2% = &H02FE
    register% = msrcom2%
    IF (INP(register%) AND 2^5) = 0 THEN dsrcom2$ = "low"
    IF (INP(register%) AND 2^5) = 2^5 THEN dsrcom2$ = "high"
END FUNCTION
```

Since a bit can only be either 1 or 0 the above function could also be written using the IF ... THEN ... ELSE construction as follows.

```
IF (INP(register%) AND 2^5) = 0 THEN
    dsrcom2$ = "low"
    ELSE
    dsrcom2$ = "high"
END IF
```

PART II
MISCELLANEOUS TOPICS

(6) Kermit

(7) Electrical safety and the PC

(8) Data analysis

6
Kermit

6.1 Introduction

Kermit is a powerful public domain communication software program which was originally developed for the IBM PC in 1981 for file transfer and VT24 terminal emulation.

The standard references for MS-DOS Kermit are those by Da Cruz (1987), Gianone *et al.* (1988), and Gianone (1992). Good documentation is also given in the **read.me, .hlp** and **.doc** files supplied with Kermit. A very useful Chapter on Kermit can be found in Gofton (1986).

The address for further information regarding updates, lists of currently available versions, and the newsletter Kermit News is as follows.

Kermit distribution,
Columbia University Center for Computing Activities,
612 West 115th Street,
New York, NY 10025,
USA.
Tel: 212-8543703.
INTERNET:info-kermit@watson.cc.columbia.edu

All the examples given in this Chapter have been written for use with the Nellcor N-200E pulse oximeter.

6.2 Setting up Kermit

Although Kermit is mostly used for file transfer between computers, it can also be used to institute terminal emulation, and so capture data output from monitoring devices, e.g. pulse oximeters.

Having invoked the Kermit program (type 'Kermit' at the DOS

prompt) both the protocol and the filename (and path) for saving the data need to be entered.

6.2.1 Setting the protocol

The SET command establishes or modifies parameters required for data transfer. The protocol to be used is established using SET PORT (for the COM port number), SET BAUD (for the bit-rate), and SET PARITY (for parity). Details of the SET commands are as follows.

- SET PORT COMn   This statement defines the COM port to be used. Thus SET PORT COM2 selects COM2 etc. The default parameter is COM1. Since Kermit clears hardware parity on COM1 on startup, it is not recommended that COM1 is used for a serial printer unless the printer works with no parity (see Gianone *et al.* (1988), under SET PARITY on Page 43).
- SET BAUD n   This statement defines the bit-rate to be used. Thus SET BAUD 1200 selects a bit-rate of 1200 bps. The bit-rate can also be SET using the SET SPEED command which is exactly equivalent.
- SET PARITY x   This statement defines the parity option to be used. The parity options are EVEN, ODD, MARK, SPACE, NONE. Thus the statement SET PARITY NONE selects for no parity bit being used. Note that the number of data bits being used is inferred from the parity setting. Thus the option NONE implies that 8 data bits are being used. All other options imply that only 7 data bits are used.

6.2.2 Specifying a file to receive data

Two commands define how the captured data is saved.

- LOG SESSION   This command saves all the incoming data in a specified file. Note that the LOG SESSION command does *not* overwrite the old file, but always adds the new data to the end of the old file. For example, the following command directs Kermit to save all received data into a file called nelldata.dat on a disk in drive B.

  LOG SESSION b:nelldata.dat

- CAPTURE   Unlike the LOG SESSION command, the CAPTURE command automatically overwrites the old file with the new data. The format is as follows.

  CAPTURE b:nelldata.dat

6.3 Running Kermit

Kermit is run by entering the CONNECT command which invokes terminal emulation. From then on, characters received from a peripheral device via the serial port will be echoed to the screen, and all characters typed from the keyboard will be transmitted to the device.

For example, typing the following statements at the MS-Kermit> prompt will save data from a Nellcor N-200E pulse oximeter via COM port 2 into a file called nelldata.dat in drive B using the following protocol: 1200 baud, no parity, 8 bit data, 1 stop bit. Note that the underlined statements are typed from the keyboard.

MS-Kermit>SET PORT COM2
MS-Kermit>SET BAUD 1200
MS-Kermit>SET PARITY NONE
MS-Kermit>LOG SESSION b:nelldata.dat
MS-Kermit>CONNECT

In this particular case each line of data from the Nellcor pulse oximeter appears on the screen as follows, and is saved on disk in the same format.

R064S096L045H154O090A005M015T182432Q100
R066S097L045H154O090A005M015T182437Q100
...

6.3.1 The initialisation file

Where a list of statements is frequently used for an application, it is often convenient to run Kermit by putting the statements into a file (the **initialisation file**), which Kermit specifies must have the filename extension **.ini**. Read the **mskermit.ini** file for help regarding initialisation files.

The initialisation routine is then invoked by the -f command at the DOS prompt as in the following example, where nellcor.ini is the name of the customised initialisation file.

C:\KERMIT> kermit -f nellcor.ini

Alternatively, the program could be run from a batch file (e.g. nellcor.bat) containing only the above -f command to call the initialisation file (nellcor.ini). The Kermit program could then be run simply by typing the command **nellcor** at the DOS prompt, as follows.

C:\KERMIT> nellcor

6.3.2 Sending commands and control characters

If the peripheral device supports the sending of software control codes to enable the output of data, Kermit can be used to send the necessary codes and then collect the data, providing that hardware handshaking is *not* also required to control the flow of data.

The control codes to be used are usually placed in an ASCII text file, which is then sent to the peripheral device using Kermit's TRANSMIT command. Note that in this situation it is generally best to have the initial command code sent using an initialisation file, in which case the TRANSMIT command must be placed immediately before the LOG SESSION or the CAPTURE command.

For example, the Nellcor N-200E pulse oximeter can be enabled to output Trend data by sending the command code W followed by the ⟨CR⟩⟨LF⟩ pair as follows.

W⟨CR⟩⟨LF⟩

In order to transmit the control characters ⟨CR⟩⟨LF⟩ in a text file, they have to be transmitted as their decimal values within anglebrackets, since only characters whose ASCII decimal code is between 32 and 126 (inclusive) can be sent using the character itself (see Harvey & Nelson, 1990; Page 353).

Since the ASCII codes for ⟨CR⟩ and ⟨LF⟩ are 13 and 10 respectively, the codes W⟨CR⟩⟨LF⟩ would be put into a text file (say, sendtren.txt) as the following line.

W<13><10>

In order to send this line of code the TRANSMIT command must be included in the initialisation file (say, nellcor.ini) as follows.

```
SET PORT COM2
SET BAUD 1200
SET PARITY NONE
TRANSMIT sendtren.txt
LOG SESSION b:nelldata.dat
CONNECT
```

6.3.3 End of session

The Kermit Escape command ^]C is used to escape from the program, and returns the user to the prompt MS-Kermit>. This should then be followed by the CLOSE SESSION command which closes the log file. To exit Kermit altogether, type the command QUIT.

For example, a typical session to access data from a Nellcor N-200E oximeter, using a customised initialisation file (`nellcor.ini`), might be as follows (the statements underlined are those typed from the keyboard).

```
C:\KERMIT> kermit -f nellcor.ini    ' this runs the
                                    ' program using the
                                    ' initialising file
                                    ' nellcor.ini
...
...
^]C                                 ' escapes from the prog
MS-Kermit> close session            ' ends the session
Closing session log
MS-Kermit> quit                     ' returns to DOS
C:\KERMIT>
```

6.4 Problems with Kermit

Although Kermit will access data from a variety of monitoring devices, there are some serious practical limitations when using Kermit for collecting data.

One of the problems is that Kermit saves all data on disk exactly as it appears on the screen. Thus if the output from a peripheral device does not include the time of data sampling, Kermit does not allow this information to be added *en route* in real-time by the computer before the data is stored on disk. Furthermore, any editing to extract particular data items from the peripheral device's output data-string, for example saturation or heart rate values, has to be done later by recalling the data-file and then editing the data.

Another problem is that Kermit cannot be used where hardware handshaking is necessary to access the data. For example, when accessing Trend data from the Pulsox-7 oximeter, intermittent hardware handshaking is required to toggle the oximeter's CTS line *in addition* to sending software control codes.

However, while these problems make Kermit less than ideal for communicating with monitoring equipment, Kermit can often be useful for looking at the general format of data output by a peripheral device.

7

Electrical safety and the PC

by

J. P. McCarthy and R. J. Hall

7.1 Introduction

This chapter seeks to provide an overview of medical electrical safety relevant to PC users, covers the electrical safety categories for Medical Electrical Equipment, and suggests guidelines for the safe use of PCs in a medical environment.

Electrical safety problems associated with interfacing PCs to Medical Electrical Equipment arise from the fact that PCs are not designed to meet the more demanding constructional and safety standard that applies to medical equipment. In view of this, a number of restrictions on the use of PCs are necessary when they are interfaced to Medical Electrical Equipment, particularly those having a Patient Connection (see Section 7.1.3).

The 601 series of International Standards relates to the electrical safety of medical equipment. The two Standards of particular relevance are as follows.

- IEC 601-1:1988 (BS EN 60601-1:1993). Medical electrical equipment. General requirements for safety. International Electrotechnical Commission.†
- IEC 601-1-1:1992 (BS 5724 Section 1.1:1992). Collateral standard. Safety requirements for medical electrical systems. International Electrotechnical Commission.

Other relevant Standards are as follows.

- IEC 950:1991 (BS EN 60950:1991). Specification for safety of information technology equipment, including electrical business equipment. International Electrotechnical Commission.
- EN 60742:1990 (BS 3535 Part 1:1990). Isolating transformers and safety isolating transformers. General requirements. CENELEC.‡

† International Electrotechnical Commission, 3 rue de Varembe, Geneva, Switzerland.
‡ CENELEC, rue de Stassart 35, B-1050 Brussels, Belgium.

The International Standard IEC 601 defines a number of terms used in this area, and these are now considered in turn.†

7.1.1 Medical Electrical Equipment

The Standard defines **Medical Electrical Equipment** as follows.

> Electrical Equipment, provided with not more than one connection to a particular supply mains and intended to diagnose, treat, or monitor the patient under medical supervision, and which makes physical or electrical contact with the patient and/or transfers energy to or from the patient and/or detects such energy transfer to or from the patient. The Medical Electrical Equipment includes those accessories which are necessary to enable the intended use of the equipment.

7.1.2 Applied Parts

Medical Electrical Equipment will normally have one or more **Applied Parts**, which are defined as being Parts which in normal use

- necessarily come into physical contact with the patient for the equipment to perform its function, or
- can reasonably be expected to be brought into contact with the patient, or
- need to be contacted by the patient.

Examples of commonly used Applied Parts are ECG electrodes and leads, defibrillator paddles, and pulse oximeter probes. Less obvious examples are the plastic tubing connecting an infusion device to the patient; the breathing circuit connecting the ventilator to the patient; and a non-invasive blood pressure (NIBP) measuring cuff. Very few types of Medical Electrical Equipment have no Applied Part; an example would be an infra-red treatment lamp.

7.1.3 Patient Connection

Some Applied Parts constitute a **Patient Connection**, which is defined as follows.

† This material is reproduced with permission from the British Standards Institution. Copies of the standard can be purchased from BSI Sales, Linford Wood, Milton Keynes, MK14 6LE, UK. Tel: +44–(0)181-996-7000.

> Every individual part of the Applied Part through which current can flow between the patient and equipment in normal condition and in single fault condition.

Examples of a Patient Connection are the ECG electrodes and the defibrillator paddles connections quoted above, but *not* the plastic infusion tubing or the NIBP cuff. Note that while most pulse oximeter probes do not form a Patient Connection, some might under certain circumstances.

7.1.4 Patient Circuit

Where a Patient Connection exists, a **Patient Circuit** will also exist. This is defined as follows.

> Any electrical circuit which contains one or more Patient Connections. Patient Circuits include all conductive parts not insulated from the Patient Connections to the extent necessary to comply with the relevant parts of the Standard.

7.1.5 Patient Environment

When a PC is interfaced to Medical Electrical Equipment, it is likely to be physically placed in what is known as the **Patient Environment**, in which case there are additional safety implications. The Patient Environment as defined in the Standard may be summarised as follows.

> Any space within which it is possible to simultaneously touch electrical equipment *and* either the patient, or another person who may be touching the patient.

Practical considerations suggest that *any* equipment in the same room as the patient may come into the Patient Environment. Consequently, a PC should probably not be used in the same room as the patient, *unless* it can be used safely within the Patient Environment.

7.2 General aspects of electrical safety

All electrical equipment, both medical and non-medical, must be safe for users/operators both in normal use, and when a so-called **Single Fault Condition** exists (a condition in which either a single means for protection against a safety hazard in equipment is defective, or a single external abnormal condition is present).

Medical equipment is made electrically safe by incorporating a number of design precautions, some of which are as follows.

- Insulation of all live parts to provide basic protection against electric shock, together with either the earthing of external metal cases, or an additional layer of insulation, or a single reinforced layer of equivalent electrical strength.
- The incorporation of fuses or excess current trip-switches to isolate the equipment in the event of a fault leading to excessive current flow.

All *mains* powered equipment, both medical and non-medical, is classified as being either **Class I** or **Class II** equipment depending on the means used to provide protection against electric shock to the user. These two groups are now described in turn.

7.2.1 Class I

This class covers equipment in which protection does not rely solely on basic insulation of live parts, but includes the additional safety precaution of connecting the equipment to a protective earth conductor in the fixed wiring of the supply system, in such a way that accessible metal parts cannot become live in the event of a failure of the basic insulation. The connection point for the protective earth conductor must be marked on the equipment, either internally or externally. Most domestic electrical appliances fall into this class. Note that there is no symbol for this class of equipment.

7.2.2 Class II

This class covers equipment in which protection against electric shock does not rely solely on basic insulation of live parts, but includes an additional layer of insulation (**double insulation**) between the live parts and the user. No provision is made for connection of a protective earth conductor. Class II equipment must be marked with the double-box symbol shown above.

Note that an item of equipment may incorporate parts built to a Class II standard in combination with parts built to a Class I standard. In such cases the equipment as a whole must be classified as Class I.

7.3 Safety of Medical Electrical Equipment

Electrical safety requirements specific to Medical Electrical Equipment are concerned with isolating the patient from any currents which could be harmful if applied to the patient.

Such currents include so-called **Patient Leakage Currents** from the supply mains, since these can find a route to earth through the patient both in normal circumstances, and in single fault conditions such as an open circuit protective earth conductor on Class I equipment.

The level of Leakage Current that can safely be allowed depends on whether the Applied Part is or is not intended for direct cardiac application, as it may take only a few tens of microamps connected directly across heart muscle to cause a cardiac arrest.

7.3.1 Insulation/isolation of the Applied Part

Additional protection for the patient is generally achieved by either incorporating **double insulation** or using **isolation circuits** as follows.

Double insulation. This involves constructing the Applied Part with insulating materials to such a degree that it is effectively double insulated, with the effect that the patient is completely isolated from the equipment.† An ultrasound probe is an example where double insulation is necessary, since although it does not constitute a Patient Connection, the probe does require voltages in excess of 100 volts DC to excite the piezo-electric crystals which generate the ultrasound wave-front. A pulse oximeter probe would be another example.

Isolation circuits. These are used in cases where a Patient Connection exists. The isolation circuits built into the Patient Circuits prevent the patient being earthed by the connections to the equipment, and prevent the flow of earth leakage currents or earth fault currents to the patient. An ECG monitor is an example of equipment in which isolation circuits are used.

F-type isolation. A high degree of isolation known as F-type isolation is defined in the Standard. This requires that the Applied Part is sufficiently isolated from other parts of the Medical Electrical Equipment and from earth, so that the patient leakage current allowable in a single fault condition is not exceeded, even when a voltage equal to 1.1 times the highest rated mains voltage is applied between the Applied Part and earth.

An Applied Part which does not provide isolation, or one in which the

† Alternatively a single layer of sufficient physical and electrical strength as to be equivalent to double insulation may be employed (reinforced insulation).

Electrical safety and the PC 93

degree of isolation does not meet this strict additional requirement, must be classified as being Type B (see Section 7.3.2).

7.3.2 Applied Part Types

The Applied Parts of Medical Electrical Equipment are categorised into three **Types** (B, BF, CF) according to the degree of protection provided to the patient. Each Type has a specific symbol which is usually displayed at the outlet of the Applied Part.

Type BF and CF Applied Parts both provide F-type isolation, but the maximum allowed patient leakage current for Type CF is one tenth of that allowed for Type BF (i.e. $50\,\mu A$ compared to $500\,\mu A$). For direct cardiac connections a high specification F-type isolated Applied Part is mandatory, hence the classification CF (i.e. suitable for Cardiac connection and F-type isolation).

Type B. This Type provides the specified degree of protection against electric shock, particularly regarding allowable leakage currents. However, the degree of isolation provided by Type B Applied Parts is not as stringent as for Type BF and Type CF, and *may* earth the patient. Type B Applied Parts are not suitable for direct cardiac connection.

Note that while a Type B Applied Part will not necessarily earth a patient, nevertheless, it will not incorporate sufficient isolation to fully protect a patient in the event of mains potential being applied to the patient.

Type BF. This Type provides F-type isolation, isolating the patient from live parts and from earth, and in addition provides a high degree of protection against electric shock in the event of mains potential being applied to the patient, as might happen owing to a fault in another item of equipment. Type BF Applied Parts are not suitable for direct cardiac connection.

Type CF. Equipment of this Type provides a considerably greater degree of protection than Type BF, particularly in respect of allowable leakage currents in normal and single fault conditions. The isolation is such that Type CF Applied Parts are suitable for direct cardiac connection.

Table 7.1. *Applied Parts and their Types.*

Product	Applied Part	Type
Ohmeda 3700	Pulse oximeter probe	BF
Ohmeda 3740	Pulse oximeter probe	BF
Nellcor N-200E	Pulse oximeter probe	BF
Novametrix 515A	Pulse oximeter probe	BF
Minolta Pulsox-7	Pulse oximeter probe	BF
Datex Cardiocap™ II	ECG	CF
	NIBP	BF
	Invasive BP	CF
	Temperature probe	CF
Datex Ultima™	Pulse oximeter probe	BF
	Gas sampling probe	B
	Spirometry probe	B
Graseby 3400 pump	Infusion tubing	CF
Ohmeda 9000 pump	Infusion tubing	BF
Vitalograph Compact II	Flowhead and tubing	BF
Ohmeda 7800 ventilator	Breathing circuit	BF
Dräger Evita ventilator	Breathing circuit	B

Table of Applied Parts. A list of the various items of medical equipment described in Part III of this book, together with the Applied Parts and Types, is shown in Table 7.1.

Note that an item of medical equipment may have more than one Applied Part, in which case each connection must be individually Type marked.

7.3.3 Compatibility with flammable anaesthetic gases

Medical Electrical Equipment is further categorised regarding whether or not the equipment is safe to use in the vicinity of flammable anaesthetic gases. Equipment or equipment parts complying with specified requirements regarding construction, marking, and documentation, in order to avoid sources of ignition in a flammable anaesthetic mixture with air, are categorised and marked **AP** in a circular symbol as shown above. Equipment or parts suitable for use with flammable agents mixed with oxygen or nitrous oxide are categorised **APG**. Equipment not suitable for use in the vicinity of flammable anaesthetic gases is unclassified in this respect, and carries no AP or APG marking.

7.4 General precautions when using PCs

In view of the fact that PCs do not meet the standard for Medical Electrical Equipment, the principles of safe practice when using a PC in a medical environment focus on two issues; firstly, the danger of by-passing the carefully designed protective and isolation circuitry associated with all Medical Electrical Equipment, particularly those having a Patient Connection and secondly, the danger of igniting a flammable or explosive gas/vapour mixture.

The precautions to be taken when interfacing a PC to Medical Electrical Equipment also depend on whether it is intended to place the PC within the Patient Environment, or to keep it outside this area.

Definitive standards for connecting medical and non-medical equipment to form a system are laid down in IEC 601-1-1 (1992), and the following guidelines are based on this Standard (see also McCarthy & Potter, 1985; Slater, 1985).

7.4.1 Basic principles for safe practice

Prior to interfacing a PC to Medical Electrical Equipment, the user should check that the latter equipment meets the IEC 601-1 electrical safety Standard. The user must be aware of the Type classification of all of the Applied Parts that will be attached to the patient.

The patient. Patients must only be connected to equipment complying with medical Standards. Medical Electrical Equipment complying with the IEC 601 Standard will display one of the following symbols at the connection of each Applied Part.

The PC. The PC should comply with the IEC 950 Standard. PCs are not suitable for use in potentially explosive atmospheres.

Leakage current. All equipment placed within the Patient Environment must have enclosure leakage currents in single fault conditions of less than 0.5 mA. For Class I equipment, this usually equates to normal earth leakage current.

Individual items of Medical Electrical Equipment will meet this requirement, which is the limit allowed by the IEC 601 standard. Combinations of Medical Electrical Equipment using a *common* mains lead may not, and many PCs and display monitors will not. The standard for PCs quoted above allows 3.5 mA; most colour monitors have at least 1mA leakage. A battery-powered laptop PC *without* its mains charger pack will usually meet the 0.5 mA requirement. The mains charger pack for a battery-powered laptop PC *may* provide the low leakage isolation required by the Standard, but checks will be required.

If the PC is positioned outside the Patient Environment but within the same room, then no additional measures to limit its enclosure leakage current to 0.5 mA need be taken, with the exception that the PC must be plugged in separately from the Medical Electrical Equipment. However, practical considerations suggest that any movable equipment in the same room as the patient is likely come into the Patient Environment, and consequently this practice cannot be recommended.

By far the most satisfactory method of ensuring the low leakage required by the Standard in fault conditions is to supply the PC from an **isolating transformer** constructed in accordance with EN 60742 (BS 3535 Part 1:1990). In practice a range of medical and non-medical equipment housed on one trolley can all be collectively powered from a single isolating transformer.

Type B Applied Part. Interfacing to Medical Electrical Equipment with a Type B Applied Part requires a careful investigation of the nature of the Applied Part. It is important to determine whether or not it constitutes a Patient Connection. For example, interfacing a PC to an EEG monitor classified as Type B is potentially dangerous, since the Applied Part in this case constitutes a Patient Connection, which *may* earth the patient.

Similarly, interfacing to a combination monitor having a Type CF ECG and a Type B pulse oximeter probe may also be hazardous. In this case specialist advice should be sought regarding the conductivity to earth of the pulse oximeter probe, with a view to determining whether or not it constitutes a Patient Connection, and if not, whether it provides sufficient isolation to withstand mains voltage on the Applied Part.

Interfacing to a Type B ventilator presents a similar potential hazard, particularly with wet patient tubing, and again specialist advice should be sought.

Electrical safety and the PC 97

7.4.2 Suggested guidelines

In view of the various factors discussed above, it is suggested that in the absence of Medical Physics/Engineering advice to the contrary, the following guidelines should be adhered to when interfacing a PC to Medical Electrical Equipment.

- Do not use a PC in an environment where flammable or explosive gas mixtures are used.
- Only interface a PC to Medical Electrical Equipment displaying one of the following symbols, and so indicating that it meets the IEC 601 Standard.

- Do not interface a PC to Medical Electrical Equipment having any Type B Applied Parts attached to a patient. They may earth the patient.
- If a PC is used in the *same* room as the Medical Electrical Equipment to which it is interfaced, the PC should be powered from an isolating transformer.
- If a PC is used in a *separate* room from the Medical Electrical Equipment to which it is interfaced, then isolation of the interfacing connections must be provided (e.g. opto-isolation). This is because the protective earths in different rooms could be at different potentials, and so give rise to a ground loop current.

8
Data analysis

8.1 General aspects

Although data gathered from monitoring devices may be subjected to many different types of analysis, the particular approach used depends largely on the nature of the problem being studied. However, in general, 'data analysis is largely a search for patterns—that is, for meaningful relations among the various items observed' (Godfrey, 1985). In practice, data analysis can be considered to be a process incorporating the following procedures.

- Descriptive procedures
- Inferential procedures
- Predictive procedures

8.1.1 Descriptive procedures (graphical analysis)

During the initial stage of data analysis the aim is to describe the main features of the data being studied. Calculation of mean, median, standard deviation, variance, and frequency distribution fall into this category. The results from these and many other related procedures can then be displayed graphically in a form that aids the process of understanding.

Tukey (1977) has stressed both the importance and benefits of a graphical description of the experimental data. His proposals, collectively known as Exploratory Data Analysis, aim to facilitate the process of understanding numerical data. In his view 'the greatest value of a picture is when it forces us to notice what we never expected to see' (Tukey, 1977). The same view is echoed by Tufte who points out that 'graphics reveal data' (Tufte, 1983).

The graphical approach to data description is often referred to as **data visualisation**, and is greatly facilitated by powerful software tools, for example spreadsheets, statistical packages, presentation graphics and dedicated visualisation packages.

A major advance in data visualisation software is the ability to link independent variables in a data set to attributes of a plot like colour, height, shape etc. However, while adopting this approach to data display, it is important to keep in mind Weber's warning about data visualisation, namely that 'data visualisation is about comprehension, not graphics' (Weber, 1993).

For general aspects of data visualisation see Beard (1992), Wayner (1993), Gershon & Dozier (1993). Visualising multi-dimensional data is discussed in detail by Ribarsky (1993).

8.1.2 Inferential procedures (statistical analysis)

Inferential procedures use statistical techniques with a view to hypothesis testing. As an example, Table 8.1 indicates the range of inferential procedures used in the analysis of pulse oximetry data.

8.1.3 Predictive procedures (modelling)

Much of the data gathered from monitoring equipment are sequential measurements related in time, and may therefore be viewed as a **time series**. Since time series are one of the most commonly encountered forms of data structure, many techniques have been developed for extracting information from them. A good introduction to the study of these analytical procedures including the **autoregressive integrated moving average** (ARIMA), and **autocorrelation**, is given by Chatfield (1975).

An interesting Bayesian technique for analysing a time series is the **Kalman filter** (Harrison & Stevens, 1976; Knapp et al., 1986), a modified version of which has been used in Renal medicine to indicate early signs of transplant rejection (Trimble et al., 1983).

Techniques for detecting changes in a time series include **Pettitt's non-parametric test** (Pettitt, 1979), **piecewise linear regression** (Freedman et al., 1979), and the **cumulative sum** test—CUSUM (Stoodley & Mirnia, 1979; Chaput de Saintonge & Vere, 1974; Wohl, 1977).

Analytical techniques for predicting the trend of a time series include the **tracking function** described by Trigg. This function and other related procedures are discussed in detail by Endresen & Hill (1977) and Avent

& Charlton (1990). For a general overview of computer modelling see the series of articles by Bedford (1993a).

8.2 Software tools

Most analytical procedures can be performed with relative ease with the software packages available for PCs. This section therefore offers a brief overview of some of the relevant software tools and their role in data analysis. A useful overview of data analysis and presentation tools for scientists is that by Beard (1993).

The various software packages may be classified as follows.

- Spreadsheet
- Database
- Graphics
- Statistics
- Mathematics

8.2.1 Spreadsheet packages

Spreadsheets consist of rows and columns of data partitioned into **cells**, and are well suited for handling numerical data. A typical DOS spreadsheet can handle up to 256 columns and 8192 rows, with each cell being identified by an **address** consisting of its column letter and row number.

Spreadsheets are generally well equipped with mathematical, statistical and financial functions for manipulating numbers or text strings which occupy the cells. One of the major advantages of spreadsheets is their ability to present numerical data as a graphical display, and while their graph formats vary somewhat, most spreadsheet packages include the usual bar-graphs, pie-charts, and x-y plots.

DOS packages include Quattro Pro, Lotus 1-2-3, and SuperCalc. Those for the Microsoft Windows environment include Quattro Pro for Windows, Excel, Lotus 1-2-3 for Windows, CA SuperCalc for Windows, CleanSheet, and Lotus Improv.

8.2.2 Database packages

Database packages generally require the formulation of a structure for data organisation before the data can be input. For example, the user may need to specify the type of data (i.e. text, currency, date, memo etc.)

Data analysis

that will be stored, as well as the format of various data fields. The capacity for holding data is generally larger than that of spreadsheets.

It is important to appreciate the various technical terms and concepts used in association with databases; for example **field, record, table, index, query, form, sort**. There are also different forms of database; for example there are **relational** databases as well as **flat file** databases. For an overview of the various terms and concepts see Townsend (1992).

DOS databases include Dbase IV, FoxPro, Rbase, and Paradox. Windows users can choose from Paradox for Windows, FoxPro for Windows, Access, SuperBase, FileMaker Pro, Approach, WindowBase, DataEase, Omnis, dbFast, and Idealist.

8.2.3 Graphics packages

Graphics packages offer a much wider variety of graph types than either spreadsheets or databases, but their analytical capacity is generally not as extensive. However, some graphics packages (e.g. DeltaGraph Professional, Stanford Graphics, Spyglass†) have remedied this deficiency and offer a variety of analytical procedures in addition to a range of graph types.

It is worth emphasising that the mainstream spreadsheet and database packages have, until recently, provided only the commonly used graph types such as bar, pie, and line graphs, the needs of the technical and scientific users being met by a handful of specialist graphics packages. However this is a rapidly developing area, and the conventional spreadsheets are now offering graph types that are specifically aimed at the technical and scientific users (e.g. QuattroPro for Windows version 5).

DOS graphics packages include Harvard Graphics, WordPerfect Presentations, Freelance, EasyPlot, Graph, Axum, and GNUPLOT.‡ Packages for the Windows environment include Powerpoint, CA-Cricket Graph, CA-Cricket Presents, Aldus Persuasion, Corel Draw, Harvard Graphics for Windows, Freelance for Windows, EasyPlot, Enplot, Stanford Graphics, Spyglass, DeltaGraph Professional, and Charisma.

8.2.4 Statistics packages

In addition to their ability to perform advanced statistical analysis most dedicated statistical packages have a good graphics capability.

† For information on Spyglass contact the Internet address **info@spyglass.com**.
‡ GNUPLOT is a freeware package—see Appendix 7.

DOS packages include Minitab, SPSS, C-Stat, Statistica, Systat, and UniStat. Packages for Windows include Minitab, SPSS, C-Stat, Systat, and UniStat.

8.2.5 Mathematics

A number of very sophisticated mathematical and engineering packages are available for PCs. The main contenders in this area are Maple, Mathcad, Mathematica, MatLab, and Diffeq. For an overview of their abilities see Beard (1993), and Bedford (1992b, part II).

8.3 Analysis of pulse oximetry data

In view of the increasing use of pulse oximeters in a wide range of fields, this section outlines some of the procedures used in the display and analysis of pulse oximetry data.

8.3.1 Display and analysis of pulse oximetry data

The aim of data display in studies of oxygen saturation should be, as stressed by Slutsky & Strohl (1980), to present the complete saturation profile during the period of observation with accurate quantification of episodes of hypoxaemia. The main problems here are the large volume of data generated and episodic nature of desaturation.

Several approaches to this problem have been discussed in the literature with a view to determining a useful index of severity, and displaying the data in a convenient way (Slutsky & Strohl, 1980; Evans *et al.*, 1984; Pasterkamp & Daien, 1988; Wheatley *et al.*, 1990; Taylor, 1991). The following measurements are commonly used as an index of severity.

- The lowest saturation during the period of observation.
- The average of the lowest saturation value recorded for each desaturation episode.
- The percentage of time that the saturation was less than a given value.

The following graphical displays are commonly used.

- Time plot
- Frequency distribution plot
- Cumulative distribution plot
- Compressed spectral array plot

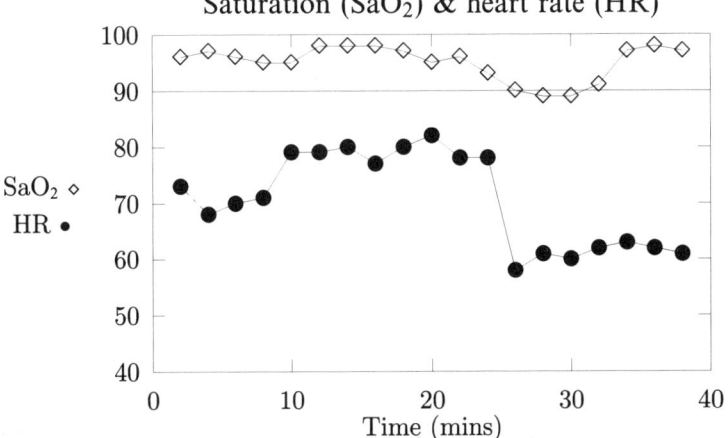

Fig. 8.1. Example of a time plot using GNUPLOT 3.4.

Since some of these plots are quite difficult to generate, a number of programs have been developed to facilitate the acquisition, display and analysis of oximetry data (see Pasterkamp & Daien, 1988; Taylor, 1991; Evans *et al.*, 1984).

Pasterkamp & Daien (1988) have published details of a spreadsheet macro package written in the Lotus 1-2-3 macro language, which generates all the above plots except the compressed spectral array plot.† Examples of plots generated by running their program on data from an Ohmeda 3700 pulse oximeter are shown in Figures 8.2, 8.3, 8.4. Taylor (1991) has published details of a GW-BASIC program which performs graphical trending and statistical analysis of oximetry data. Evans *et al.* (1984) describe a program for analysing oximetry data which determines a desaturation index, and generates a cumulative distribution plot.

Time plot. A simple plot of saturation against time is often all that is necessary to indicate an association between certain events and episodes of desaturation (see Figure 8.1). There are numerous examples in the anaesthetic literature where a simple time plot is the primary method of assessing the data (Marjot & Valentine, 1990; Wheatley *et al.*, 1990; Madej *et al.*, 1992; Wheatley *et al.*, 1992; Reeder *et al.*, 1991; Reeder *et al.*, 1992; Rosenberg *et al.*, 1990; Rosenberg *et al.*, 1992; Al-Shaikh, 1991).

† This macro package (O2SAT.COM) can be downloaded from the CompuServe MEDSIG forum (library 12).

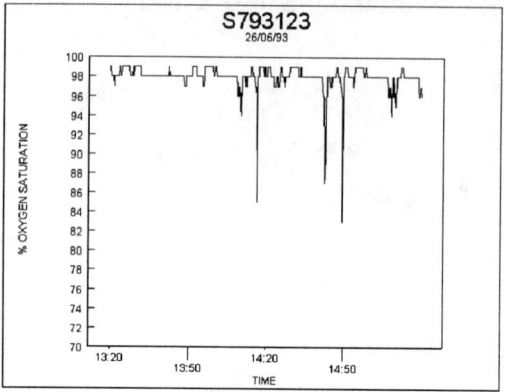

Fig. 8.2. Example of a time plot generated by the macro package described by Pasterkamp & Daien (1988).

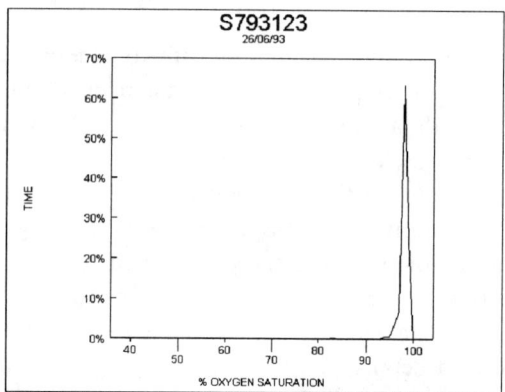

Fig. 8.3. Example of a frequency distribution plot generated by the macro package described by Pasterkamp & Daien (1988).

A time plot generated by the macro package described by Pasterkamp & Daien (1988) is shown in Figure 8.2.

Frequency distribution plot. The frequency of occurrence of measured oxygen saturation values during the study period may be plotted as a distribution plot, as shown by Wheatley *et al.* (1990). A frequency distribution generated by the macro package described by Pasterkamp & Daien (1988) is shown in Figure 8.3.

Data analysis 105

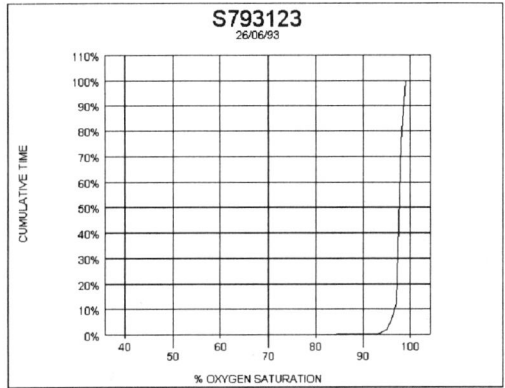

Fig. 8.4. Example of a cumulative distribution plot generated by the macro package described by Pasterkamp & Daien (1988).

Cumulative distribution plot. A plot of the cumulative percentage of time spent below given values of oxygen saturation is known as a cumulative distribution plot. An example of this plot generated by the macro package described by Pasterkamp & Daien (1988) is shown in Figure 8.4.

Compressed spectral array. When oxygen saturation is monitored over several hours, as is the case in intraoperative or postoperative studies, there is a need for displaying vast amounts of data in a meaningful way. One approach is to stack the frequency distribution plots of data collected each hour, to produce a 'compressed array' of curves as shown in Figure 8.5. Recent examples of the use of compressed spectral array plots to display oxygen saturation data are those published by Wheatley *et al.* (1990); Entwistle *et al.* (1991); Jones *et al.* (1992).

8.3.2 Inferential procedures and pulse oximetry data

Deciding how best to analyse pulse oximetry data is not easy, and this is reflected in the wide variety of inferential statistical procedures that have been used. This Chapter concludes therefore with a survey of the recent oximetry literature, indicating both the aspects studied and the method of analysis used, as shown in Table 8.1.

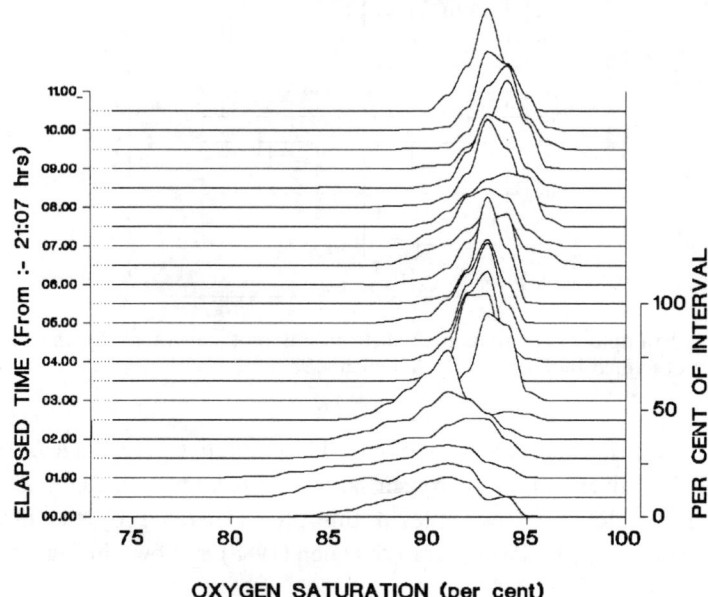

Fig. 8.5. Compressed spectral array plot, courtesy of I.D. Somerville, D.J. Sapsford and J.G. Jones. The y-axis on the left indicates the the hours during which the component curves of the compressed array plot were recorded. The y-axis on the right indicates the percentage of each hour spent at a given oxygen saturation value.

Data analysis 107

Table 8.1. *Types of inferential procedures used to analyse oximetry data*

Study	Aspects studied	Analysis
Marjot & Valentine (1990)	SaO_2 after premedication	Student's paired t-test
Wheatley et al. (1990)	Median value of SaO_2, predefined values of hypoxaemia	Kolmogorov-Smirnoff test
Al-Shaikh (1991)	Persistent decrease in SaO_2 of 2% or greater, maximum decrease in SaO_2, time of occurrence of decrease in SaO_2	Chi-square with Yates' correction & Mann-Whitney U test
Suresh et al. (1991)	Median baseline & median least SaO_2, incidence of predefined levels of hypoxaemia & its relation to the grade of the surgeons and the anaesthetists, non-parametric 95% confidence intervals	Mann-Whitney U test & three-way analysis of variance
Moller et al. (1991)	Incidence and duration of predefined levels of hypoxaemia, patient-related and operative risk factors of hypoxaemia	Chi-square test, Goodman-Kruskal's gamma test, Stepwise multiple logistic regression
Entwistle et al. (1991)	Median and 50th and 20th centile of hourly SaO_2 values, predefined levels of hypoxaemia, duration of hypoxaemia	Least square linear regression
Madej et al. (1992)	Percentage of time spent at various predefined SaO_2 levels, hourly mode SaO_2, number & duration of episodes of moderate & severe hypoxaemia (predefined)	ANOVA, Welch's test, Fisher's exact test
Wheatley et al. (1992)	Percentage and distribution of recorded SaO_2 values, number & duration of episodes of severe hypoxaemia (predefined)	Unpaired t-test, Welch's test, Chi-square with Yates' correction

Table 8.1. *(cont.)*

Study	Aspects studied	Analysis
Haynes et al. (1992)	Median, range, inter-quartile & 95% confidence interval of SaO_2 values	Kruskal-Wallis test, Mann-Whitney U test
Gill et al. (1992)	Pre & postoperative SaO_2, mean and least SaO_2, duration of desaturation, ST segment elevation or depression	Chi-square test, ANOVA and correlation
Rosenberg et al. (1992)	Median, range, & minimum SaO_2 values, number of episodes of desaturation, 95% confidence limits of median difference	Mann-Whitney test, Fisher's exact test and Spearman's rank correlation
Reeder et al. (1992)	Mean and standard deviation of pre and postoperative SaO_2 values & percent of time spent with $SaO_2 < 90\%$ and 85%	Correlation
Lanigan (1992)	Frequency distribution of SaO_2 values observed during recovery, median smallest SaO_2, frequency of desaturation	Mann-Whitney, Kruskal-Wallis & Chi-square (with Yates's correction) tests
Moller et al. (1992)	Mean, median & range of cumulative duration of predefined levels of hypoxaemia, lowest SaO_2 values	Chi-square (with Yates's correction), Mann-Whitney test
Beydon et al. (1992)	Mode of SaO_2 distribution, standard deviation of SaO_2, % of total time at $SaO_2 < 90\%$, number of episodes of $SaO_2 < 90\%$, mean of lowest SaO_2 values observed, % time spent at $SaO_2 < 85\%$	Two-way ANOVA, Tukey's Multiple range tests, Wilcoxon tests, Pearson's linear regression, Multiple linear correlations
Dottrens et al. (1992)	Mean, standard deviation, & range of SaO_2	One-way analysis of variance followed by Student's t-test with Bonferroni's correction
Pollock & Kenny (1993)	Baseline & minimum $SaO_2\%$ & % of time spent at $SaO_2 >$ & $< 90\%$	Student's t-test & Spearman's rank correlation
Crawford et al. (1993)	Median of least SaO_2 observed & mean of SaO_2	Chi-square & Student's t-test

PART III
THE EQUIPMENT

(9) The Ohmeda 3700 and 3740 pulse oximeters

(10) The Nellcor N-200E pulse oximeter

(11) The Novametrix 515A pulse oximeter

(12) The Minolta Pulsox-7 pulse oximeter

(13) The Datex Cardiocap™ II and Capnomac Ultima™ series

(14) The Graseby 3400 syringe pump

(15) The Ohmeda 9000 syringe pump

(16) The Vitalograph Compact II spirometer

(17) The Ohmeda 7800 ventilator

(18) The Dräger Evita intensive care ventilator

9

The Ohmeda 3700 and 3740 pulse oximeters

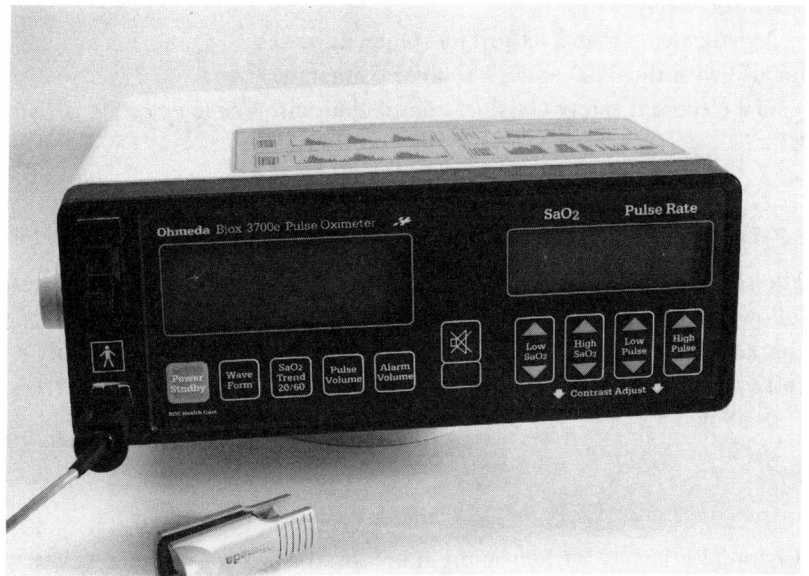

9.1 Introduction

The two models currently available from Ohmeda† are the Biox 3700 and 3740. Both models have internal batteries and Trend data output capability. The main differences are indicated below.

- **3700** This model has an integral mains transformer, but Trend data has no time-stamp associated with it.

- **3740** This model requires an external mains transformer. Trend data is time-stamped at 5-minute intervals.

---

† Ohmeda Monitoring Systems, 1315 West Century Drive, Louisville, Colorado 80027, USA. Tel: +1-303-6667001. Fax: +1-303-6659175.

Table 9.1. *Software level codes.*

A	B	C	D	E	F	G	H	..
1	2	3	4	5	6	7	8	..

The batteries recharge irrespective of whether the pulse oximeter is switched on or not. Charging to 80 and 100% capacity takes 4 and 6.5 hrs respectively.

A dedicated dot-matrix printer (Ohmeda series 37 printer) is available for use with the 3700 and 3740 pulse oximeters.

The electrical safety classification of the pulse oximeter probe is Type BF.†

9.1.1 Software version

The software revision is shown in the front display window immediately following power on. Note that Ohmeda has recently changed from *alpha* characters (letters) to *numeric* characters (numbers) when identifying software revision levels. Thus revision level F will be followed by revision 7, as shown in Table 9.1.

9.1.2 Available software

Taylor (1991) has written a program for the 3700e oximeter covering retrieval, storage, and numerical/graphical trending.

Ohmeda have produced a software package called COMMANDER‡ which accesses and stores data from the 3700 and 3740 oximeters. It comes with two disks and a user manual, and requires a minimum of 512 K bytes of RAM. Note that there are various versions of COMMANDER, so it is important, when ordering, to specify the particular oximeter.

Pasterkamp & Daien (1988) have written a macro program for processing Ohmeda 3700 Trend data. This involves a two step process, which first makes use of Intelpro's printer emulation package (PEP) for accessing the data and saving it as an ASCII file, and then uses the

† See Chapter 7 for further details.
‡ COMMANDER: a software package for the Ohmeda pulse oximeters. Published by Ohmeda, Ohmeda House, 71 Great North Road, Hatfield, Hertfordshire, England, AL9 5EN, UK. Tel: +44–(0)1707–263570. Fax: +44–(0)1707–260191.

The Ohmeda 3700 and 3740 pulse oximeters 113

Lotus 1-2-3 spreadsheet package for IBM compatible PCs to perform data distribution and statistical analysis.

Pasterkamp and Daien have also put together a macro package called O2SAT.COM, which is written in the Lotus 1-2-3 macro language. The package can be downloaded from CompuServe, where it can be found by searching in the MEDSIG forum (library 12).

9.1.3 Communication modes

The two oximeters have a number of modes of communication as follows.

- **Auto-output** Outputs real-time saturation and heart rate data every 2 seconds. This is the default mode which the oximeter is in following power-on. Both Trend mode and Waveform mode are accessed from Auto-output mode.
- **Control** This mode is enabled by the ⟨ESC⟩C sequence, and allows the computer to control the various alarm limits and averaging times, and access both Trend and Waveform data.
- **Trend** Outputs data since the last power on (Recent Trend), or data from the last 8 hours (8-hr Trend). Trend mode is accessed via Auto-output mode. Both groups of Trend data can be output either **manually**, by operating the buttons on the front of the oximeter, or initiated **remotely** using software codes sent by the computer using the Control mode.
- **Waveform** Outputs the shape of the pulse waveform as amplitude data sampled at either every 1/25 sec (50 Hz mains) or every 1/30 sec (60 Hz mains). Waveform mode is accessed via Auto-output mode.
- **Slave** This mode is enabled by the ⟨ESC⟩S sequence, and suspends the regular heart rate and saturation data output associated with the Auto-output mode. In Slave mode data is only output in response to a command-code from the computer, and consists of a single string giving saturation, heart rate and oximeter status.

9.2 Serial port

Both Ohmeda oximeters have a 25-pin D-type female serial port located on the rear panel. The pin-outs for the serial port are shown in Table 9.2. No more than ± 15 volts should be applied to the pins.

Note that on both oximeters the TxD and RxD pins are reversed

Table 9.2. *Ohmeda 3700 & 3740 serial port.*

Pin No.	Name	Function
1		Chassis ground
2	RxD	Receives data
3	TxD	Transmits data
7	GND	Signal ground

Table 9.3. *Ohmeda 3700 & 3740 protocol.*

Bit rate	1200
Data bits	7
Parity	Odd
Stop bits	1

compared to the RS-232 specification. Thus both oximeters transmit data via pin-3 instead of pin-2 as is usual for 25-pin connectors.

Only four pins are available for interfacing, namely pins 1, 2, 3, 7. The remaining pins are not connected internally on the 3700 model. However, on the 3740 model, pins 11, 18, and 25 are connected directly to TTL circuits (0–5 volts), and are used by Ohmeda for factory testing purposes. Care must therefore be taken when making RS-232 connections to the 3740, as the oximeter may be permanently damaged if the TTL pins come into contact with RS-232 voltage levels (± 15 volts).

9.2.1 Protocol options

Both the Ohmeda 3700 and 3740 oximeters have a fixed serial protocol as shown in Table 9.3.

9.2.2 Cable connections

Figure 9.1 shows the wiring configuration for interfacing to a PC. Since hardware handshaking is not used with either oximeter, the options CS and DS need to be used in the QuickBASIC OPEN COM statement in order to disable CTS and DSR checking respectively (see Chapter 5).

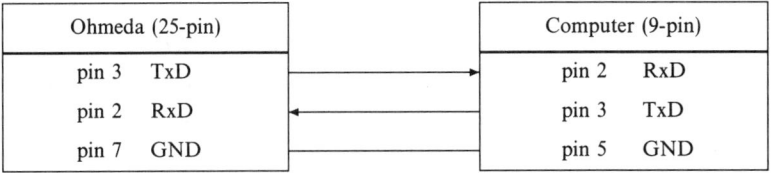

Fig. 9.1. Ohmeda 3700 & 3740 wiring diagram. Note that the TxD and RxD pins are reversed on both the 3700 and 3740 oximeters compared to the EIA/TIA-232 Standard.

Table 9.4. *Error messages and codes used by the Ohmeda oximeters.*

Codes		Message	Oximeter model	
CF	02	Circuit failure	—	3740
PF	04	Probe failure	—	3740
NP	06	No probe	3700	3740
IN	08	Interference detected	3700	3740
CK	09	Check probe site	—	3740
PO	10	Probe off patient	3700	3740
NS	11	No pulse	—	3740
IL	12	Insufficient light	3700	3740
ID	13	Probe ID error	—	3740
LQ	14	Low quality signal	3700	3740

9.3 Auto-output mode

This is the default mode which the oximeter is in when switched on in the usual way. In this mode both oximeters output real-time data every 2 seconds, and allow access to both Trend and Waveform data.

The format of the real-time data varies slightly depending on whether an error message is present or not. The two formats, together with examples, are shown below. The error messages used by the two oximeters are given in Table 9.4. The symbol ␣ represents a space.

:SaO2=nnn␣PR=nnn␣␣␣⟨CR⟩⟨LF⟩

:SaO2=nnn␣PR=nnn␣⟨error message⟩⟨CR⟩⟨LF⟩

Note that neither of the Ohmeda oximeters gives the time of data sampling (time-stamp) with the real-time data output (Auto-output mode). In view of this, if date and time are required, then these must be added to each data-string by the computer.

9.3.1 Program for accessing real-time data

An example QuickBASIC 4.5 program which will access real-time data from either oximeter, and save it to a file (datafile.dat), is given below. Pressing <Q> will quit the program.

Program points

- The input routine used by the example program extracts the data from the Receive buffer and adds it to the end of the string a$. The program then removes strings which end in ⟨CR⟩ from the string a$ and places them in the variable data$. Each time the condition L% > 0 is satisfied (except usually the first) the string a$ will therefore start with ⟨LF⟩ and contain a ⟨CR⟩. A typical a$ when L% > 0 is as follows.

⟨LF⟩:SaO2=␣98␣PR=␣64␣␣␣⟨CR⟩⟨LF⟩...

Note that when data is passed to the string data$ the initial ⟨LF⟩ control character is removed. This is achieved by starting data$ at the second character of a$, and removing L%-2 characters. This is performed by the following QuickBASIC statement.

data$ = MID$(a$, 2, L% - 2)

- Since only three lines are used for communications, there is no hand-shaking, and so the CS and DS options should be used in the OPEN COM statement.
- Since there is no time-stamp with the data, both date (DATE$) and time (TIME$) are added by the computer.
- The program will capture real-time data from both the 3700 and 3740 oximeters. It will also capture Trend data initiated manually.

Example program

```
REM [ohm374-r.bas]
REM to access real-time data from Ohmeda 3740 and 3700
CLEAR
CLS
OPEN "COM1:1200,0,7,1,CS,DS,OP2000" FOR INPUT AS #1
OPEN "c:datafile.dat" FOR OUTPUT AS #2
DO
    DO
```

```
        a$ = a$ + INPUT$(LOC(1), #1)
        L% = INSTR(1, a$, CHR$(13))
        key$ = INKEY$
        IF UCASE$(key$) = "Q" THEN
            CLOSE #1, #2
            END
        END IF
    LOOP UNTIL L% > 0
    data$ = MID$(a$, 2, L% - 2)
    PRINT data$; SPACE$(2); DATE$; SPACE$(2); TIME$
    PRINT #2, data$; SPACE$(2); DATE$; SPACE$(2); TIME$
    a$ = RIGHT$(a$, LEN(a$) - L%)
LOOP
END
```

An example of data saved using the above program is shown below.

:SaO2=␣97␣PR=␣72␣␣6-29-1993␣␣14:33:15
:SaO2=␣97␣PR=␣73␣**␣LOW␣QUALITY␣SIGNAL␣␣6-29-1993␣␣14:33:17
:SaO2=---␣PR=---␣**␣PROBE␣OFF␣PATIENT␣␣6-29-1993␣␣14:33:19

9.4 Control mode

Both oximeters allow the various modes (e.g. Waveform, Trend, etc.) and oximeter settings (e.g. alarm volume, pulse volume etc.) to be controlled directly by computer using software control codes.

The Control mode is first enabled by sending the codes ⟨ESC⟩⟨C⟩ to the oximeter. The oximeter function or mode can then be changed by sending a single letter command-code followed (where appropriate) by a variable parameter followed by ⟨CR⟩ as follows.

⟨ESC⟩C⟨command-code⟩⟨CR⟩

The full list of command-codes used by the 3700 and 3740 pulse oximeters is shown in Table 9.5.

For example, the pulse volume function code is H, for which the parameter option range is 0 (silent) to 10 (very loud) in steps of 1. The following code would therefore silence the pulse volume beep.

⟨ESC⟩CH0⟨CR⟩

Since the ASCII code for ⟨ESC⟩ is 27, and that for ⟨CR⟩ is 13, the above sequence of codes could be sent by using the following lines of

Table 9.5. *Command-codes for Ohmeda oximeters.*

Code	Meaning	Range (step)	Oximeter	
A	Alarm silence	no parameter	3700	3740
B	SaO2 low alarm limit	50–100 (1) [0 = off]	3700	3740
C	SaO2 high alarm limit	70–100 (1) [0 = off]	3700	3740
D	Pulse rate low alarm	40–200 (5) [0 = off]	3700	3740
E	Pulse rate high alarm	70–250 (5) [0 = off]	3700	3740
F	Fast response mode	no parameter	3700	3740
G	Slow response mode	no parameter	3700	3740
N	Normal response mode	no parameter	3700	3740
H	Pulse volume	0–10 (1) [0 = off]	3700	3740
I	Alarm volume	0–10 (1)	3700	3740
J	Start trend output	no parameter	3700	3740
K	Stop trend output	no parameter	3700	3740
O	Enable 8-hr trend data	no parameter	—	3740
P	Enable recent trend data	no parameter	—	3740
L	Start waveform mode	no parameter	3700	3740
M	Stop waveform mode	no parameter	3700	3740

QuickBASIC where, in this example, the above sequence of codes is placed in a string called `pulsevolumezero$`.

```
pulsevolumezero$ = CHR$(27) + "CH0" + CHR$(13)
PRINT #1, pulsevolumezero$
```

Note that when QuickBASIC executes a PRINT statement without a terminal semicolon, an additional ⟨CR⟩ is added (see Section 5.3.1), and so the above CHR$(13) could be omitted. In practice however, both oximeters do not mind an additional ⟨CR⟩ in Control mode.

9.5 Trend mode (manual operation)

This mode outputs Trend data (sampled at 12-second intervals) via the serial port, and is accessed from the Auto-output mode. There are two forms of Trend data as follows.

- **Recent Trend data**   All data since the machine was last switched on (i.e. all data for the current session).
- **8-hr Trend data**   All data saved during the last eight hours of oximeter use.

The method for manually accessing both Trend modes for each machine is as follows.

9.5.1 3700 oximeter

Recent Trend. With the 3700 oximeter the Recent Trend data is accessed manually by pressing the 'Trend' button for at least three seconds, whereupon the following message appears in the oximeter's graphic display window.

```
TREND OUTPUT MODE
HIT TREND TO START OUTPUT
```

Pressing the 'Trend' button once more starts the output. Pressing the 'Trend' button again stops the Recent Trend output, and returns the oximeter to the normal Auto-output mode, outputting real-time data.

8-hr Trend. With the 3700 oximeter the stored 8-hr Trend data is accessed manually by first switching the oximeter on *while* pressing the 'Trend' button. Following this, the oximeter displays the following message in the display window.

```
8-HR TREND DATA AVAILABLE
```

Now when the Trend mode is accessed (by pressing the 'Trend' button for 3 seconds, and then pressing it again) the 8-hr Trend data will be output via the RS-232 port. The example program given earlier for accessing real-time data can also be used for accessing the 3700 Trend data if it is initiated manually.

9.5.2 3740 oximeter

With the 3740 oximeter the Trend mode is obtained manually by first entering the options menu (by pressing the 'menu/enter' button on the front panel), and selecting the TREND OUTPUT option. This results in the following message appearing in the display window.

```
CURRENT DATA
8 HOURS OF DATA

- -TREND OUTPUT- -
```

When one of the two Trend data options is selected (current data or 8 hours of data), the oximeter then shows the following message in the display window.

> -TREND OUTPUT MODE -
> START CHART RECORDER
> THEN HIT UP ARROW
> TO START OUTPUT

At this point make sure that the computer program is running, and then press the 'up' arrow. The oximeter then starts outputting the Trend data via the serial port, and simultaneously displays the following message indicating the time remaining (mm:ss).

> - OUTPUTTING TREND -
> TIME REMAINING: 2:06
> HIT MENU/ENTER
> TO STOP

The example program given earlier for accessing real-time data can also be used for accessing the 3740 Trend data if it is initiated manually.

9.5.3 Trend data format

Both the Recent Trend and the 8-hr Trend data are output in essentially the same format for both the 3700 and 3740 oximeters. An important difference, however, is that the 3700 oximeter does *not* give the date and time of data sampling. This omission was corrected in the more recent 3740 model which gives a time-stamp (hh:mm mm/dd/yy) every 5 minutes. Since Trend data is sampled every 12 seconds, there are therefore 25 data-string items between time-stamps.

Dashes are used in place of the data when the pulse rate and calculated SaO2 are considered to be invalid, and error messages (where appropriate) are condensed into a two letter code (see Table 9.4) in order to save memory. For example, the 'probe off patient' message is condensed to the error code PO. Note that the Trend output starts with the ⟨CR⟩⟨LF⟩ pair.

An example of the beginning of the Trend data output of the 3740 oximeter is as follows.

⟨CR⟩⟨LF⟩
OHMEDA␣BIOX␣3740␣PULSE␣OXIMETER⟨CR⟩⟨LF⟩
TREND␣ DATA␣OUTPUT⟨CR⟩⟨LF⟩
12␣SECONDS␣PER␣DATA␣POINT⟨CR⟩⟨LF⟩
⟨LF⟩⟨LF⟩
:SaO2=␣98␣PR=␣64␣␣␣␣␣15:48␣04/23/92⟨CR⟩⟨LF⟩

:SaO2=⎵98⎵PR=⎵65⟨CR⟩⟨LF⟩
:SaO2=⎵98⎵PR=⎵64⟨CR⟩⟨LF⟩
:SaO2=---⎵PR=---⎵PO⟨CR⟩⟨LF⟩
...
...

9.6 Trend mode (initiated by computer)

Accessing either the Recent Trend or 8-hr Trend data directly by the computer is achieved in two stages. Firstly, access to the Trend data must be enabled. Secondly, the command to start transmitting Trend data must be sent. The exact procedure varies slightly between the two oximeters, and so in the following each oximeter is considered separately.

- **3700 oximeter** Access to the Recent Trend data does not have to be enabled since it is immediately available by default. Access to the 8-hr Trend data is enabled manually, by switching the oximeter on *while pressing the 'Trend' button*. Trend data output is started by sending the command-code J.
- **3740 oximeter** Access to both the Recent Trend and 8-hr Trend data is enabled by sending a command-code, which is P for the Recent Trend, and O for the 8-hr Trend data (see Table 9.5). Trend data output is started by sending the command-code J.

For example, access to the Recent Trend data in the 3740 oximeter would be enabled by using the following statements. Note that a short pause between the commands is necessary.

```
enablerecenttrend$ = CHR$(27) + "CP" + CHR$(13)
PRINT #1, enablerecenttrend$
SLEEP 1
sendtrend$ = CHR$(27) + "CJ" + CHR$(13)
PRINT #1, sendtrend$
```

The output of Trend data can be stopped at any stage by sending the 'stop Trend' command-code K as follows.

```
stoptrend$ = CHR$(27) + "CK" + CHR$(13)
PRINT #1, stoptrend$
```

Following this command the oximeter reverts to the default Auto-output mode, and outputs real-time data at 2-second intervals.

9.6.1 Program for accessing Trend data

The following example QuickBASIC 4.5 program for the 3740 oximeter will initiate Trend output, and save the data on disk. Pressing E (Escape) will stop Trend output, and return the oximeter to its default Auto-output mode, whereupon data will continue to be output every 2 seconds. Pressing <Q> will quit the program altogether.

Program points

- Note that the serial port is opened FOR RANDOM ACCESS READ WRITE since the program is both sending control codes and receiving data through the same port.
- The 3740 oximeter seems to require a short pause between receiving the 'enable Trend' command and the 'start Trend output' command, hence the SLEEP 1 statement between the two commands.
- After the 3740 oximeter receives the 'enable Trend data' command, the usual real-time data is still output every two seconds. In view of this, several real-time data messages usually arrive in the computer's input buffer before the Trend data arrives, and will be printed immediately before the Trend data. The following program therefore empties the buffer, stopping when it finds the ⟨CR⟩⟨LF⟩⟨CR⟩ sequence which is transmitted to the PC immediately before the Trend data heading. Since the program inputs data up to and including the ⟨CR⟩, this sequence is identified by finding a string consisting of only two characters (i.e. when B% = 2). The DO...LOOP UNTIL B% = 2 section which empties the buffer is therefore only required if it is necessary to remove the preceding data.
- Pressing <Q> will terminate the output of Trend data, and exit the program. Pressing <E> will terminate the output of Trend data, and then continue to access real-time data.
- In order to use the following program to access Trend data from a 3700 oximeter it is necessary to delete the statements which enable the two Trend modes in the CASE "R" and CASE "8" sections.

Example program

```
REM [ohm374-T.bas]
REM program to access trend data from Ohmeda 3740
```

```
CLS
CLEAR
OPEN "COM1:1200,0,7,1,CS,DS" FOR RANDOM ACCESS READ WRITE
                                                        AS #1
OPEN "c:datafile.dat" FOR OUTPUT AS #2
LOCATE 5, 5: PRINT "enter R for Recent trend data"
LOCATE 7, 5: PRINT "enter 8 for 8-hr trend data"
SLEEP: key$ = INKEY$
LOCATE 9, 5: PRINT "waiting for oximeter to send data"
SELECT CASE UCASE$(key$)
    CASE "R"
        REM enable Recent trend data
        PRINT #1, CHR$(27) + "CP"
        SLEEP 1
        REM start trend data output
        PRINT #1, CHR$(27) + "CJ"
        PRINT #2, "Recent Trend data", TIME$, DATE$
    CASE "8"
        REM enable 8-hr trend data
        PRINT #1, CHR$(27) + "CO"
        SLEEP 1
        REM start trend data output
        PRINT #1, CHR$(27) + "CJ"
        PRINT #2, "8-hr Trend data", TIME$, DATE$
END SELECT
REM empty buffer; stop when find <CR><LF><CR> sequence
DO
    buff$ = buff$ + INPUT$(LOC(1), #1)
    B% = INSTR(1, buff$, CHR$(13))
    buff$ = RIGHT$(buff$, LEN(buff$) - B%)
LOOP UNTIL B% = 2
REM now collect Trend data from buffer
DO
    DO
        a$ = a$ + INPUT$(LOC(1), #1)
        L% = INSTR(1, a$, CHR$(13))
        key$ = INKEY$
        SELECT CASE UCASE$(key$)
            CASE "Q"
                stoptrend$ = CHR$(27) + "CK"
```

```
                PRINT #1, stoptrend$
                CLOSE #1, #2
                END
            CASE "E"
                stoptrend$ = CHR$(27) + "CK"
                PRINT #1, stoptrend$
        END SELECT
    LOOP UNTIL L% > 1
    data$ = MID$(a$, 2, L% - 2)
    PRINT data$
    PRINT #2, data$
    a$ = RIGHT$(a$, LEN(a$) - L%)
LOOP
END
```

9.7 Waveform mode

The Waveform mode outputs real-time data which describes the pulse waveform shown in the oximeter's display window. The waveform data comprises the **waveform amplitude**, which is sampled at either 1/25 or 1/30 sec intervals depending on the frequency of the power source (50 or 60 Hz respectively), and **signal strength** (sampled once per second). In addition, saturation and pulse rate are given every two seconds. Error codes (when appropriate) are added to the end of the saturation/heart rate string.

9.7.1 Amplitude

The waveform amplitude is output as a two digit decimal number (nn) in the range 00–31, with 00 indicating an error condition. The format is as follows.

nn⟨CR⟩⟨LF⟩

9.7.2 Signal strength (S)

The signal strength is expressed as a two-digit decimal number in the range 00–31, with 00 indicating an error condition. The format is as follows.

Snn⟨CR⟩⟨LF⟩

9.7.3 Waveform data

An example of typical waveform data is shown below.

09⟨CR⟩⟨LF⟩
17⟨CR⟩⟨LF⟩
28⟨CR⟩⟨LF⟩
30⟨CR⟩⟨LF⟩
28⟨CR⟩⟨LF⟩
26⟨CR⟩⟨LF⟩
22⟨CR⟩⟨LF⟩
17⟨CR⟩⟨LF⟩
16⟨CR⟩⟨LF⟩
15⟨CR⟩⟨LF⟩
13⟨CR⟩⟨LF⟩
11⟨CR⟩⟨LF⟩
10⟨CR⟩⟨LF⟩
S31⟨CR⟩⟨LF⟩
09⟨CR⟩⟨LF⟩
08⟨CR⟩⟨LF⟩
08⟨CR⟩⟨LF⟩
:SaO2=␣98␣PR=␣57⟨CR⟩⟨LF⟩
09⟨CR⟩⟨LF⟩

9.7.4 Program for accessing Waveform data

The method of extracting Waveform data is the same for both oximeters, and is achieved by sending the command-code L using the ⟨ESC⟩ format as follows.

⟨ESC⟩CL⟨CR⟩

The following example QuickBASIC 4.5 program will initiate the output of Waveform data from either oximeter and save it to a disk. When the program is run the usual real-time Auto-output data will be received. Waveform data is accessed by pressing <W>. Pressing <E> will return to real-time data. Pressing <Q> will quit the program altogether.

The program is essentially similar to that for accessing Trend data, except that in this case the INPUT# routine is used for inputting the data, in order to illustrate the alternative method which can be used when all the data-strings are terminated by ⟨CR⟩⟨LF⟩. Although this method is simpler and could be used for all the programs in this Chapter, it does lack the flexibility of the INPUT$ routine (see Chapter 5).

Program points

- Since data is being sent and received via the same serial port, the port must be opened FOR RANDOM ACCESS READ WRITE.
- In this example, the codes initiating the Waveform mode are placed in a string called startwaveform$.
- The Waveform data stream can be terminated by sending the control code M. This occurs when either <Q> or <E> is pressed. Note that there is no CHR$(13) at the end of the line to be transmitted as this is added by the PRINT statement (see Section 5.3.1).

Example program

```
REM [ohm374-W.bas]
REM program for Waveform data from Ohmeda 3740 and 3700
CLEAR
CLS
OPEN "COM1:1200,0,7,1,CS,DS" FOR RANDOM ACCESS READ WRITE
                                                            AS #1
OPEN "c:datafile.dat" FOR OUTPUT AS #2
DO
    INPUT #1, data$
    PRINT data$
    PRINT #2, data$
    key$ = INKEY$
    SELECT CASE UCASE$(key$)
        CASE "Q"
            stopwaveform$ = CHR$(27) + "CM"
            PRINT #1, stopwaveform$
            CLOSE #1, #2
            END
        CASE "E"
            stopwaveform$ = CHR$(27) + "CM"
            PRINT #1, stopwaveform$
        CASE "W"
            startwaveform$ = CHR$(27) + "CL"
            PRINT #1, startwaveform$
```

```
        END SELECT
LOOP
END
```

9.8 Slave mode

Slave mode is enabled by the ⟨ESC⟩S command from the Auto-output mode, and disabled by ⟨ESC⟩X. The Slave mode commands are shown in Table 9.6. While in Slave mode the usual real-time data output is suspended, and data is output only in response to the ⟨ESC⟩? command.

Table 9.6. *Slave mode commands.*

Command	Meaning
⟨ESC⟩?	Requests Slave mode data-string
⟨ESC⟩S	Enables Slave mode
⟨ESC⟩X	Disables Slave mode

9.8.1 Commands

The Slave mode command string must *not* include the ⟨CR⟩, and therefore the PRINT# statement must be terminated with a semicolon as shown in the following examples (see Section 5.3.1).

```
PRINT #1, CHR$(27) + "S";
PRINT #1, CHR$(27) + "?";
PRINT #1, CHR$(27) + "X";
```

9.8.2 Data format

The Slave mode data-string returns saturation, heart rate, and status information. The format, and some examples, are shown below. Table 9.7 indicates the coding, and Table 9.4 lists the error codes.

:aaa␣bbb␣ccc␣ddd␣eee␣fff␣g␣hh␣ii␣jj⟨CR⟩⟨LF⟩
:␣98␣␣69␣␣90␣OFF␣␣50*OFF␣N␣31␣50⟨CR⟩⟨LF⟩
:---␣---␣␣90␣OFF␣OFF␣OFF␣N␣␣0␣50␣10⟨CR⟩⟨LF⟩

If the command syntax is incorrect, then the oximeters reply with

Table 9.7. *Slave mode data format.*

Code	Meaning
aaa	Saturation
bbb	Heart rate
ccc	Low saturation alarm limit
ddd	High saturation alarm limit
eee	Low heart rate alarm
fff	High heart rate alarm
g	Response mode; F (fast), N (normal), S (slow)
hh	Signal strength
ii	Power source; 50 (Hz), 60 (Hz), BT (battery)
jj	Alarm message code
*	Alarm limit violated

WHAT? and a beep. The format, and an example showing the symbol used for the control character ⟨BEL⟩, are as follows.

WHAT?⟨BEL⟩⟨CR⟩⟨LF⟩
WHAT?•⟨CR⟩⟨LF⟩

10
The Nellcor N-200E pulse oximeter

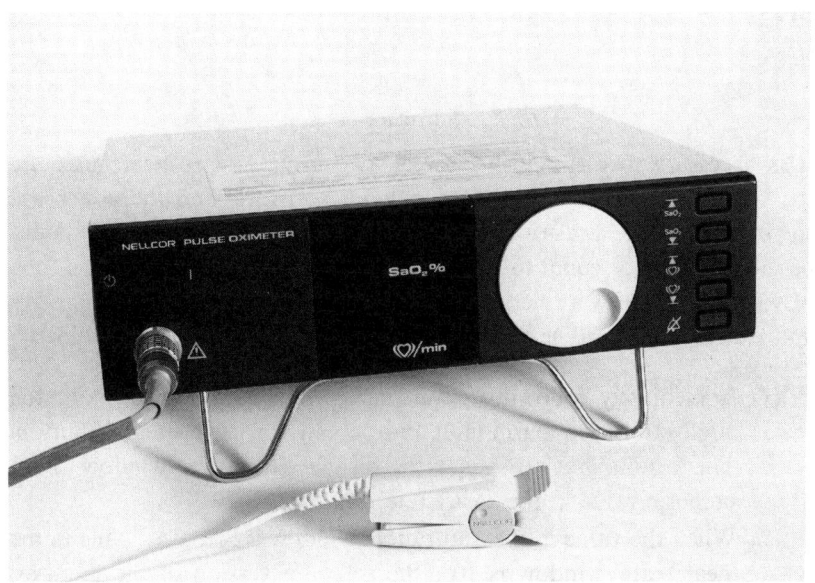

10.1 Introduction

The Nellcor N-200E pulse oximeter† consists of three components: the monitor, the powerbase, and the patient module (receives input from the oximeter probe and ECG leads). The oximeter displays heart rate and oxygen saturation, as well as a qualitative display of pulse amplitude. Saturation measurements made in a high-motion environment can be made more reliable by using the Nellcor C-LOCK ECG synchronisation feature.

The powerbase is a detachable AC power supply, and is the external interface for the N-200E. It also contains the circuitry required for

† Nellcor Incorporated, 4280 Hacienda Drive, Pleasanton, California 94588, USA.
Tel: +1–510–4634000. Fax: +1–510–4634420.
Nellcor Europe B.V., Hambakenwetering 1, 5231 DD's-Hertogenbosch, The Netherlands. Tel: +31–(0)73–426565. Fax: +31–(0)73–410915.

communicating with the computer. The N-200E is portable, and can operate for up to two hours on internal batteries.

In addition to the serial interface, the N-200E has analog outputs for pulse rate, saturation, pulse waveform, and ECG. As well as real-time data, the Nellcor N-200E can also output stored Trend and Event data. The internal clock, which can only be set to the nearest minute, should be set to the correct time before storing data.

The electrical safety classification of the pulse oximeter probe is Type BF.†

10.1.1 Software version

It is necessary to distinguish between two groups of software used by the N-200E oximeter, namely the **monitor** software, and the **powerbase** software. As a general rule the software version of the monitor should be greater than or equal to that of the powerbase software. At the time of writing the software versions for the monitor and powerbase are 2.9 and 2.7 respectively. The two software versions are accessed as follows.

(1) Immediately following power-on simultaneously press both the 'high saturation alarm limit' button and the 'silence alarm' button. This results in a zero appearing in the 'saturation' window and a numeric value in the 'heart rate' window.
(2) When the value in the 'saturation' window is zero, the value in the 'heart rate' window is 10× the software version of the monitor. For example, if the value is 27, then the software version is 2.7.
(3) Now rotate the wheel anticlockwise until the value in the 'saturation' window changes to Pb; then read the value in the 'heart rate' window. This value is 10× the software version of the powerbase.

10.1.2 Available software

A software package for PCs called FORNOX (version 2.3, June 1992) is available for accessing data from Nellcor products. It is available from Nellcor Inc., and is compatible with those Nellcor N-200 oximeters for which the software version of the powerbase is 2.7 or higher. FORNOX is multi-lingual, and can be run in either English, French, German, Spanish or Italian.

† See Chapter 7 for further details.

Table 10.1. *Switch settings for the various communication modes. X indicates that switch position is not important.*

Mode	DIP switches			
	2	3	4	5
Beat-to-beat	X	up	down	up
Computer (normal)	down	down	up	down
Computer (alternative)	up	down	up	down
Conversation	X	down	up	up

10.1.3 Silencing the beep/alarms

When testing the oximeter it is often useful to silence both the pulse 'beep' and the alarms. The pulse 'beep' is silenced by rotating the wheel anticlockwise. The alarms are permanently silenced by simultaneously pressing the 'audio alarm off' button and rotating the wheel clockwise until the word 'off' appears in the 'saturation' window.

10.1.4 Communication modes

The N-200E has nine different communication modes, each outputting data in different formats. However only three of the available modes, namely the **Beat-to-beat**, **Computer**, and **Conversation** modes, will be described here since only these modes seem particularly useful when interfacing the oximeter to a PC. Note that *two* Computer modes are available, namely a **normal** mode, and an **alternative** mode.

The various communication modes are set using the DIP switches located on the back of the powerbase module, as shown in Table 10.1.

10.2 Serial port

A 9-pin female D-type serial port is located on the rear panel of the powerbase. The pin-outs for the serial port are shown in Table 10.2.

The powerbase contains the optically-isolated digital interface for the oximeter. For data communication to occur between the oximeter and computer, the powerbase module must be mains powered *and* switched on.

Table 10.2. *Nellcor N-200E serial port.*

Pin No.	Name	Comments
1	—	Not connected
2	RxD	Receives data
3	TxD	Transmits data
4	DTR	Set HIGH (positive) when powered up
5	GND	Signal ground
6	DSR	This pin must be held HIGH (positive) to enable Trend and Event data to be output to the computer using the Conversation mode
7	RTS	Set HIGH (positive) when powered up
8	CTS	This pin can be used to control data flow
9	RI	This pin is set HIGH (positive) whenever an alarm state exists

Table 10.3. *Nellcor N-200E protocol.*

Bit rate	1200, 2400, 9600, 19200
Data bits	8
Parity	None
Stop bits	1

10.2.1 Protocol options

The serial protocol options are shown in Table 10.3. A wide range of bit-rates is available, and these are set using DIP switches 7 and 8 as shown in Table 10.4.

10.2.2 Cable connections

Once the powerbase is mains powered *and* switched on, an RS-232 line-checker connected only to the N-200E will indicate the following line voltage states: TxD—negative, RTS—positive, DTR—positive. Figure 10.1 shows the recommended wiring configuration for interfacing to a PC.

- **DSR** The N-200E oximeter requires its DSR pin to be held HIGH (positive) to enable Trend and Event data output when using the Conversation mode. However, for both Beat-to-beat and Computer modes, it does *not* matter whether DSR is held HIGH or LOW. In practice, therefore, it is best to wire the N-200E's DSR pin to either

Table 10.4. *Switch settings for the bit-rate.*

Bit-rate	DIP switches	
	7	8
1200	down	down
2400	down	up
9600	up	down
19200	up	up

Nellcor N-200E (9-pin)		Computer (9-pin)	
pin 2	RxD	pin 3	TxD
pin 3	TxD	pin 2	RxD
pin 4	DTR	pin 6	DSR
pin 5	GND	pin 5	GND
pin 6	DSR	pin 7	RTS
pin 7	RTS	pin 8	CTS
pin 8	CTS	pin 4	DTR
pin 9	RI	pin 9	RI

Fig. 10.1. Nellcor N-200E wiring diagram.

the PC's RTS or DTR pin, since both of these are automatically set positive by QuickBASIC on executing the OPEN COM statement (unless the RS option is used—see Chapter 5).

- **CTS** Data transmission is enabled whenever the oximeter's CTS is either positive or not connected.† When CTS is made LOW (negative), transmission in all modes is halted, and data for output accumulates in the oximeter's output buffer. When CTS is next made NOT LOW (i.e. either HIGH or not connected), all the data stored in the oximeter's buffer is transmitted as a block, following which the usual transmission frequency is resumed.
- **RI** When no alarms are set this pin is LOW (negative). When an alarm state exists this pin is set HIGH. This pin can therefore be used for detecting alarm states, by connecting it to one of the computer's

† When CTS is not connected, internal circuitry forces the state of the line HIGH, i.e. the line is said to 'float' HIGH.

input control lines (e.g. RI), and monitoring the status of this line (see Section 5.17).

10.3 Beat-to-beat mode

When in Beat-to-beat mode, the N-200E transmits saturation (S) and pulse rate (R) data once per beat. No data is transmitted if the finger probe is not attached. Three Operating modes are available which provide for three different averaging times; mode 1 (5–7 secs), mode 2 (2–3 secs), and mode 3 (10–15 secs). The default Operating mode at power-on is Mode 1.

The format, and an example of Beat-to-beat data, is as follows.

RnnnSnnn⟨CR⟩⟨LF⟩

Note that neither the date nor time of data sampling is included in the Beat-to-beat data-string. If these are required they can be added during data collection by the computer using the DATE$ and TIME$ functions.

10.3.1 Program for accessing Beat-to-beat data

An example QuickBASIC program which will access real-time data using the Beat-to-beat mode and save it to a file (datafile.dat) is given below. Pressing <Q> will quit the program.

Program points

- The powerbase must be mains powered and switched on.
- The program assumes that the oximeter is in Beat-to-beat mode (see Table 10.1), and is attached to serial port 1 (COM1). Both DSR and CTS checking by the computer are disabled using the CS and DS options in the OPEN COM statement.
- Since each data-string is terminated by ⟨CR⟩⟨LF⟩, the INPUT# command can be used which inputs all data up to the next carriage return. However, if there is no data output the program will simply continue to wait at this line, and pressing <Q> to quit will not be effective. Ctrl-break will then have to be used to exit. A more flexible alternative is to use INPUT$ as shown in Section 5.4.1 (see also the program **ohm374-r.bas** in Section 9.3.1).

- There is no data output from the N-200E *unless* the finger probe is on and generating a sufficient amplitude. Each 'beep' from the oximeter is associated with the output of a Beat-to-beat data-string.
- In this example program, both date (DATE$) and time (TIME$) have been added by the computer, and are printed at the end of each data-string.

Example program

```
REM [nel-bk-r.bas]
REM Nellcor N-200E pulse oximeter
REM program to access Beat-to-beat data
REM monitor software = 2.7
REM powerbase software = 2.7
CLEAR
CLS
OPEN "COM1:1200,N,8,1,CS,DS,OP10000" FOR INPUT AS #1
OPEN "b:datafile.dat" FOR OUTPUT AS #2
PRINT "communications open"
PRINT "waiting for data"
DO
    INPUT #1, data$
    key$ = INKEY$
    IF UCASE$(key$) = "Q" THEN
        CLOSE #1, #2
        END
    END IF
    PRINT data$; SPACE$(8); TIME$; SPACE$(3); DATE$
    PRINT #2, data$; SPACE$(8); TIME$; SPACE$(3); DATE$
LOOP
END
```

An example of the data output when using the above Beat-to-beat program is shown below. The data is output at 1-second intervals.

```
R065S097      18:41:10    01-14-1992
R065S097      18:41:11    01-14-1992
R065S097      18:41:12    01-14-1992
```

10.4 Computer mode

When in Computer mode, the N-200E outputs the following comprehensive data every 10 seconds; saturation and heart rate with both high and low alarm settings; time (hrs/mins/secs); an index of pulse amplitude; the alarm status (on or off); and monitor status. Note that the N-200E codes the low saturation alarm setting using the letter O, which unfortunately is easily misread for the number 0.

Although the Computer format gives the time of data sampling to the nearest second, it is actually only possible to set the N-200E's clock to the nearest minute. Furthermore, the date of data sampling is not included in the data-string. If the date is required it can be added by the computer using the DATE$ function.

There are two Computer data formats which are called **Normal** (for outputting to a PC), and **Alternative** (used for interfacing to a Spacelabs printer). The only difference between these two formats is that the checksum is placed between two ⟨ETX⟩ control characters in the Alternative format. Examples of the two formats are shown below (see Table 10.5 for details of the codes).

10.4.1 Normal format

The Normal format for data output is as follows.

⟨STX⟩RnnnSnnnPnnnLnnnHnnnOnnnAnnnMnnnTnnnnnnQnnn⟨CR⟩⟨LF⟩⟨checksum⟩⟨ETX⟩

In practice, because of the position of the ⟨CR⟩⟨LF⟩ pair, the string occupies two lines when displayed by the computer. Furthermore, since the control codes ⟨STX⟩ and ⟨ETX⟩ are commonly represented on the screen by ☻ and ♥ respectively (see Appendix 1), PCs will usually show the *complete* data-string as follows.

☻R065S098P102L050H110O090A005M015T163455Q100
⟨checksum⟩♥

10.4.2 Alternative format

The Alternative format for data output is as follows.

⟨STX⟩RnnnSnnnPnnnLnnnHnnnOnnnAnnnMnnnTnnnnnnQnnn⟨CR⟩⟨LF⟩⟨ETX⟩⟨checksum⟩⟨ETX⟩

Table 10.5. *N-200E data-string codes.*

⟨STX⟩	Start of data
R	Heart rate
L	Low rate alarm setting
H	High rate alarm setting
S	Saturation
O	Low saturation alarm setting
Q	High saturation alarm setting
P	Pulse amplitude
A	Alarm status
M	Monitor status
T	Time (hhmmss)
⟨CR⟩	Carriage return
⟨LF⟩	Line feed
checksum	1-byte Σ-checksum (*modulo* 128)
⟨ETX⟩	End of data

The *complete* string is usually displayed occupying two lines as follows.

☻R065S098P102L050H110O090A005M015T163455Q100
♥⟨checksum⟩♥

Note that some PCs will show the ASCII control characters using the alternative Ctrl notation which represents ⟨STX⟩ by ^B and ⟨ETX⟩ by ^C (see Appendix 1). The codes used in the data-strings are listed in Table 10.5.

10.4.3 Alarm status (code Annn)

The value **nnn** following the alarm status code A in the Computer data format represents a decimal value which is bit-encoded (4 bits), as shown in Figure 10.2.

For example, suppose the alarm status code is A005. Since 005 (decimal) is equivalent to 0101b, this would indicate that both LoSat and HiPR alarms were on (see Figure 10.2).

10.4.4 Monitor status (code Mnnn)

The value **nnn** following the monitor status code M in the Computer data format represents the decimal value of a bit-encoded 8-bit byte, as shown in Table 10.6.

For example, suppose the monitor status code is M015. Since 015

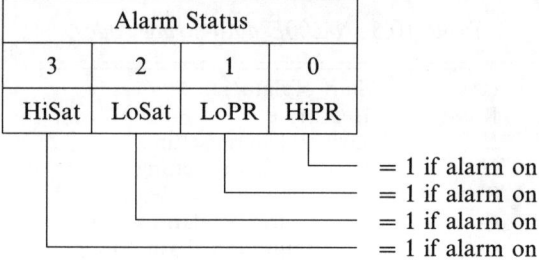

Fig. 10.2. Alarm status.

Table 10.6. *Monitor status byte.*

Bit No.		Meaning	
Bit-0	Pulse search status	0 = searching	1 = locked
Bit-1	Sensor status	0 = off	1 = attached
Bit-2	Audio alarm status	0 = disabled	1 = enabled
Bit-3	ECG status	0 = in use	1 = not in use
Bit-4	Not used—set to 0		
Bit-5	Not used—set to 0		
Bit-6	Not used—set to 0		
Bit-7	Communications status	0 = intact	1 = lost

(decimal) is equivalent to 00001111b, this would indicate the following state: pulse locked on; sensor attached; audio alarms enabled; ECG not in use; and communications intact.

10.4.5 *Checksum*

The Nellcor N-200E uses a *modulo*128 Σ-checksum which is the value represented by the lowest 7 bits of the sum of the relevant characters (see Chapter 3). The checksum includes all characters (letters and integers) and the ⟨CR⟩⟨LF⟩ but *not* the ⟨STX⟩ or ⟨ETX⟩ control characters, as follows.

⟨STX⟩ RnnnSnnn....TnnnnnnQnnn⟨CR⟩⟨LF⟩ ⟨checksum⟩⟨ETX⟩
         checksum

In the following example (Normal computer mode) the arithmetic sum of the relevant characters and control codes is 2463. The remainder after dividing by 128 is 31, and so the checksum is 31. This checksum is then

The Nellcor N-200E pulse oximeter 139

transmitted as the character whose ASCII code is 31, namely ▼, as shown below.

⟨STX⟩R065S098P102L050H110O090A005M015T163455Q100
⟨CR⟩⟨LF⟩▼⟨ETX⟩

arithmetic sum = 2463
Σ-checksum (*modulo*128) = 31   (▼)

10.4.6 Program for accessing Computer mode data

An example of a QuickBASIC program which will access the Computer format data using the Normal computer mode, and save it to a file (datafile.dat) is given below. Pressing <Q> will quit the program.

Program points

- The powerbase must be mains powered and switched on.
- The example program is for the **normal computer** mode (see Table 10.1), and assumes that the oximeter is attached to serial port 1 (COM1). Both CTS and DSR checking by the computer are disabled using the CS and DS options in the OPEN COM statement.
- The example program inputs all characters up to and including the ⟨ETX⟩ control character (ASCII 3) into a string called data$. The number of characters (L%) in data$ up to and including the ⟨ETX⟩ control character is given by

L% = INSTR(1, data$, CHR$(3))

Once the number of characters up to and including the next ⟨ETX⟩ is known, then the required data (oximdata$) and checksum (check$) can be extracted as follows.

oximdata$ = MID$(data$, 2, L% - 5)
check$ = MID$(data$, L% - 1, 1)

- In order to view the complete data-string, include the following line immediately after the statement IF L% < 5 THEN GOTO endloop

PRINT data$

- Both the date (DATE$) and time (TIME$) are printed with the data-string.

Example program

```
REM [nel-bknc.bas]
REM Nellcor N-200E pulse oximeter
REM program to access NORMAL computer mode data
REM monitor software 2.7, powerbase software 2.7
CLEAR
CLS
OPEN "COM1:1200,N,8,1,CS,DS,OP10000" FOR INPUT AS #1
OPEN "b:datafile.dat" FOR OUTPUT AS #2
PRINT "communications open"
DO
    DO
        data$ = data$ + INPUT$(LOC(1), #1)
        key$ = INKEY$
        IF UCASE$(key$) = "Q" THEN
            CLOSE #1, #2
            END
        END IF
        L% = INSTR(1, data$, CHR$(3))
    LOOP UNTIL L% > 0
    IF L% < 5 THEN GOTO endloop
    oximdata$ = MID$(data$, 2, L% - 5)
    check$ = MID$(data$, L% - 1, 1)
    PRINT "time/date"; " "; TIME$; "    "; DATE$
    PRINT oximdata$; "   "; "checksum = "; ASC(check$)
    PRINT
    PRINT #2, "time/date"; " "; TIME$; "    "; DATE$
    PRINT #2, oximdata$; "   "; "checksum = "; ASC(check$)
    endloop:
    data$ = RIGHT$(data$, LEN(data$) - L%)
LOOP
END
```

An example of the data output when using this example program is shown below. Note that the time-stamp shows that Computer mode data is output at 10-second intervals.

```
time/date    19:23:59      02-28-1992
R060S098P100L055H1400085A000M015T192359Q100   checksum = 42
```

The Nellcor N-200E pulse oximeter 141

```
time/date      19:24:09      02-28-1992
R067S098P100L055H1400085A000M015T192409Q100   checksum =   45
```

Since Computer mode data fields are fixed (i.e. leading zeros are transmitted), the value of any particular parameter can be extracted from oximdata$ using straightforward string manipulation. For example, since the saturation data-string (say, saturation$) is three integers long and starts at position 6, it would be given by the following statement.

```
saturation$ = MID$(oximdata$, 6, 3)
```

If the numeric value is required for mathematical manipulation (say, satdata), then this would be given by the following statement.

```
satdata = VAL(MID$(oximdata$, 6, 3))
```

See Chapter 5 for further details of string manipulation.

10.5 Conversation mode

When in Conversation mode (see Table 10.1) the N-200E only outputs data in response to a command message from the computer requesting data. Note that the N-200E requires its DSR to be held HIGH (positive) to enable data output when using the Conversation mode.

10.5.1 Command format

A command message consists of the command-code (a single uppercase letter) followed by the ⟨CR⟩⟨LF⟩ pair, as follows.

⟨command-code⟩⟨CR⟩⟨LF⟩

The command-codes are the same uppercase letters as used in the Computer mode data-string, with the addition of W (request Trend data), X (request Event data), and V (stop Trend/Event data output), as shown in Table 10.7.

10.5.2 Reply format

A reply message includes the initiating command-code followed by the data. With the exception of Trend and Event data, the reply format for Conversation mode, together with an example, is as follows.

⟨STX⟩⟨command-code⟩⟨data⟩⟨CR⟩⟨LF⟩
⟨STX⟩R073⟨CR⟩⟨LF⟩

Table 10.7. *N-200E Conversation mode command-codes.*

Command-code	Data requested
R	Heart rate
L	Low rate alarm setting
H	High rate alarm setting
S	Saturation
O	Low saturation alarm setting
Q	High saturation alarm setting
P	Pulse amplitude
A	Alarm status
M	Monitor status
T	Time (hhmmss)
W	Trend data
X	Event data
V	Stop Trend/Event data output

Trend/Event data. The reply format for both Trend and Event data differs from all other replies in that there is a terminal ⟨ETX⟩. Accessing Trend and Event data is therefore dealt with in a later section.

10.5.3 Interactive program for accessing Conversation mode data

An example QuickBASIC program which indicates how to send the command message interactively from the keyboard, collect the reply, and save it to a file, is given below.

The example program prompts the operator for a command-code from Table 10.7, and then sends it to the N-200E on pressing <enter>. The program then displays the reply, and saves it to a log file called datafile.log.

Program points

- The powerbase must be mains powered and switched on.
- The example program is for the **Conversation** mode (see Table 10.1), and assumes that the oximeter is attached to serial port 1 (COM1). The oximeter's DSR is held HIGH by being connected to the computer's RTS. Both DSR and CTS checking by the computer are disabled using the CS and DS options in the OPEN COM statement.
- If there is no reply after 2 seconds, then the program stops waiting and asks for another command.

The Nellcor N-200E pulse oximeter

- Typing 'END' will quit the program. <Q> can not be used here as Q is a command-code (see Table 10.7).

Example program

```
REM [nel-bk-c.bas]
REM Nellcor N-200E pulse oximeter
REM interactive program for testing CONVERSATION mode
REM monitor software 2.7, powerbase software 2.7
CLEAR
CLS
OPEN "COM1:1200,N,8,1,CS,DS,OP2000" FOR RANDOM ACCESS
                                            READ WRITE AS #1
OPEN "b:datafile.log" FOR RANDOM AS #2
LOCATE 5
PRINT "check N-200E is in conversation mode"
PRINT "press any key when ready"
PRINT
DO: LOOP WHILE INKEY$ = ""
DO
    PRINT
    INPUT "enter code (type END to quit)   "; code$
    IF UCASE$(code$) = "END" THEN
        CLOSE #1, #2
        END
    END IF
    REM send code to oximeter
    PRINT #1, UCASE$(code$)
    timenow = TIMER
    DO
        data$ = data$ + INPUT$(LOC(1), #1)
        REM look for the next LF character
        L% = INSTR(1, data$, CHR$(10))
        IF TIMER > timenow + 2 THEN
            PRINT "No Reply - code error"
            PRINT #2, "No Reply - code error"
            GOTO endloop
        END IF
    LOOP UNTIL L% > 0
```

```
        REM remove the <STX>, <CR>, <LF> characters from data$
        reply$ = MID$(data$, 2, L% - 3)
        PRINT "reply = "; reply$
        PRINT #2, "reply = "; reply$
        data$ = ""
        endloop:
LOOP
END
```

10.6 Accessing stored data

The transmission of stored data from the oximeter's memory (either Trend or Event data) can be initiated either manually, or by the computer.

Before outputting Trend or Event data using the Conversation mode, the Nellcor N-200E checks to see if its DSR is held HIGH (positive). If the oximeter's DSR is *not* held HIGH, then no data will be transmitted.

10.6.1 Memory

The N-200E has two memories, a **Trend** memory for Trend data, and an **Event** memory for Event data.

Trend memory. Up to 12 hours of data (pulse rate, saturation, and time-stamp) can be stored in the machine's Trend memory. Trend data is stored every 5 seconds; each data point being the average for the previous 5 seconds.

Event memory. Event data (pulse rate, pulse amplitude, saturation, and sampling time) is data which is collected for specified periods of time before and after a so-called 'event' occurs. The Event data is sampled and stored once a second.

There are two types of events: (a) **Alarm-limit** events (i.e. when a parameter value triggers an alarm setting), and (b) **User-defined** events (i.e. initiated by the user—see the Operator's manual for details).

For an Alarm-limit event, data is stored during the period from 30 seconds before the event until 30 seconds after the event. For a User-defined event, data is collected during the period from 30 seconds before the event until a defined period (maximum of 60 minutes) after the event.

10.6.2 Data packets

The stored data is output in a series of data packets, each made up of data-strings bracketed by the control characters ⟨STX⟩ (start of data) and ⟨ETX⟩ (end of data). Dispersed among the Trend and Event data packets are a number of statements indicating such things as the end of data output (E packet), reason for transmission stopping (V packet), and descriptions of the various events (Y packet).

Trend data (W packet). Each Trend data packet is prefixed by Wn...n which gives the number of the data packet. This is followed by the saturation (Snnn) and pulse rate (Rnnn). The format of the W packet, and an example, is as follows.

⟨STX⟩Wn...nSnnnRnnn⟨CR⟩⟨LF⟩⟨ETX⟩
⟨STX⟩W62S97R61⟨CR⟩⟨LF⟩⟨ETX⟩

Trend data is sampled once every second, and each Trend data packet gives the average of the last five data points for both saturation and pulse rate.

Event data (X packet). Each Event data packet is prefixed by Xn...n which gives the number of the data packet. This is followed by the saturation (Snnn), pulse rate (Rnnn), and pulse amplitude data (Pnn). The format of the X packet, and an example, is as follows.

⟨STX⟩Xn...nSnnnRnnnPnn⟨CR⟩⟨LF⟩⟨ETX⟩
⟨STX⟩X62S97R61P58⟨CR⟩⟨LF⟩⟨ETX⟩

Each Event data packet is sampled at one-second intervals, and there is no averaging.

End of data (E packet). The code E is used to indicate that all the data has been sent. The actual data-string sent by the N-200E is as follows.

⟨STX⟩E⟨CR⟩⟨LF⟩⟨ETX⟩

Transmission failure (V packet). The code Vnnn is sent only if transmission terminates before it is complete. The value following the letter V is a decimal code indicating the cause of the transmission failure. The V packet codes are shown in Table 10.8.

For example, a data-recall error would be transmitted by the N-200E as follows.

⟨STX⟩V64⟨CR⟩⟨LF⟩⟨ETX⟩

Table 10.8. *V packet codes.*

Value	Meaning
4	Time out error
8	Data error
16	Timed out error
32	Communications lost
64	Data-recall error
128	By operator request

Table 10.9. *Y event codes.*

Value	Meaning
0	User defined
1	Alarm defined
2	Patient signal lost
3	Not used
4	Time-stamp (after each hour for Trend data, and after each minute for Event data)
5	Power turned off
6	Patient signal acquired
7	Clock reset
8	Start new event

Event description (Y packet). The code Y is used to indicate the occurrence of an event, the nature of the event, and the time and date of the event. The format of the Y packet, and an example, is as follows.

⟨STX⟩YnDnnnnnnnn⟨CR⟩⟨LF⟩⟨ETX⟩
⟨STX⟩Y5D34082907⟨CR⟩⟨LF⟩⟨ETX⟩

Yn indicates the nature of the event (see Table 10.9). The time/date string is prefixed with D; the format, and an example, is as follows.

Dmmhhddmm (time/date).
Y5D34082907

For example, the typical Y packet shown above would therefore represent the event of power being turned off (code Y5), at the time 34m 08h 29d July.

Number and range of data (Z packet). The code Z is used to indicate how many data packages there are to be sent. The maximum and

The Nellcor N-200E pulse oximeter

minimum values of the saturation and pulse rate data are also given. The format of the Z packet, and an example, is as follows.

⟨STX⟩Zn...nSnnnsnnnRnnnrnnn⟨CR⟩⟨LF⟩⟨ETX⟩
⟨STX⟩Z163S100s89R114r55⟨CR⟩⟨LF⟩⟨ETX⟩

where

Zn...n	=	number of data packets to be sent
Snnn	=	maximum saturation
snnn	=	minimum saturation
Rnnn	=	maximum pulse rate
rnnn	=	minimum pulse rate

10.6.3 Manual operation

Both Trend and Event data are most easily accessed by selecting the Beat-to-beat mode, and then pressing the Trend or Event button on the back of the powerbase module. In this case the data can be captured and saved to a datafile using the example program given above for accessing Beat-to-beat data. Once the program has been started, then the relevant button can be pressed. The datafile can then be tidied up using a text editor if necessary.†

10.6.4 Computer operation (Conversation mode)

The recommended communication mode for accessing stored data is the Conversation mode, which allows the N-200E to respond to certain software control codes (sent by the computer) by transmitting either Trend or Event data.

To output stored data. The code which instructs the N-200E to transmit Trend data is the uppercase letter W. The equivalent code for Event data is the uppercase letter X. The letter code must be followed by the ⟨CR⟩ and ⟨LF⟩ control characters. The format and an example is as follows.

⟨command-code⟩⟨CR⟩⟨LF⟩
W⟨CR⟩⟨LF⟩

---

† When the stored data is accessed using Beat-to-beat mode in this way, it will necessarily be preceded and followed by some beat-to-beat data which may need to be removed. In practice this is not a problem since there are usually only a few additional lines of such data.

Since the ASCII codes for ⟨CR⟩ and ⟨LF⟩ are 13 and 10 respectively, an example of QuickBASIC statements which will initiate the output of Trend data is shown below. Note the use of the semicolon at the end of the PRINT# statement to stop an extra ⟨CR⟩⟨LF⟩ pair being sent by the PRINT# statement.

```
sendtrenddata$ = "W" + CHR$(13) + CHR$(1Ø)
PRINT #1, sendtrenddata$;
```

Alternatively, this command could be sent simply using the following statement.

```
PRINT #1, "W"
```

Similarly the following statements will initiate the output of Event data.

```
sendeventdata$ = "X" + CHR$(13) + CHR$(1Ø)
PRINT #1, sendeventdata$;
```

To stop the output of stored data. The letter code V is used to instruct the N-200E to stop the output of either Trend or Event data. Thus the program could send the code V⟨CR⟩⟨LF⟩ in response to pressing <Q> (to Quit). Example QuickBASIC statements which would do this are as follows.

```
stopdata$ = "V" + CHR$(13) + CHR$(1Ø)
PRINT #1, stopdata$;
```

or alternatively

```
stopdata$ = "V"
PRINT #1, stopdata$
```

since the PRINT# statement automatically adds a ⟨CR⟩⟨LF⟩ pair.†

10.6.5 Trend data output

Once the N-200E receives the code W (to output trend data), it responds by returning the code W, then a Z packet, and then a series of Trend data packets (W packets), interspersed with a number of event description packets (Y packets). A time-stamp (Y4 packet) is given at 1-hr intervals.

An extract from a typical Trend data output is shown in Figure 10.3 together with comments.

† See Chapter 5 for further details regarding the PRINT# statement.

The Nellcor N-200E pulse oximeter

```
W                        start of Trend data
Z2613S100s0R126r0        2613 data packets to follow
                         max Sat=100; min Sat=0
                         max PR = 126; min PR = 0
Y1D381701111             alarm event (Y1)
                         time = 38m 17h 01d Nov
Y4D381701111             time marker (Y4) for beginning of
                         the hour: time = 38m 17h 01d Nov
W1S95R55                 data No 1: Sat = 95; PR = 55
W2S96R55                 data No 2: Sat = 96; PR = 55
W3S96R56                 data No 3: Sat = 96; PR = 56
...
...
W720S93R77               data No 720: Sat = 93; PR = 77
Y4D381801111             time marker (Y4)
                         time = 38m 18h 01d Nov
W721S94R78               data No 721: Sat = 94; PR = 78
...
...
W2613S99R84              data No 2613: Sat = 99; PR = 84
E                        end of Trend data
```

Fig. 10.3. An extract of a typical Trend data output, together with comments.

10.6.6 Event data output

Once the N-200E receives the code X (to output Event data), it responds by returning the code X, then a Z packet, and then a series of Trend data packets (X packets), interspersed with a number of event description packets (Y packets). The event for which the Event data have been saved is defined by a Y packet after the first 30 Event data packets. A time-stamp (Y4 packet) is given at 1-minute intervals.

An extract from a typical Event data output is shown in Figure 10.4, with comments.

10.6.7 Program for accessing Trend/Event data

An example QuickBASIC program which will access either Trend or Event data using the Conversation mode, and save it to a file (e.g. trend.dat) is given below. Pressing <S> will stop the data output; pressing <Q> will quit the program.

The operator is prompted to select either <E> (for Event data) or <T> (for Trend data).

X	start of Event data output.
Z359S99s0R90r0	359 data packets to follow
	max Sat = 99; min Sat = 0
	max PR = 90; min PR = 0
	(=1st packet for 1st Event)
X1S95R55P49	data No 1: Sat = 95; PR = 55
X2S96R55P51	data No 2: Sat = 96; PR = 55
X3S96R56P52	data No 3: Sat = 96; PR = 56
...	
...	
X30S96R56P51	data No 30: Sat = 96; PR = 56
Y1D45151606	alarm event (Y1)
	time = 45m 15h 16d June
Y4D45151606	time marker (Y4)
	time = 45m 15h 16d June
X31S94R57P51	data No 31: Sat = 94; PR = 57
X32S93R58P51	data No 32: Sat = 93; PR = 58
X33S93R55P52	data No 33: Sat = 93; PR = 55
...	
...	
X89S99R50P52	data No 89: Sat = 99; PR = 50
Y4D46151606	time marker (Y4)
	time = 46m 15h 16d June
X90S98R52P51	data No 90: Sat = 98; PR = 52
...	
...	
X359S95R50P62	data No 359: Sat = 95; PR = 50
X360S95R50P62	data No 360: Sat = 95; PR = 50
	(=last packet for 1st Event)
Z60S100s95R71r49	60 data packets to follow
	max Sat = 100; min Sat = 95
	max PR = 71; min PR = 49
	(=1st packet for 2nd Event)
X1S97R67P60	data No 1: Sat = 97; PR = 67
X2S97R67P61	data No 2: Sat = 97; PR = 67
X3S97R66P63	data No 3: Sat = 97; PR = 66
...	
...	
E	end of Trend data

Fig. 10.4. An extract from a typical Event data output, together with comments. Note that although the initial Z packet indicates that 359 data packets will be transmitted, 360 are actually sent.

Program points

- The example program is for the **Conversation** mode (Table 10.1), and assumes that the oximeter is attached to serial port 1 (COM1). The oximeter's DSR is held HIGH by being connected to the computer's

The Nellcor N-200E pulse oximeter 151

RTS as shown in Figure 10.1. Both CTS and DSR checking by the computer are disabled using the CS and DS options in the OPEN COM statement.
- Note that after running the program, a slight delay of about 30 seconds is necessary before the data can be accessed from the oximeter again. This is to allow the oximeter to reorganise its data. Alternatively, the oximeter can be simply switched off and then powered on again, as this will automatically reset the oximeter's software.
- The program gives the download time for the Trend/Event data.
- The program terminates when the final E code is detected.

10.6.8 Example program

```
REM [nel-bk-t.bas]
REM Nellcor N-200E pulse oximeter
REM program for accessing Trend/Event data
REM using CONVERSATION mode
REM monitor software 2.7, powerbase software 2.7
CLEAR
OPEN "COM1:1200,N,8,1,CS,DS,OP2000" FOR RANDOM ACCESS
                                   READ WRITE AS #1
CLS
LOCATE 5
PRINT "check N-200E is in conversation mode"
PRINT "press any key when ready"
DO: LOOP WHILE INKEY$ = ""
startloop:
CLS
LOCATE 5
PRINT "press <E> for EVENT data (saved to event.dat)"
LOCATE 6
PRINT "press <T> for TREND data (saved to trend.dat)"
LOCATE 8
PRINT "press <Q> to quit"
LOCATE 9
PRINT "press <S> to stop data output"
SLEEP
key$ = INKEY$
REM empty the input buffer
```

```
DO: buff$ = INPUT$(LOC(1), #1): LOOP UNTIL EOF(1)
timenow = TIMER
SELECT CASE UCASE$(key$)
    CASE "E"
        OPEN "c:event.dat" FOR OUTPUT AS #2
        REM get EVENT data
        PRINT #1, "X"
    CASE "T"
        OPEN "c:trend.dat" FOR OUTPUT AS #2
        REM get TREND data
        PRINT #1, "W"
    CASE "Q"
        CLOSE #1, #2
        END
    CASE ELSE
        GOTO startloop
END SELECT
DO
    DO
        key$ = INKEY$
        SELECT CASE UCASE$(key$)
            CASE "Q"
                stopdata$ = "V"
                PRINT #1, stopdata$
                CLOSE #1, #2
                END
            CASE "S"
                stopdata$ = "V"
                PRINT #1, stopdata$
                CLOSE #2
                data$ = ""
                PRINT
                PRINT "data output terminated"
                GOTO endloop2
        END SELECT
        data$ = data$ + INPUT$(LOC(1), #1)
        REM look for <ETX> character
        L% = INSTR(1, data$, CHR$(3))
    LOOP UNTIL L% > 0
    IF L% < 4 THEN GOTO endloop
```

```
          storeddata$ = MID$(data$, 2, L% - 4)
          PRINT storeddata$
          PRINT #2, storeddata$
          IF storeddata$ = "E" THEN EXIT DO
          endloop:
          data$ = RIGHT$(data$, LEN(data$) - L%)
LOOP
PRINT
PRINT "END OF STORED DATA"
PRINT "time taken = "; TIMER - timenow ; " secs"
endloop2:
PRINT
PRINT "press <C> (continue) or <Q> (quit)"
SLEEP
key$ = INKEY$
IF UCASE$(key$) = "C" THEN GOTO startloop
CLOSE #1, #2
END
```

11
The Novametrix 515A pulse oximeter

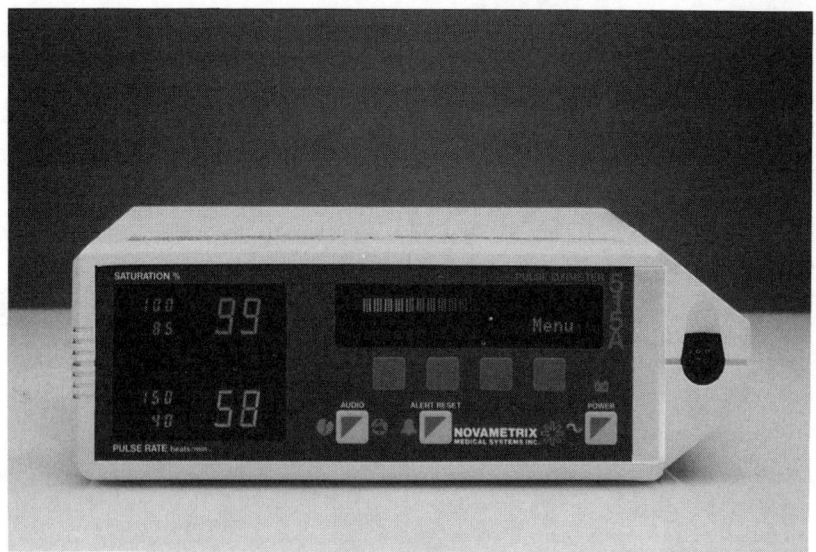

11.1 Introduction

The Novametrix 515A pulse oximeter† displays both saturation and heart rate, and can be powered by either mains AC or internal batteries.

Real-time heart rate and saturation data is output at one second-intervals via the serial port in a format suitable for PCs. A variable duration Trend Memory allows data to be saved up to a maximum of 24 hours. However, stored Trend data is not accessible by PCs since it is output in a graphic format which is only compatible with certain serial printers.‡

Analog data for heart rate, saturation and plethysmogram is also

---

† Novametrix Medical Systems Inc., One Barnes Industrial Park Road,
P.O. Box 690, Wallingford, Connecticut 06492, USA. Tel: +1-203-265-7701.
Fax: +1-203-284-0753.

‡ At the time of writing the compatible printers are: Novametrix 315; Seiko DPU-411; Hewlett-Packard ThinkJet.

available via the serial port, but can only be accessed using a special signal processing unit (Analog Output Module) available from Novametrix.

The electrical safety classification of the pulse oximeter probe is Type BF.†

11.1.1 Other Novametrix oximeters

While this Chapter is primarily directed towards the 515A pulse oximeter, it is worth noting that the 520A and the earlier 500 and 505 Models are interfaced in essentially the same way. Where the differences are significant, these will be described briefly.

For example, although all Novametrix 500 oximeters have a 25-pin D-type serial connector on the rear-panel, the 2335 CPU Board which contains the serial interface circuitry was not included as standard. Those Model 500 oximeters which do have a functioning serial interface can be identified by the presence of either a J, R, S, M or W serial number suffix.‡

11.1.2 Software version

The EPROM Revision level and data is displayed in the right-hand display window when the oximeter is switched on while the 'audio' button is also pressed (see below). Note that the message remains displayed only while both buttons remain pressed.

```
Revision 2.03
MAR/27/92
```

Revision 2.0 introduced a number of new and improved features which are described in **Model 515A User's Manual Addendum-B**. At the time of writing the current Revision level is 2.03.

The EPROM checksum is given in the right-hand display window when the oximeter is switched on while the leftmost soft key is also pressed.

```
Checksum = 436F Hex
```

† See Chapter 7 for further details.
‡ See Novametrix 500 Service Manual (Dec. 1987), Section 8.8.

Table 11.1. *Novametrix serial port; Models 515A, 520A.*

Pin No.	Name	Comments
2	RxD	Receives data
3	TxD	Transmits data
6	CTS	Output enable
7	GND	Signal ground
20	DTR	Always set HIGH (positive)
21	GND	Signal ground
22	GND	Signal ground
24	+5 volts	
25	+5 volts	

11.1.3 Communication modes

The 515A oximeter supports a number of communication modes which allow interfacing to a PC (**Full Format** mode) and certain serial printers, as well as to Saracap, Dräger, and Telesat equipment.

Only the Full Format mode (for interfacing to a PC) is described in this Chapter.

11.2 Serial port

A 25-pin female D-type serial port is located on the rear-panel of the oximeter. The serial port pin-outs for both the 515A and the 520A oximeters are shown in Table 11.1.

The serial ports for the 500 and 505 Models have an additional output on pin-4 (always set HIGH) which is labelled RTS. In addition, both these Models have pin-6 labelled as DSR, although functionally this is the same as pin-6 for the 515A.

11.2.1 Protocol options

The serial protocol options are shown in Table 11.2. The protocol is set using the **Options** menu to access the Full Format mode, and then stepping through the protocol options. Once the protocol options have been set, they are retained in memory until changed again.

Setting the protocol options. The Options menu is accessed by switching the oximeter on while pressing the right-hand soft key, which results in the following message.

The Novametrix 515A pulse oximeter 157

OPTIONS MENU 1
Run   Ser.   Clock   Next

Select the **Serial** option which accesses a Mode menu; now cycle through the menu until 'Full Format mode' appears in the window as follows.

Full Format Mode
Next   Prev.   Enter

When the Full Format mode is entered (select 'enter') the oximeter then cycles through the protocol options (Baud, Parity, Data bits, Stop bits).

Table 11.2. *Novametrix protocol; Models 500, 505, 515A and 520A. The default options are underlined.*

Bit rate	300, <u>1200</u>, 2400, 4800, 9600
Data bits	7, <u>8</u>
Parity	Odd, Even, <u>None</u>
Stop bits	<u>1</u>, 2

11.2.2 Cable connections

Figure 11.1 indicates a suitable wiring configuration for interfacing the 515A and 520A Models to a PC. The same configuration will also serve the 500 and 505 Models, although pin-6 in these Models is labelled DSR.

Note that the Novametrix oximeters have TxD on pin-3 and RxD on pin-2, which are *reversed* compared to the RS-232 Standard for 25-pin D-type connectors.

- **CTS** This is an 'output enable' pin, and must be maintained HIGH (positive) to enable data output from the oximeter. This is most conveniently done by wiring it to one of the PC's output control lines (DTR and RTS)† since both of these are set HIGH when QuickBASIC executes the OPEN COM statement.‡ In Figure 11.1 CTS is wired to the PC's DTR.

  Alternatively, CTS could be held HIGH by wiring it to the oximeter's pin-20 (DTR) since this pin is always set HIGH. In this case only two wires would be needed to interface the oximeter to a PC.

† See Chapter 1 for details of the output control lines.
‡ See Chapter 5 for details of opening the serial port.

158   *Chapter 11*

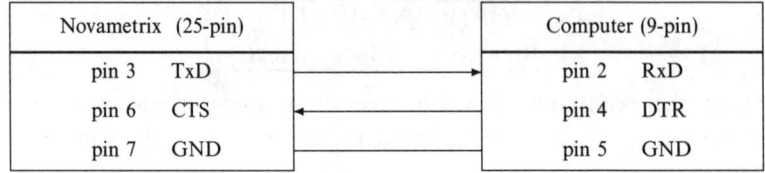

Fig. 11.1. Novametrix wiring configuration; Models 515A, 520A.

11.3 Accessing real-time data

Real-time oximetry data is output once per second, and consists of saturation, heart rate, and a status message when applicable. The format of data generated by the 515A oximeter, including spaces ␣ and control characters, is as follows.

:␣SpO2␣=␣nnn␣␣Rate␣=␣nnn␣␣Status␣:␣⟨status message⟩⟨CR⟩⟨LF⟩

Note that neither the date nor time of data sampling is included in the data-string. If these are required they can be added during data collection by the computer using the QuickBASIC DATE$ and TIME$ functions.

11.3.1 *Program for accessing real-time data*

An example QuickBASIC program which will access the data and save it to a file (novadata.dat) is given below. Pressing <Q> will quit the program.

Program points

- Check that the oximeter and program protocols are the same.
- The example program uses COM1. If a different COM port is used then an appropriate change will have to be made to the OPEN COM statement.
- Since no handshaking is used both CTS and DSR checking by the computer are disabled using the CS and DS options in the OPEN COM statement.
- In this example program, both date (DATE$) and time (TIME$) have been added by the computer.

Example program

```
REM [nova515A.bas]
REM Novametrix 515A pulse oximeter
REM program for real-time data
PRINT "opening serial port"
OPEN "COM1:1200,N,8,1,RS,DS,CD" FOR INPUT AS #1
OPEN "c:novadata.dat" FOR OUTPUT AS #2
CLS
PRINT "port open OK -- waiting for data"
PRINT "press <Q> to quit"
PRINT "Date = "; DATE$
PRINT #2, "Date = "; DATE$
DO
    DO
        key$ = INKEY$
        IF UCASE$(key$) = "Q" THEN
            CLOSE
            END
        END IF
        REM: collect all characters up to and including LF
        a$ = a$ + INPUT$(LOC(1), #1)
        L% = INSTR(1, a$, CHR$(10))
    LOOP UNTIL L% > 0
    data$ = MID$(a$, 1, L% - 2)
    PRINT TIME$; data$
    PRINT #2, TIME$; data$
    a$ = RIGHT$(a$, LEN(a$) - L%)
LOOP
END
```

An example of the data output when using the above program for accessing real-time data is shown below. The data is output at 1-second intervals.

```
Date = 09-22-1992
16:41:23: SpO2 = 097   Rate = 072   Status :
16:41:24: SpO2 = 000   Rate = 000   Status : PROBE OFF PATIENT
```

12
The Minolta Pulsox-7 pulse oximeter

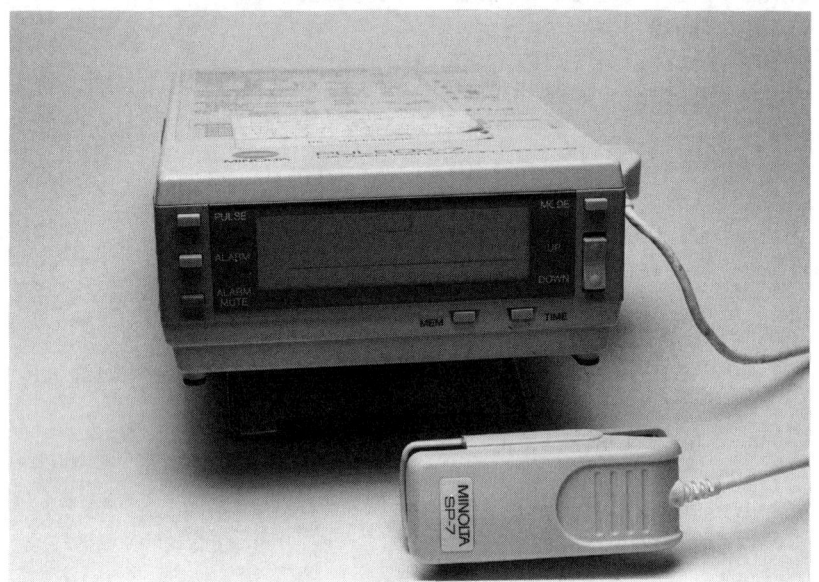

12.1 Introduction

The Minolta Pulsox-7† is a portable pulse oximeter, which displays heart rate and oxygen saturation, as well as the alarm limit settings. Both real-time (heart rate and saturation) and Trend data (heart rate, saturation, and sampling time) can be accessed by computer via the serial interface and stored on disk. A total of 13.5 hrs of Trend data can be stored by the oximeter.

In addition to the serial interface, the Pulsox-7 has analog outputs for both heart rate and oxygen saturation. An optional plug-in printer module is available (Pulsox DP-7).

† Minolta Camera Co. Ltd., Radiometric Instrument Operations, 2–30 Toyozu-Cho, 564 Suita-Chi, Osaka, Japan. Tel: +81-6-3863617, Fax: +81-6-3863618.

Table 12.1. *Pulsox-7 serial port.*

Pin No.	Name	Comments
1		Protective ground (shield)
2	TxD	Transmits data
3	RxD	Receives data
4	RTS	Normally held LOW (negative). Goes HIGH with each data output
5	CTS	Must be held HIGH (positive) by the PC to enable data output
6–8		Reserved for use with Pulsox-7 printer module
9–12	GND	Signal ground
13–15		Reserved for use with Pulsox-7 printer module

The electrical safety classification of the pulse oximeter probe is Type BF.†

12.2 Serial port

A 15-pin female D-type serial port is located on the rear panel of the oximeter. Details of the pin-outs are shown in Table 12.1. Note that pins 6–8 and 13–15 are reserved for use with the Pulsox DP-7 printer, and cannot be used for computer interfacing.

Placing a line checker on the oximeter's serial port following power-on shows that both RxD and RTS are initially held LOW (negative) by the oximeter. If CTS is now made HIGH then RTS will start to go HIGH once per second, coinciding with the output of data from TxD.

12.2.1 Protocol options

The Pulsox-7 oximeter has a fixed protocol as shown in Table 12.2.

12.2.2 Cable connections

Figure 12.1 shows a suitable wiring configuration for connecting the Pulsox-7 to a PC running QuickBASIC. Note that this configuration requires the PC's DSR checking to be disabled by using the DS option in the OPEN COM statement.

† See Chapter 7 for further details.

Table 12.2. *Pulsox-7 protocol.*

Bit rate	4800
Start bit	1
Data bits	7
Parity	Even
Stop bits	1

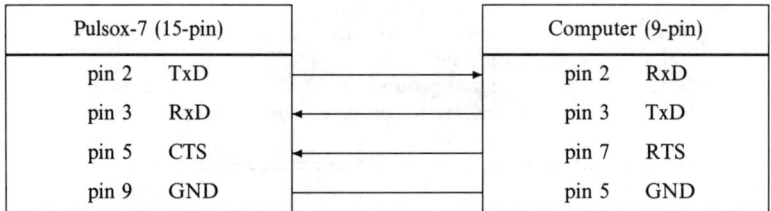

Fig. 12.1. Pulsox-7 wiring diagram.

- **CTS** The Pulsox-7 requires its CTS to be held HIGH (positive) to enable data output. This is most conveniently arranged by wiring the oximeter's CTS to one of the PC's two output control lines (RTS or DTR), since both of these can be programmed to either remain HIGH in order to enable real-time data output, or to toggle LOW/HIGH as required by the Pulsox-7 in order to access Trend data.

- **RTS** Although the oximeter's RTS line goes HIGH (positive) when data is being output, this information is not required by the computer when simply accessing data. The oximeter's RTS line does not, therefore, need to be connected to the computer.

12.3 Real-time data

Following power-on, real-time data is automatically output via the serial port at 1-second intervals, providing the oximeter's CTS is made HIGH (positive). The format of real-time data, together with some examples, is shown below. The alarm codes used by the Pulsox-7 are shown in Table 12.3. Note that while the saturation and heart rate data occupy

Table 12.3. *Pulsox-7 alarm codes.*

Code	Meaning
INOP	Probe not in operation (e.g. probe off finger)
INOPC	Probe not connected to oximeter
INOPL	Problem with light: too much or too little
INOPP	Weak pulse signal
INOPA	Motion artifact
LS	Low saturation alarm
HS	High saturation alarm
LP	Low pulse rate alarm
HP	High pulse rate alarm

fixed fields within the data-string, the number of alarm codes transmitted is variable. Spaces are indicated by the symbol ␣.

month/day␣hr:min␣SAO2:nnn␣PR:nnn␣⟨alarm code⟩⟨CR⟩

12.3.1 Program for accessing real-time data

An example QuickBASIC program which will access real-time data from the Pulsox-7 and save it to a file (datafile.dat) is given below.

Program points

- The program assumes that the oximeter is attached to serial port 1 (COM1), and that the oximeter's CTS is maintained HIGH as shown in Figure 12.1. Both CTS and DSR checking are disabled using the CS and DS options in the OPEN COM statement.
- As each real-time data-string output by the Pulsox-7 is terminated by ⟨CR⟩, the simpler INPUT# command can be used to input the data-string instead of INPUT$ (see Chapter 5).
- Since the Pulsox-7 only gives the time to the nearest minute, time to the nearest second has to be added by the program if required. In this example program both the date (DATE$) and time (TIME$) are added to the end of each data-string by the computer. Note that before adding the time and date the terminal ⟨CR⟩ is removed using the following statement.

data$ = MID$(a$, 1, L% - 1)

- Pressing <Q> will quit the program.

Example program

```
REM [pul7bk-r.bas]
REM program to access real-time data from Pulsox-7
CLEAR
CLS
OPEN "COM1:4800,E,7,1,CS,DS,OP2000" FOR INPUT AS #1
OPEN "c:datafile.dat" FOR OUTPUT AS #2
PRINT "press <Q> to quit"
DO
    DO
        a$ = a$ + INPUT$(LOC(1), #1)
        L% = INSTR(1, a$, CHR$(13))
        key$ = INKEY$
        IF UCASE$(key$) = "Q" THEN
            CLOSE #1, #2
            END
        END IF
    LOOP UNTIL L% > 0
    data$ = MID$(a$, 1, L% - 1)
    PRINT data$; SPACE$(4); DATE$; SPACE$(2); TIME$
    PRINT #2, data$; SPACE$(4); DATE$; SPACE$(2); TIME$
    a$ = RIGHT$(a$, LEN(a$) - L%)
LOOP
END
```

A typical example of data saved using the above program is shown below. The times show that real-time data is output at 1-sec intervals.

 5/15 16:27 SAO2: 98 PR: 73 HP   5-15-1991 16:27: 6
 5/15 16:27 SAO2: 99 PR: 73 HP   5-15-1991 16:27: 7
 5/15 16:27 SAO2: 98 PR: 70 HP   5-15-1991 16:27: 8

12.4 Trend data

Trend data is stored in blocks known as **files**, where each file contains all the data collected during a single period from power-on to power-off. A maximum of 225 files can be stored by the Pulsox-7. Trend data is transmitted in 3-byte groups known as **data-groups**.

12.4.1 Coding system for Trend data

Each parameter value transmitted as Trend data (e.g. saturation, heart rate) is coded as a single 7-bit byte (see Table 12.2). For example, a heart rate of 64 beats per minute is transmitted as a byte having the value 64. The computer's screen and printer would then process the byte as if it were an ASCII character; the character @ in this case, since 64 is the ASCII value of this character (see Appendix 1 for details of the ASCII code).

Bytes having an ASCII value *less* than 32 will be printed using either the IBM graphics characters (e.g. ♣, ☺) or the DOS Ctrl codes (e.g. ^E, ^A), depending on the particular system being used by the computer.

Viewing the original ASCII data can be somewhat confusing, as the computer will interpret some bytes (e.g. those with the same value as some of the control codes) as an instruction instead of a character to be printed. For example, if the byte is coding for December (i.e. the 12th month), it will be coded as ASCII 12. When the computer tries to print this character, it interprets it as a command to start a new page, and does exactly that since 12 is the ASCII code for starting a new page (form feed).

In practice, therefore, if a copy of the original output data is required (say, for checking the program), it is probably best to print the data initially in hexadecimal.†

Parameter values greater than 127. Since the Pulsox-7 stores each Trend data value as a single 7-bit byte an interesting problem arises with heart rates greater than 127.

The oximeter actually stores the lowest 7 bits of the parameter. This has the effect that a *true* heart rate of 200 would be stored and subsequently transmitted as a heart rate of only 73, since 73 represents the lowest 7 bits of the number 200.

The interpretation of apparently normal heart rates in Pulsox-7 Trend data is therefore not without hazard. One easy solution is to always save Trend data with the 'high rate' alarm set to 127, as then the presence of a 'high rate' alarm indicates that the true heart rate is the displayed heart rate *plus* 127.

Data-groups. Trend data is output in 3-byte **data-groups** which represent either **Measurement** data (coding for saturation, heart rate, alarm status), or **Special** data (coding for file number, year, date, time, and number of continuous inoperative periods). The format of both the Measurement and Special data-groups are described in detail below.

† See Appendix 8 for details of hexadecimal notation.

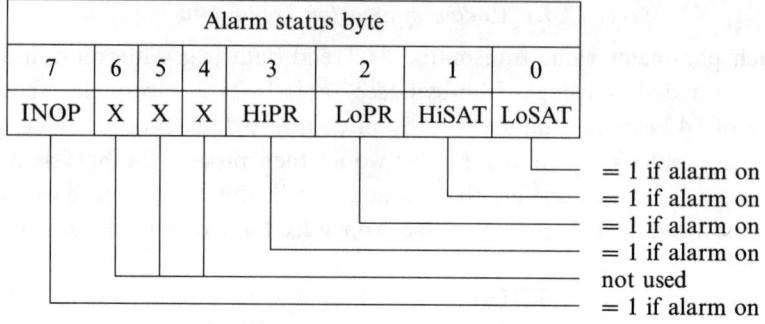

Fig. 12.2. Alarm status.

12.4.2 Measurement data-groups

The first, second and third bytes of Measurement data-groups represent saturation, heart rate and alarm status respectively, as stored every 5 seconds. The format of Measurement data-groups is as follows.

⟨saturation⟩⟨heart rate⟩⟨alarm status⟩

The screen representation of values < 32 will depend on the particular computer's software; thus the value 5 will be represented as either ♣ or ^E (see Appendix 1). A typical 3-byte data-group may therefore appear as either \ + ♣ or \ + ^E (see Table 12.4).

The ⟨alarm status⟩ byte is bit-encoded for the five alarm status codes as shown in Figure 12.2. For example, if the byte was printed as ♦, this would indicate that the 'low heart rate' alarm was active since this character is equivalent to ASCII 4, which has the binary equivalent of 00000100b.

The first two bytes of a Measurement data-group therefore need to be converted into decimal notation (in order to extract the saturation and heart rate data), while the third byte needs to be converted into binary notation (in order to determine the alarm status).†

An analysis of a typical Measurement data-group (\ + ♣) is shown in Table 12.4, which shows how this particular data-group represents saturation 92%; heart rate 43 bpm; and activated Low PR and Low Sat alarms.

† See Appendix 8 for details of binary notation.

Table 12.4. *The components of the Measurement data-string \ + ♣ in terms of their IBM, DOS, hex, decimal, and binary representations.*

	Sat.	HR	Alarm
IBM	\	+	♣
DOS	\	+	^E
Hex	5C	2B	5
Decimal	92	43	5
Binary (3rd byte)			00000101

Table 12.5. *Details of Special data codings.*

Byte 1	Byte 2	Byte 3	Example	
7F (file/year)	file no.	year	7F 08 5B 08 91	hex decimal
7E (date)	month	day	7E 0C 0F 12 15	hex decimal
7D (time)	hour	minute	7D 0D 15 13 21	hex decimal
7C (end of data)	00	00	7C 00 00 00 00	hex decimal
7B (INOP)	high byte	low byte	7B 01 FF 511	hex decimal

12.4.3 Special data-groups

In addition to Measurement data, the Pulsox-7 also sends a number of 3-byte data-groups consisting of so-called Special data which are used to indicate time, date, end of data, and number of continuous periods of inactivity. The various Special data-groups are distinguished according to the nature of the first byte of the data-group which, in hexadecimal, is either 7B, 7C, 7D, 7E, or 7F (see Appendix 8 for details of hexadecimal notation).

Depending on the hexadecimal coding of the first byte, the remaining two bytes of a Special data-group will variously code for **file**, **year**, **date**, **time** etc. as shown in Table 12.5.

End of data code (7Ch). The final data-group to be sent, which marks the end of the Trend data, is 7Ch 00h 00h.

Number of continuous inoperative periods (7Bh). The two bytes following the hex code 7B are the high and low bytes of a 16-bit number which represents the number of continuous INOP data-groups (each of 5 seconds). The hex data-group 7B 01 FF (see Table 12.5) therefore indicates that there were 511 (= 01FFh) consecutive 5-second periods when the oximeter was inoperative, i.e. a total of 2555 seconds (= 511 x 5).

Thus, the following sequence of 3-byte hexadecimal data-groups which are shown in Table 12.5 would represent file No. 8; time 13h:21m on 15th Dec, 1991.

7F 08 5B
7E 0C 0F
7D 0D 15

12.4.4 Procedure for accessing Trend data

Accessing the stored Trend data from the Pulsox-7 oximeter involves a complicated combination of both software handshaking (sending codes to the oximeter to start and terminate Trend output) and hardware handshaking (toggling the Pulsox-7's CTS line HIGH and LOW to control the flow of Trend data). The steps involved are summarised below.

(1) Open the serial communication port.
(2) Set the computer's RTS (linked to the oximeter's CTS) HIGH (positive) to enable data output from the oximeter.
(3) Send the command-code D to the oximeter. This enables the Pulsox-7 to output stored Trend data. In practice, it does not matter whether the command-code is followed by an additional ⟨CR⟩ or not. When the oximeter receives the command, it responds by replying with the uppercase letter B. Note that the oximeter will not output the letter B *unless* its CTS is held HIGH (positive). No further data is output at this stage.
(4) Trend data is now available, and its output is controlled by toggling the oximeter's CTS line LOW and then HIGH, whereupon the oximeter will transmit one data-group (three bytes) and then stop. Each time the oximeter's CTS line is switched from LOW to HIGH, read the contents of the PC's input buffer into a string (e.g.

data$) until the string is three bytes long (i.e. three characters long).
(5) Convert the three ASCII characters (three bytes) into their hexadecimal equivalent. Add leading zeros as necessary.
(6) If the hexadecimal value of the first byte is 7C (see Table 12.5), print 'end of data' and end the program. Otherwise, toggle the PC's RTS line LOW and then HIGH again, and repeat the process.

12.4.5 Typical Trend data

As an example, a typical Trend data output (converted to hexadecimal) is shown in Figure 12.3, together with a 'translation' of each data-group. Note that each new file of data begins with a block of three Special data-groups, the first bytes of which are 7Fh, 7Eh, and 7Dh. These are then followed by Measurement data-groups sampled at 5-second intervals. Each minute is marked by a 'time-stamp' data-group which begins with 7Dh. Finally, the 'end of data' marker 7Ch 00h 00h is transmitted.

There appears to be a software 'bug' in the Pulsox-7, in that if the Trend period includes midnight then the date in the 7Eh... data-group is *not* advanced at midnight. The date is not advanced correctly until the next power-on. The time given in the 7Dh... data-group, however, remains correct throughout.

12.4.6 Example program for accessing Trend data

The following example QuickBASIC program illustrates a method of accessing Trend data from the Pulsox-7, and saving it to a file (e.g. pulsox-7.dat).

The program includes two subroutines which allow the user to print the data in different ways. The subroutine PRINTHEXDATA only prints out the data in hexadecimal form, as in Figure 12.3. The subroutine PRINTALLDATA also prints out the data in hexadecimal, but also decodes the data into fixed fields of date, time, saturation, heart rate, alarm status (see Figure 12.4).

The particular data format is controlled by selected the appropriate CALL statement in the main module. Selecting the subroutine PRINTALLDATA as follows will make the program decode the data as shown in Figure 12.4.

```
REM CALL printhexdata
CALL printalldata(data$)
```

```
...
7F 08 5B     file No. 8; year 1991
7E 0C 0F     month 12 (Dec); day 15
7D 0D 15     1300 hrs; 21 mins
7F 09 5B     file No. 9; year 1991
7E 0C 0F     month 12 (Dec); day 15
7D 14 3A     2000 hrs; 58 mins
7B 00 43     67 INOP periods (i.e. 67 × 5 = 335 mins)
7D 15 04     2100 hrs; 04 mins
62 2A 04     Sat = 98%; HR = 42; low PR alarm
61 48 00     Sat = 97%; HR = 72; no alarms
61 46 00     Sat = 97%; HR = 70; no alarms
...
5A 73 09     Sat = 90%; HR = 115; alarms: Low Sat/ High PR
7D 15 05     2100 hrs; 05 mins
5B 75 09     Sat = 91%; HR = 117; alarms: Low Sat/ High PR
...
7C 00 00     end of data
```

Fig. 12.3. Pulsox-7 Trend data printed out in hexadecimal form, together with a translation.

Program points

- The example program uses COM1. If a different COM port is used, then appropriate changes will have to be made to the OPEN COM statement, and to the address used by the Modem Control Register (mcr%) in the main module (see Section 4.4.3).
- The program requires the oximeter's handshaking line (CTS) to be wired to the PC's RTS as described earlier. Details of how to program the PC's RTS to toggle LOW and then HIGH are given in Section 5.16.
- The function BIT is used to determine whether a given bit of the alarm status byte is set to 1 or not, and hence establish which alarms are set (see Figure 12.2). Note that the program uses the following four codes for high and low pulse and saturation alarms: HPA, LPA, HSA, LSA.
- The complete Trend data occupies approximately 10 Kbytes, and takes approximately 6 minutes to download. Pressing <Q> at any time will abort the download, and reset the oximeter.
- The number of INOP periods (inopvalue%) is held as a 16-bit value, which is determined by combining the high and low bytes given in a 7B data-group (see Table 12.5) using the following statement in the subroutine PRINTALLDATA.

```
inopvalue% = (ASC(highbyte$)) * 256 + ASC(lowbyte$)
```

- The program also determines both the total number of data-groups and the time taken to download all the data, and prints these values at the end.

Example program

```
REM [pul7bk-t.bas]
REM program to access Trend data from the Pulsox-7
REM program will print either just Hex data or all data
DECLARE SUB printhexdata ()
DECLARE SUB printalldata (trend$)
DECLARE SUB shutdown ()
DECLARE FUNCTION bit% (b!, n!)
COMMON SHARED pulsox7time$, timezero
COMMON SHARED year$, month$, day$, hour$, min$, n
COMMON SHARED data$, hexbyte1$, hexbyte2$, hexbyte3$
CLEAR
OPEN "COM1:4800,E,7,1,CS,DS,OP2000" FOR RANDOM ACCESS READ
                                                   WRITE AS #1
OPEN "c:pulsox-7.dat" FOR OUTPUT AS #2
PRINT #2, "TREND DATA FROM PULSOX-7:", DATE$, TIME$
CLS
LOCATE 5, 5
PRINT "Program to access Trend data from Pulsox-7"
LOCATE 7, 5:
PRINT "press any key to continue (<Q> to quit)"
SLEEP: key$ = INKEY$
IF UCASE$(key$) = "Q" THEN
    CLOSE #1, #2
    END
END IF
REM empty input buffer
DO WHILE NOT EOF(1): buff$ = INPUT$(LOC(1), #1): LOOP
REM send code to enable trend data output
PRINT #1, "D"
PRINT "sending code to get Trend data"
timezero = TIMER
DO
    a$ = a$ + INPUT$(LOC(1), #1)
```

```
        IF TIMER > timezero + 4 THEN
            PRINT "no reply - exit program"
            CLOSE #1, #2
            END
        END IF
LOOP UNTIL a$ = "B"
PRINT a$: PRINT #2, a$
REM set the correct mcr register address for the COM port
REM mcr% = &H3FC for COM1, mcr% = &H02FC for COM2
mcr% = &H3FC: REM com1
REM now toggle RTS low and then high to get first data-group
OUT mcr%, (INP(mcr%) AND (NOT 2 ^ 1)): REM sets RTS low
OUT mcr%, (INP(mcr%) OR 2 ^ 1): REM sets RTS high
REM read data arriving at the input buffer
readinputbuffer:
data$ = ""
DO
    data$ = data$ + INPUT$(LOC(1), #1)
    key$ = INKEY$
    IF UCASE$(key$) = "Q" THEN CALL shutdown
    REM continue until data$ is 3 characters long
LOOP UNTIL LEN(data$) = 3
REM add a leading zero if necessary to make hex value 2 chars
hexbyte1$ = RIGHT$("0" + HEX$(ASC(LEFT$(data$, 1))), 2)
hexbyte2$ = RIGHT$("0" + HEX$(ASC(MID$(data$, 2, 1))), 2)
hexbyte3$ = RIGHT$("0" + HEX$(ASC(RIGHT$(data$, 1))), 2)
REM CALL printhexdata
    CALL printalldata(data$)
REM toggle RTS low and then high to get next data-group
OUT mcr%, (INP(mcr%) AND (NOT 2 ^ 1)): REM makes RTS low
OUT mcr%, (INP(mcr%) OR 2 ^ 1): REM makes RTS high
n = n + 1
GOTO readinputbuffer
END



FUNCTION bit% (b, n)
    REM  b = bit no, n = integer
    x = 2 ^ (b)
    IF n AND x THEN bit% = 1
```

```
        IF x AND (NOT n) THEN bit% = 0
END FUNCTION


SUB printalldata (trend$)
    byte1 = ASC(LEFT$(trend$, 1))
    byte2 = ASC(MID$(trend$, 2, 1))
    byte3 = ASC(RIGHT$(trend$, 1))
    SELECT CASE hexbyte1$
        CASE "7F", "7E", "7D"
            SELECT CASE hexbyte1$
            CASE "7F"
                year$ = RIGHT$("19" +LTRIM$(STR$(byte3))), 4)
            CASE "7E"
                month$ = RIGHT$("0" + LTRIM$(STR$(byte2))), 2)
                day$ = RIGHT$("0" + LTRIM$(STR$(byte3))), 2)
            CASE "7D"
                hour$ = RIGHT$("0" + LTRIM$(STR$(byte2))), 2)
                min$ = RIGHT$("0" + LTRIM$(STR$(byte3))), 2)
            END SELECT
            pulsox7time$ = year$ + "-" + month$ + "-" +
day$ + SPACE$(1) + "/" + SPACE$(1) + hour$ + ":" + min$
            shortdata$ = hexbyte1$ + "*" + hexbyte2$ + "*"
+ hexbyte3$
            PRINT pulsox7time$ + SPACE$(2) + shortdata$
            PRINT #2, pulsox7time$ + SPACE$(2) + shortdata$
        CASE "7B"
            REM this is the INOP number
            highbyte$ = MID$(data$, 2, 1)
            lowbyte$ = RIGHT$(data$, 1)
            inopvalue% = (ASC(highbyte$)) * 256
+ ASC(lowbyte$)
            mediumdata$ = hexbyte1$ + "*" + hexbyte2$ + "*"
+ hexbyte3$
            inop$ = SPACE$(2) + "INOP No. = " +
LTRIM$(STR$(inopvalue%))
            PRINT pulsox7time$ + SPACE$(2) + mediumdata$ +
inop$
            PRINT #2, pulsox7time$ + SPACE$(2) + mediumdata$
+ inop$
```

```
            CASE ELSE
                so2$ = RIGHT$("ØØ" + LTRIM$(STR$(byte1)), 3)
                hr$ = RIGHT$("ØØ" + LTRIM$(STR$(byte2)), 3)
                alarm = byte3
                alarmØ$ = "": alarm1$ = "": alarm2$ = ""
                alarm3$ = "": alarm7$ = ""
                IF bit%(Ø, alarm) = 1 THEN alarmØ$ = "LSA"
                IF bit%(1, alarm) = 1 THEN alarm1$ = "HSA"
                IF bit%(2, alarm) = 1 THEN alarm2$ = "LPA"
                IF bit%(3, alarm) = 1 THEN alarm3$ = "HPA"
                IF bit%(7, alarm) = 1 THEN alarm7$ = "INOP"
                longdata$ = pulsox7time$ + SPACE$(2) + hexbyte1$
+ "*" + hexbyte2$ + "*" + hexbyte3$ + SPACE$(2) + "Sat=" +
so2$ + SPACE$(2) + "HR=" + hr$ + SPACE$(2) + alarmØ$ +
SPACE$(1) + alarm1$ + SPACE$(1) + alarm2$ + SPACE$(1) +
alarm3$ + SPACE$(1) + alarm7$
                PRINT longdata$
                PRINT #2, longdata$
        END SELECT
        REM check for code 7C (= end of data)
        IF hexbyte1$ = "7C" THEN CALL shutdown
END SUB



SUB printhexdata
    REM print the data-groups in hexadecimal
    PRINT hexbyte1$; "  "; hexbyte2$; "  "; hexbyte3$
    PRINT #2, hexbyte1$; "  "; hexbyte2$; "  "; hexbyte3$
    REM check for code 7C (= end of data)
    IF hexbyte1$ = "7C" THEN CALL shutdown
END SUB



SUB shutdown
    REM send code to stop data output
    PRINT #1, "S"
    PRINT "end of trend data"
    PRINT "no of data-groups = "; n
    PRINT "time taken = "; TIMER - timezero; "secs"
    PRINT #2, "end of trend data"
```

```
        PRINT #2, "no of data-groups = "; n
        PRINT #2, "time taken = "; TIMER - timezero; "secs"
        CLOSE #1, #2
        BEEP: BEEP
        END
END SUB
```

An example of the output of the above program when using the subroutine PRINTALLDATA is shown in Figure 12.4.

```
date(ymd)      time      hex data   sat        hr          alarm status

1991-12-20  /  20:37     7F*02*5B
1991-12-20  /  20:37     7E*0C*14
1991-12-20  /  20:37     7D*14*25
1991-12-20  /  20:37     61*4F*00   Sat = 97   HR = 79
1991-12-20  /  20:38     7D*14*26
1991-12-20  /  20:38     62*4D*00   Sat = 98   HR = 77
1991-12-20  /  20:38     63*53*00   Sat = 99   HR = 83
1991-12-20  /  20:38     63*64*08   Sat = 99   HR =100     HPA
   ...
   ...
1991-12-20  /  20:38     63*53*00   Sat = 99   HR = 83
1991-12-20  /  20:38     7B*00*43   INOP No. = 67
1991-12-20  /  20:39     7D*14*27
1991-12-20  /  20:39     62*52*00   Sat = 98   HR = 82
1991-12-20  /  20:39     63*50*00   Sat = 99   HR = 80
   ...
   ...
1991-12-20  /  20:50     7C*00*00   end of data
```

Fig. 12.4. Trend data output when using the subroutine PRINTALLDATA. HPA = high pulse alarm. The hex data-bytes are separated by an asterisk *.

13

The Datex Cardiocap™ II and Capnomac Ultima™ series of monitors

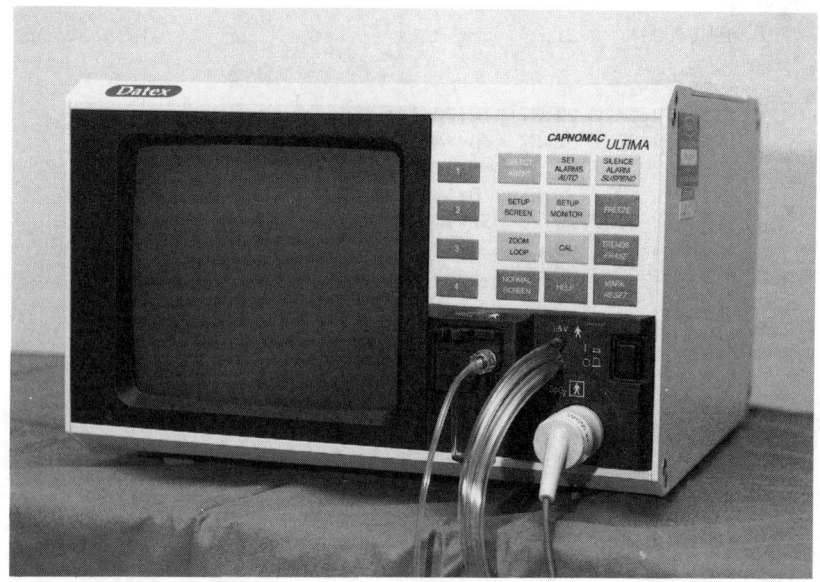

13.1 Introduction

The Datex† range of anaesthesia monitors consists of a large number of pre-configured variants which include the Cardiocap™ II and Capnomac Ultima™ series. While all the Cardiocap™ II monitors incorporate ECG, non-invasive blood pressure (NIBP) and temperature (T), the monitors in this series vary in their capability to monitor up to two invasive blood pressures (BP_1, BP_2), pulse oximetry (SaO_2), respiration, and airway gases (CO_2, O_2, N_2O).

The Capnomac Ultima™ series consists of a range of devices with varying capability to monitor the anaesthetic agent (halothane, enflurane,

---

† Datex Instrumentarium Corp., P.O. Box 466, SF-00101, Helsinki, Finland. Tel: +358-0-39411. Fax: +358-0-1463310.

Table 13.1. *Applied Parts and their Types.*

Product	Applied Part	Type
Cardiocap™ II series	ECG	CF
	NIBP	BF
	Invasive BP	CF
	Temperature probe	CF
Capnomac Ultima™ series	Pulse oximeter probe	BF
	Gas sampling probe	B
	Spirometry probe	B

isoflurane, desflurane, sevoflurane), pulse oximetry, airway gases (CO_2, O_2, N_2O), airway pressure, and gas flow.

All monitors have a serial interface and output measured data at 10-second intervals. Furthermore, the serial output from a Capnomac Ultima™ can be interfaced to monitors of the Cardiocap™ II CH series allowing data from both monitors to be accessed via the serial/analog port of the Cardiocap™. A pamphlet covering various aspects of serial communication with the Cardiocap™ II CH series of monitors is also available (Sainsbury, 1992).

Stored Trend data can be output in either a graphics or numeric format compatible with the following printers: HP ThinkJet, Epson, Seiko DPU411.

The electrical safety Type classifications of the various Applied Parts† (e.g. NIBP cuff, temperature probe) are shown in Table 13.1.

13.1.1 Software version

The current software version is indicated on the screen when the monitor is switched on. Since the launch of the Cardiocap family in 1985 there have been several software and hardware revisions, which include improvements and updates to the communication protocol. Compatibility with older revisions has been maintained throughout.

13.1.2 Available software

A program for PCs called COLLECT.EXE is available from Datex. The program collects the data-strings output by Datex monitors and saves

† See Chapter 7 for further details.

Table 13.2. Cardiocap™ CCI-104 serial/analog port.

Pin No.	Signal	Type
1	Chassis ground	
2	RxD (receives data)	RS-232
3	TxD (transmits data)	RS-232
4	Not used	
5	CTS (data enable)	RS-232
6	Gas freeze (testing purposes only)	TTL
7	GND (signal ground)	
8	Testing purposes only	TTL
9	+12 volts DC	
10	−12 volts DC	
11	+15 volts DC	
12	−15 volts DC	
13	Invasive BP$_2$ (25.5 mV/mm Hg)	analog
14	O$_2$ (10 volts ≡ 100%)	analog
15	+5 volts DC (500 mA max)	
16	Not used	
17	Invasive BP$_2$ (260 mm Hg ≡ 10 volts)	analog
18	ECG (gain = 1750)	analog
19	Invasive BP$_1$ (260 mm Hg ≡ 10 volts)	analog
20	CO$_2$ (10 volts ≡ 10%)	analog
21	+22 volts DC (1A max)	
22	Auxiliary input (ADC 7)	
23	−22 volts DC (1A max)	
24	20 volts AC (1A max)	
25	20 volts AC (1A max)	

Table 13.3. Cardiocap™ II CG-series serial/analog port.

Pin No.	Signal	Type
1	Chassis ground	
2	TxD (transmits data)	RS-232
3	RxD (receives data)	RS-232
4	RTS	RS-232
5	CTS (data enable)	RS-232
6	Gas freeze (testing purposes only)	TTL
7	GND (signal ground)	
8	Testing purposes only	TTL
9	+12 volts DC	
10	−12 volts DC	
11	+15 volts DC	
12	−15 volts DC	
13	SaO$_2$ (10 volts ≡ 100%)	analog
14	O$_2$ (10 volts ≡ 100%)	analog
15	+5 volts DC (300 mA max)	
16	Not used	
17	Invasive BP$_2$ (260 mm Hg ≡ 10 volts)	analog
18	ECG (gain = 1660)	analog
19	Invasive BP$_1$ or Pleth.	analog
20	CO$_2$ (10 volts ≡ 10%)	analog
21	+22 volts DC (500 mA max)	
22	Infra-red signal (0–10 volts)	analog
23	−22 volts DC (500 mA max)	
24	20 volts AC (500 mA max)	
25	20 volts AC (500 mA max)	

them to the hard disk of the PC either as an ASCII file or in a form compatible with LOTUS 1-2-3.

Note that since this program does not add a separate time-stamp to the data care must be taken to check the internal clock setting (hh:mm) of the monitor being used.

13.2 Serial/analog port

All Datex monitors have a female 25-pin D-type serial port which is labelled 'serial/analog I/O'. A wide range of signals and voltage supplies (often both AC and DC) is available via the serial/analog port, and care must be taken when interfacing not to inadvertently connect the TTL lines (range: 0–5 volts) to RS-232 voltages, as this may damage the monitor.

Note that the configuration of the serial/analog port varies slightly depending on the monitor and its capability. For example, the Receive (RxD) and Transmit (TxD) pins are reversed in some of the early models (e.g. Cardiocap™ CCI-104). Consequently, the monitor's manual should always be consulted before interfacing to a PC. In view of these differences the serial/analog port configurations of the Cardiocap™ CCI-104, Cardiocap™ II CG, Cardiocap™ II CH, and the Capnomac Ultima™ series are shown in Tables 13.2, 13.3, 13.4, 13.5.

Probably the most useful analog data are those for volume, flow, and pressure, which are output by the Capnomac Ultima™. These are output in pairs on pins 13 (volume or pressure) and 18 (flow or volume) as shown in Table 13.5. The particular combination is configurable, and indicated by the three-digit 'recorder output' parameter given in the U03 data-string (see Section 13.3.6).

13.2.1 Cable connections

The wiring configuration for interfacing the Cardiocap™ II and Capnomac Ultima™ series monitors to a PC is shown in Figure 13.1.

- **CTS** Hardware handshaking is via the CTS line (data enable). Data output is enabled if CTS is either held HIGH (positive) or allowed to be on 'open circuit'; i.e. data output is disabled *only* when the monitor's CTS is held LOW. For most ordinary purposes, therefore, it is not necessary to connect the Datex CTS line to anything at all.

Table 13.4. *Cardiocap*™ *II CH-series serial/analog port.*

Pin No.	Signal	Type
1	Chassis ground	
2	TxD (transmits data)	RS-232
3	RxD (receives data)	RS-232
4	RTS	RS-232
5	CTS (data enable)	RS-232
6	Testing purposes only	TTL
7	GND (signal ground)	
8	Testing purposes only	TTL
9	+12 volts DC	
10	–12 volts DC	
11	+15 volts DC	
12	–15 volts DC	
13	Invasive BP_2 (25.5 mV/mm Hg uncal.)	analog
14	Not for use	
15	+5 volts DC (500 mA max)	
16	Not for use	
17	Invasive BP_2 (255 mm Hg ≡ 10 volts)	analog
18	ECG (gain = 1660)	analog
19	Invasive BP_1 or Pleth.	analog
20	Not for use	
21	+26 volts DC (1 A max)	
22	Auxiliary input (ADC 7)	
23	–29 volts DC (1 A max)	
24	22 volts AC (1 A max)	
25	22 volts AC (1 A max)	

Table 13.5. *Capnomac Ultima*™ *serial/analog port.*

Pin No.	Signal	Type
1	Chassis ground	
2	TxD (transmits data)	RS-232
3	RxD (receives data)	RS-232
4	Not used	
5	CTS (data enable)	RS-232
6	Testing purposes	TTL
7	GND (signal ground)	
8	Testing purposes only	TTL
9	+12 volts DC	
10	–12 volts DC	
11	+15 volts DC	
12	–15 volts DC	
13	Volume or pressure	analog
14	O_2 (10 volts ≡ 100%)	analog
15	+5 volts DC (500 mA max)	
16	N_2O (10 volts ≡ 100%)	analog
17	Anaesthetic agent (10 volts ≡ 10%)	analog
18	Flow or volume	analog
19	SaO_2 (10 volts ≡ 100%)	analog
20	CO_2 (10 volts ≡ 10%)	analog
21	+26 volts DC (1 A max)	
22	Pleth. (0–10 volts)	analog
23	–26 volts DC (1 A max)	
24	22 volts AC (1 A max)	
25	22 volts AC (1 A max)	

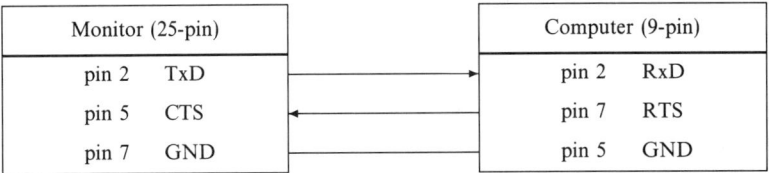

Fig. 13.1. Wiring configuration for the Cardiocap™ II and Capnomac Ultima™ series of monitors.

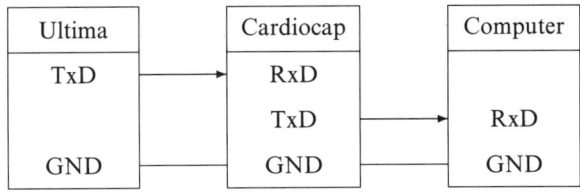

Fig. 13.2. The wiring configuration for simultaneously linking a Capnomac Ultima™ and a Cardiocap™ II CH-series monitor to a PC. Note that the connection at both Datex monitors is to the serial/analog port.

However, if it is necessary to use hardware handshaking to control data output, then it is probably best to connect the Datex CTS line to the computer's RTS line, which can then be used to control data output by setting the status of the computer's RTS line HIGH or LOW as necessary (see Section 5.16).

Note that the Datex CTS is 'edge sensitive' from LOW to HIGH. Thus a transition from LOW to HIGH triggers the release of the latest set of data from the monitor, following which the usual 10-second data output is resumed.

Linking two monitors together. The output from two Datex monitors can be combined and interfaced jointly to a PC. For example, the combined data from an Ultima™ and a Cardiocap™ II CH-series monitor can be accessed by linking the two monitors together via their serial/analog ports as shown in Figure 13.2. Note that it is not necessary to connect the Datex CTS line unless hardware handshaking is required to control data outflow, as shown in Figure 13.1.

When these two monitors are linked in this way, the B00 data-string from the Ultima™ is *not* transmitted, since its data is transferred to the C03 and C04 data-strings generated by the Cardiocap™ II CH monitor.

Table 13.6. *Protocol for the Datex series of monitors.*

Bit rate	1200
Data bits	8
Parity	None
Stop bits	1

See Section 13.3 for details of data output under these circumstances. Data collected in this way is shown in Figure 13.5.

13.2.2 Protocol

The serial protocol is fixed for the Datex series of monitors, as shown in Table 13.6.

13.3 Data format

Serial data is output from the serial/analog port every 10 seconds, and consists of a number of data-strings, each of which has a similar general structure. Each data-string starts with an alphanumeric string-code (Cxx, Uxx, Bxx) which identifies the data-string; the letter C is associated with the Cardiocap™ series; the letters B and U are associated with the Capnomac Ultima™ series. The string-code is followed by a number of three-character fields (xxx) which are separated by commas. Each data-string is terminated by ⟨CR⟩⟨LF⟩.

An example of the general structure of a data-string is as follows where x represents a character; in this example the letter C in the initial string-code indicates that the data-string is from a Cardiocap™ monitor.

Cxx, xxx, xxx, xxx, xxx, ..., xxx ⟨CR⟩⟨LF⟩

There are a number of data-string formats, which are identified by their string-codes as follows.

- Cardiocap™ II NIBP data-string (C01).
- Cardiocap™ II basic data-string (C00, C02, C03).
- Cardiocap™ II oximetry data-string (C04).
- Ultima™ B00 data-string.
- Ultima™ U01 data-string.
- Ultima™ U03 data-string.
- Alarm activation (B99, C99, U99) and deactivation (B98, C98, U98).

Cardiocap™ *II.* When a Cardiocap™ II monitor is interfaced three data-strings are output, namely C01, C04, and one of either C00, C02, or C03, depending on the particular model—see Section 13.3.2.

Capnomac Ultima™. When a Capnomac Ultima™ monitor is interfaced, three data-strings are output, namely B00, U01, U03, as shown in Figure 13.4.

Combined Cardiocap™ *II CH and Ultima*™. When these two monitors are combined (see Figure 13.2), the B00 data-string from the Ultima™ is *not* transmitted, since its data is transferred to the C03 and C04 data-strings generated by the Cardiocap™ II CH monitor. Consequently, a total of only five data-strings are transmitted, namely U01, U03, C01, C03, C04, as shown in Figure 13.5. The precise combination of transmitted data-strings will vary slightly depending on the particular combination of monitors.

```
Program to access data from the Capnomac Ultima.           18:39:41
All data saved to file <ultima.dat>                waiting for data (6)
Press <Q> to QUIT; <V> to view stored data

B00,017,053,042,001,034,038,058,083,108,ENF,011,7300ALL,200
U00,000,339,376,999,999,000,000,000,000,000,069,098,026,014,005,700
U03,049,054,000,444,000,489,085,035,015,003,015,000,000,000,001,000,900

Time = 17:53                    Resp Rate = 11 /min
HR = 069                        Insp TV = 0.489 L
FiO2 = 37.6 %                   Exp TV = 0.444 L
EtO2 = 33.9 %                   Exp MV = 04.9 L
Sat = 98 %                      Insp MV = 05.4 L
EtCO2 = 04.2 %                  Compliance = 35 mls/cm H20
Agent = ENFLURANE               V(1.0) = 85 %
Insp agent = 1.08 %             Peak pressure = 15 cm H20
Exp agent = 0.83 %              Plat. pressure = 15 cm H20
                                PEEP = 03 cms H20
B00 status = 200                I:E ratio = 1 : 1.5
U01 status = 700
U03 status = 900
```

Fig. 13.3. Example of the screen while running program **ultima.bas**. See Section 13.5

```
SAVING CAPNOMAC ULTIMA DATA 11-13-1993
20:11:31
B00,018,013,042,001,034,037,058,058,071,096,ENF,011,733,ALL,200
U01,000,335,374,999,999,000,000,000,000,000,071,098,029,016,005,700
U03,049,053,000,446,000,485,083,033,016,016,003,016,000,000,001,000,900
20:11:41
B00,018,013,042,001,034,037,058,058,071,097,ENF,011,732,ALL,100
U01,000,334,374,999,999,000,000,000,000,000,072,098,031,017,005,610
U03,049,053,000,445,000,485,084,032,016,016,003,016,000,000,001,000,900
20:11:51
B00,018,013,042,001,033,037,058,058,071,096,ENF,011,730,ALL,200
U01,000,335,374,999,999,000,000,000,000,000,073,098,030,016,005,700
U03,049,054,000,447,000,486,083,033,016,016,003,016,000,000,001,000,900
20:12:01
B00,018,013,043,001,034,037,058,058,071,096,ENF,011,729,ALL,100
U01,000,334,374,999,999,000,000,000,000,000,072,098,028,016,005,610
U03,049,053,000,445,000,484,083,033,016,016,003,016,000,000,001,000,900
20:12:11
B00,018,013,042,001,033,037,058,058,071,095,ENF,011,730,ALL,200
U01,000,335,374,999,999,000,000,000,000,000,073,098,029,016,005,700
U03,049,053,000,446,000,485,084,033,016,016,003,016,000,000,001,000,900
20:12:21
B00,018,014,043,001,034,037,058,058,071,097,ENF,011,730,ALL,100
U01,000,335,374,999,999,000,000,000,000,000,073,098,031,017,005,610
U03,049,053,000,445,000,486,084,033,016,016,003,016,000,000,001,000,900
```

Fig. 13.4. An example of how data from a Capnomac Ultima™ is saved to a file (ultima.dat) when running the program **ultima.bas**. Note the discrepancy between the monitor's time-stamp in the B00 data-string (e.g. 18.14) and that supplied by the computer (e.g. 20:12:21).

```
COMBINED ULTIMA AND CARDIOCAP II DATA
11:25:19
C03,000,011,027,061,002,031,026,063,062,013,056,000,000,000,000,000,000,500
C04,084,117,ALL,056,000,000,000,000,000
U01,000,261,314,999,999,000,000,000,000,000,056,096,060,040,012,700
U03,032,040,000,279,000,321,079,-01,001,-01,000,020,000,000,001,000,900
11:25:30
C03,000,011,027,061,002,031,026,063,062,012,056,000,000,000,000,000,000,600
C04,084,116,ENF,056,000,000,000,000,000
U01,000,261,314,999,999,000,000,000,000,000,056,096,059,039,012,620
U03,032,040,000,241,000,301,075,-01,001,-01,000,024,000,000,001,000,900
11:25:40
C03,000,011,028,062,002,031,026,063,062,012,054,000,000,000,000,000,000,100
C04,084,117,ALL,054,000,000,000,000,000
U01,000,259,313,999,999,000,000,000,000,000,055,096,059,039,012,700
U03,029,036,000,226,000,277,073,-01,001,-01,000,028,000,000,001,000,900
11:25:50
C03,000,011,028,062,002,031,026,063,062,013,056,000,000,000,000,000,000,200
C04,083,116,ENF,056,000,000,000,000,000
C01,002,091,064,055,055,018,000
U01,000,259,313,999,999,000,000,000,000,000,056,096,061,041,012,620
U03,029,037,000,226,000,287,076,-01,001,-01,000,027,000,000,001,000,900
```

Fig. 13.5. An example of how data is output when a Capnomac Ultima™ and a Cardiocap™ II CH monitor are combined using the wiring configuration shown in Figure 13.2. The C01 data-string is only output following a NIBP measurement. The above data was saved using the program **ultima.bas**. Note the discrepancy between the monitor's time-stamp in the C03 data-string (e.g. 11.28) and that supplied by the computer (e.g. 11:25:50).

13.3.1 Cardiocap™ II NIBP data-string (C01)

The non-invasive blood pressure (NIBP) data-string consists of 8 fields, starting with the string-code C01, and ending with ⟨CR⟩⟨LF⟩, as shown in the following example.

C01, 002, 129, 099, 084, 069, 019, 000 ⟨CR⟩ ⟨LF⟩

The NIBP parameters and their order in the data-string, are given in Table 13.7. Note that because NIBP measurements are made relatively infrequently (only every few minutes or so), the NIBP data-string is only output during the 10 seconds following the NIBP measurement.

Table 13.7. *NIBP data-string (C01)*.

Data	Order	Example
String-code	1	C01
NIBP status; for test purposes only	2	002
NIBP (systolic; mm Hg)	3	129
NIBP (mean; mm Hg)	4	099
NIBP (diastolic; mm Hg)	5	084
HR (heart rate; min^{-1})	6	069
Pzero	7	019
000	8	000
⟨CR⟩		⟨CR⟩
⟨LF⟩		⟨LF⟩

13.3.2 Cardiocap™ II basic data-string (C00, C02, C03)

The basic data-string varies slightly depending on the particular model. For example the Cardiocap™ II CG-2G, CG-2GS, CG-2CS, and CH-series of monitors output a data-string consisting of 20 fields, starting with the string-code C03, and ending with ⟨CR⟩⟨LF⟩, as shown in the example below. Note that the gas data is not available from a Cardiocap™ II CH-series monitor unless it is interfaced with a Capnomac Ultima™, Capnomac™ II, Multicap™ or Normocap™ (see Section 13.2.1). The parameters and their order in the C03 data-string are given in Table 13.8.

C03, 000, 012, 030, 042, 000, 034, 028, 066, 066, 012, 064, 120, 087, 063, 371, 025, 017, 012, 420 ⟨CR⟩ ⟨LF⟩

The status code cycles through all the status groups except for 7xx (e.g. 100, 200, 300, 412, 510, 600) with successive transmissions of the data-string.

Table 13.8. Cardiocap™ II basic data-string (C00, C03).

Data (C03)	Order	Examples		Data (C00)
String-code	1	C03	C00	String-code
Marker No.	2	000	000	Marker No.
Hours	3	012	012	Hours
Minutes	4	030	030	Minutes
EtCO$_2$ (%×10)	5	042	042	EtCO$_2$
FiCO$_2$ (%×10)	6	000	000	FiCO$_2$
FiO$_2$ (%)	7	034	034	FiO$_2$
EtO$_2$ (%)	8	028	028	EtO$_2$
FiN$_2$O (%)	9	066	066	FiN$_2$O
EtN$_2$O (%)	10	066	066	EtN$_2$O
RR (respiratory rate; min^{-1})	11	012	012	RR
HR (heart rate; min^{-1})	12	064	064	HR
Invasive BP$_1$ (systolic)	13	120	120	BP$_1$ (systolic)
Invasive BP$_1$ (mean)	14	087	087	BP$_1$ (mean)
Invasive BP$_1$ (diastolic)	15	063	063	BP$_1$ (diastolic)
Temperature (deg. C ×10)	16	371	371	Temp 1
Invasive BP$_2$ (systolic)	17	025	378	Temp 2
Invasive BP$_2$ (mean)	18	017	420	Status code
Invasive BP$_2$ (diastolic)	19	012	⟨CR⟩	⟨CR⟩
Status code	20	420	⟨LF⟩	⟨LF⟩
⟨CR⟩		⟨CR⟩		
⟨LF⟩		⟨LF⟩		

The Cardiocap™ II CG-1G and CG-1GS monitors measure only one invasive blood pressure, and so output a slightly modified data-string consisting of only 18 fields, starting with the string-code C00. The earlier Cardiocap™ CCI-104 outputs a 20 field data-string (string-code C02) which differs from the C03 data-string only in the order of the inspired and expired gases.

13.3.3 Cardiocap™ II oximetry data-string (C04)

The oximetry data-string consists of 10 fields, starting with the string-code C04, and ending with $\langle$CR$\rangle\langle$LF$\rangle$. The content of the data-string varies depending on the capability of the monitor (CH or CG series) and on whether it is interfaced to a Capnomac Ultima™.

For example, when a Cardiocap™ II CH-2S monitor operates alone (i.e. not interfaced to an Ultima™) the C04 data-string contains only the heart rate and saturation data as follows.

C04, 000, 000, 000, 063, 098, 026, 019, 027, 700 $\langle$CR$\rangle$ $\langle$LF$\rangle$

However, when a Capnomac Ultima™ is interfaced to a Cardiocap™ II monitor the C04 data-string includes details of the anaesthetic agent (AA) and which anaesthetic gas is represented at the analog output. Note that in this case the fourth and the tenth fields vary with alternate transmissions of the C04 data-string as follows.

C04, 095, 114, HAL, 063, 098, 026, 019, 027, 700 $\langle$CR$\rangle$ $\langle$LF$\rangle$
C04, 095, 114, CO2, 063, 098, 026, 019, 027, 612 $\langle$CR$\rangle$ $\langle$LF$\rangle$

The fourth field alternates between the code for the anaesthetic agent (e.g. HAL) and the code for the gas represented at the analog output (e.g. CO2). If the device is outputting analog voltages for all three gases at the same time (O_2, CO_2, N_2O) then the analog gas code ALL is used. If the analog output is for the anaesthetic agent, then the analog gas code AA is used. The tenth field is the status code, and alternates between the

Table 13.9. *Cardiocap™ II oximetry data-string (C04)*.

Data	Order	Example
String-code	1	C04
EtAA (%×100)	2	095
FiAA (%×100)	3	114
AA (anaesthetic agent)/analog output (gas)	4	HAL/CO2
HR (heart rate; min^{-1})	5	063
SaO_2 (%)	6	098
Infra-red amplitude modulation (×10)	7	026
Red amplitude modulation (×10)	8	019
Gain	9	027
Status code (6xx/7xx)	10	612/700
$\langle$CR$\rangle$		$\langle$CR$\rangle$
$\langle$LF$\rangle$		$\langle$LF$\rangle$

two status code groups which relate to pulse oximetry, i.e. those where the first character is either 6 or 7 (see Table 13.18).

The C04 parameters and their order in the data-string are given in Table 13.9.

13.3.4 Capnomac Ultima™ B00 data-string

The B00 data-string contains information regarding time and concentration of the anaesthetic gases. An example is as follows.

B00, 012, 030, 042, 000, 028, 034, 066, 066, 012, 064, ISO, 012, 087, ALL, 200 ⟨CR⟩ ⟨LF⟩

The B00 parameters and their order in the data-string are given in Table 13.10. The status code alternates between 1xx and 2xx in consecutive B00 data-strings. In the example shown in Table 13.10 the two alternating status codes are 110 (rebreathing alarm) and 200 (no alarm).†

Note that when a Capnomac Ultima™ is interfaced to a Cardiocap™ II monitor, the B00 data-string is not transmitted to the PC since the B00 data is transferred to the Cardiocap's C03 and C04 data-strings.

Table 13.10. *Capnomac Ultima*™ *B00 data-string.*

Data	Order	Example
String-code	1	B00
Hours	2	012
Minutes	3	030
$EtCO_2$ (×10)	4	042
$FiCO_2$ (×10)	5	000
EtO_2 (%)	6	028
FiO_2 (%)	7	034
EtN_2O (%)	8	066
FiN_2O (%)	9	066
EtAA (% ×100)	10	012
FiAA (% ×100)	11	064
AA selection	12	ISO
RR (respiratory rate; min^{-1})	13	012
Gas pressure (mm Hg)	14	087
Recorder output (analog)	15	ALL
Status code	16	110/200
⟨CR⟩		⟨CR⟩
⟨LF⟩		⟨LF⟩

† Capnomac Ultima™ status codes are detailed in Table 13.17.

13.3.5 Capnomac Ultima™ U01 data-string

The U01 data-string contains the pulse oximetry data, and consists of 20 fields ending with ⟨CR⟩⟨LF⟩, as shown in the following example.

U01, 000, 328, 371, 999, 999, 000, 000, 000, 000, 000, 000, 000, 000, 076, 098, 029, 016, 005, 700 ⟨CR⟩ ⟨LF⟩

The U01 parameters and their order in the data-string are given in Table 13.11. The status code alternates between the two pulse oximetry codes (6xx and 7xx) in successive U01 data-strings. In the example shown in Table 13.11 the two alternating status codes are 610 (plethysmogram modulation = 10%) and 740 (pulse oximeter probe off).†

Table 13.11. Capnomac Ultima™ U01 data-string.

Data	Order	Example
String-code	1	U01
Marker number	2	000
EtO_2 (%×10)	3	328
FiO_2 (%×10)	4	371
EtBalance gas	5	999
FiBalance gas	6	999
ASX status	7	000
Automatically identified gas	8	000
Reserved	9	000
EtPrimary gas (10 ≡ 1%)	10	000
FiPrimary gas	11	000
EtSecondary gas	12	000
FiSecondary gas	13	000
Reserved	14	000
HR (heart rate; min^{-1})	15	076
SaO_2 (%)	16	098
Infra-red amplitude	17	029
Red amplitude	18	016
Gain	19	005
Status code	20	610/740
⟨CR⟩		⟨CR⟩
⟨LF⟩		⟨LF⟩

† Capnomac Ultima™ status codes are detailed in Table 13.17.

13.3.6 Capnomac Ultima™ U03 data-string

The U03 data-string contains the ventilation data, and consists of 20 fields ending with ⟨CR⟩⟨LF⟩, as shown in the following example.

U03, 048, 052, 000, 434, 000, 476, 085, 030, 017, 017, 003, 016, 000, 000, 000, 000, 001, 000, 900 ⟨CR⟩ ⟨LF⟩

The U03 parameters and their order in the data-string are given in Table 13.12.

The pressure unit. The **units status** code (field 19) indicates the pressure units being used, as shown in Table 13.13.

Analog data configuration. The **recorder output** code (field 18) indicates which of the three parameters flow, volume, and pressure are output at pins 13 and 18 of the serial/analog port of the Capnomac Ultima™ as shown in Table 13.14.

Table 13.12. *Capnomac Ultima™ U03 data-string.*

Data	Order	Example
String-code	1	U03
Expired MV (L/min ×10)	2	048
Inspired MV (L/min ×10)	3	052
Expired TV (L)	4	000
Expired TV (mls)	5	434
Inspired TV (L)	6	000
Inspired TV (mls)	7	476
V(1.0) (%)	8	085
Compliance	9	030
Peak pressure	10	017
Plateau pressure	11	017
PEEP	12	003
I:E ratio (×10)	13	016
Reserved	14	000
Reserved	15	000
Reserved	16	000
Reserved	17	000
Recorder output (analog data config.)	18	001
Units status	19	000
Status code	20	900
⟨CR⟩		⟨CR⟩
⟨LF⟩		⟨LF⟩

Table 13.13. *Capnomac Ultima*™ *units status code in the U03 data-string.*

Units status code	Unit	Pressure	Compliance
000	cm H_2O	cm H_2O	ml/cm H_2O
001	kPa	kPa ×0.1	ml/kPa ×10
010	mm Hg	mm Hg	ml/mm Hg

Table 13.14. *Capnomac Ultima*™ *flow, volume, pressure analog data output from serial/analog port.*

Recorder output code in U03 data-string	Analog configuration	
	Pin 13	Pin 18
000	Volume	Flow
001	Pressure	Flow
002	Pressure	Volume

Table 13.15. *Some of the alarm codes used by Datex monitors.*

Code	Meaning	Code	Meaning
CO2	Carbon dioxide	ZER	Gas zeroing started
O2	Oxygen	NOR	Gases to normal state
O2?	Oxygen transducer error	PRO	Probe off
APN	Apnoea	PUS	Pulse search
REB	Rebreathing	PRE	Pressure
OCC	Occlusion	EEP	End expiratory pressure
HAL	Halothane	AWP	Airway pressure
ENF	Enflurane	MVL	Minute volume
ISO	Isoflurane	SAO	Oxygen saturation
DES	Desflurane	P1	Invasive pressure 1
SEV	Sevoflurane		

13.3.7 Alarm/information data-strings

Alarm data-strings are output whenever alarms are either activated or deactivated, providing the alarms have not been temporarily suspended by pressing the appropriate button on the front panel. The alarm data-string consists of up to 5 fields separated by commas, starting with the string-code and ending with ⟨CR⟩⟨LF⟩, as follows.

⟨string-code⟩,⟨parameter⟩,⟨current value⟩,⟨violation⟩,⟨alarm setting⟩ ⟨CR⟩⟨LF⟩

String-code. The string-code numbers 99 and 98 are used for alarm data-strings, and 97 for information data-strings, as follows.

99 — alarm activation.
98 — alarm deactivation.
97 — information.

Parameters. The alarm codes are shown in Table 13.15.

Type of limit violation. Whether a parameter has become greater (>) or less (<) than the set alarm limit is indicated by the usual symbols as follows.

> — greater than the high alarm limit
< — less than the low alarm limit

Examples. Typical examples of alarm/information data-strings are as follows.

C99,P1,178, >,170 ⟨CR⟩⟨LF⟩
C98,P1 ⟨CR⟩⟨LF⟩
C99,OCC ⟨CR⟩⟨LF⟩
C99,APN ⟨CR⟩⟨LF⟩
B97,ZER ⟨CR⟩⟨LF⟩
B97,PRE,790 ⟨CR⟩⟨LF⟩
B97,NOR ⟨CR⟩⟨LF⟩
U99,EEP,013, >,009 ⟨CR⟩⟨LF⟩

13.4 Status codes

A large amount of useful information is encoded in the three-character status code which occurs at the end of each data-string (e.g. 423, 1?=). However, the encoding scheme is fairly complicated, and involves the binary representation of ASCII characters.

The characters used in the status code are drawn from the set of 16 ASCII characters shown in Table 13.16. Note that the Datex documentation refers to the three characters making up the status code as the 1st character, 2nd character, and 3rd character, counting from the left.

Table 13.16. *Decimal, hex and binary equivalents of ASCII characters.*

Char	Dec	Hex	Binary
0	48	30h	0011 0000
1	49	31h	0011 0001
2	50	32h	0011 0010
3	51	33h	0011 0011
4	52	34h	0011 0100
5	53	35h	0011 0101
6	54	36h	0011 0110
7	55	37h	0011 0111
8	56	38h	0011 1000
9	57	39h	0011 1001
:	58	3Ah	0011 1010
;	59	3Bh	0011 1011
<	60	3Ch	0011 1100
=	61	3Dh	0011 1101
>	62	3Eh	0011 1110
?	63	3Fh	0011 1111

Table 13.17. *Status codes for Capnomac Ultima™ series.*

1st Digit	2nd Digit	3rd Digit	Coding
0	not used	not used	
1	(bit-0) rebreathing (bit-1) apnoea (bit-2) air leak (bit-3) occlusion	CO_2 zero error O_2 zero error N_2O zero error AA zero error	binary
2	(bit-0) O_2 low (bit-1) O_2 high (bit-2) CO_2 low (bit-3) CO_2 high	insp. AA low insp. AA high exp. AA low exp. AA high	binary
6	modulation (%) 02, 05, 10, 20 or 50		decimal
7	(bit-0) low pleth. signal (bit-1) pulse search (bit-2) probe off (bit-3) no probe	HR low HR high SaO_2 low SaO_2 high	binary
9	(bit-0) exp MV low (bit-1) exp MV high (bit-2) peak pressure low (bit-3) peak pressure high	obstruction disconnection leak PEEP high	binary

The 1st character indicates the status group that the status code refers to (see Tables 13.17 and 13.18). There are 6 such groups (1–7) for the Cardiocap™ II series, and 5 groups (1, 2, 6, 7, 9) for the Capnomac Ultima™ series.

The 2nd and 3rd characters are either bit-encoded (binary) and considered individually, or decimal values which are considered either individually or combined depending on the parameters they represent. How the 2nd and 3rd characters are to be interpreted (binary or decimal) is indicated in the right-hand column of Tables 13.17 and 13.18.

13.4.1 Decimal coding

When the right-hand column of Tables 13.17 and 13.18 indicates that the coding is *decimal*, then the 2nd and 3rd characters are taken to be decimal values, and therefore must be in the range 0–9. For example, when the 1st character of a Cardiocap™ II status code is 4 (ECG size) then the 2nd and 3rd characters are taken to be a two digit decimal value (e.g. 32) which is then used to determine the calibration from the formula

Table 13.18. *Status codes for Cardiocap™ II series.*

1st Digit	2nd Digit	3rd Digit	Coding
0	not used	not used	
1	(bit-0) air leak (bit-1) zero valve error (bit-2) O_2 inop. (bit-3) occlusion	AA zero error N_2O zero error O_2 zero error CO_2 error	binary
2	(bit-0) CO_2 low (bit-1) CO_2 high (bit-2) rebreathing (bit-3) apnoea	AA low AA high O_2 low O_2 high	binary
3	(bit-0) HR low (bit-1) HR high (bit-2) ECG leads off (bit-3) asystole	BP_2 syst./mean low BP_2 syst./mean high BP_1/NIBP low BP_1/NIBP high	binary
4	ECG size number N; range 1–99 calib. = $1/(0.051 \times (N - 5) + 0.25)$ mV/cm		decimal
5	invasive BP_1 range 0 = BP_1 not used 1 = 0–100 mm Hg 2 = 0–50 mm Hg 3 = 0–25 mm Hg 4 = zero error 5 = 150 mm Hg ref. 6 = 12.5 mm Hg ref.	invasive BP_2 range 0 = BP_2 not used 1 = 0–100 mm Hg 2 = 0–50 mm Hg 3 = 0–25 mm Hg 4 = zero error 5 = 150 mm Hg ref. 6 = 12.5 mm Hg ref.	decimal
6	pleth. size; range 1–99		decimal
7	(bit-0) poor signal quality (bit-1) no pulse (bit-2) no finger (bit-3) no probe	HR low HR high SaO_2 low SaO_2 high	binary

given in Table 13.18. However, if the 1st character of a Cardiocap™ II status code is 5 then it is clear from Table 13.18 that the 2nd and 3rd characters must be taken individually.

13.4.2 Binary coding

When the right-hand column of Tables 13.17 and 13.18 indicates that the coding is *binary*, then the 2nd and 3rd characters are bit-encoded. The Datex encoding system uses the lowest 4 bits of the 2nd and 3rd characters to code for the four status messages associated with each binary status group. It is therefore convenient to use the hexadecimal notation, since the lowest 4 bits of an ASCII character are represented by the lowest (rightmost) character of its hexadecimal equivalent.†

For example, if the 2nd or 3rd character is < then Table 13.16 indicates that this character is equivalent to 3Ch. Since the binary equivalent of Ch is 1100, this indicates that the status code character < refers to the status messages associated with bit-2 and bit-3.

13.4.3 Examples

The following three examples of status codes from a Cardiocap™ II monitor illustrate the encoding process.

- **Status code 425** The first character is 4, and so the 2nd and 3rd characters are regarded as being decimal. Table 13.18 shows that in this case the 2nd and 3rd characters are to be taken together, and therefore represent the decimal value 25. Thus $N = 25$, and substituting this value into the equation gives the ECG calibration as 0.78 mV/cm.
- **Status code 22:** The first digit is 2, and Table 13.18 indicates that the 2nd and 3rd characters (2:) are bit-encoded (binary). The hexadecimal equivalent of the 2nd character (2) is 32h, and the lowest 4 bits are therefore represented by 2h, which is equivalent to 0010, which therefore codes for bit-1, which relates to the status message 'CO_2 high' (see Table 13.18). Similarly, the hexadecimal equivalent of the 3rd character (:) is 3Ah, and the lowest 4 bits are therefore represented by Ah, which is equivalent to 1010. This therefore codes for bit-1 and bit-3, which relate to the status messages 'AA high' and 'O_2 high'.
- **Status code 513** The first character is 5, and so the 2nd and 3rd characters are regarding as being decimal. Table 13.18 shows that in this case the 2nd and 3rd characters are considered separately. Thus the 2nd character (1) indicates that the range of the BP_1 scale is 0–100 mm Hg, and the 3rd character (3) indicates that the range of the BP_2 scale is 0–25 mm Hg.

13.5 Example program

The following example QuickBASIC 4.5 program demonstrates how to access the various data-strings and save them to a file (`datafile.dat`).

† See Appendix 8 for details of binary and hexadecimal notation.

The Datex Cardiocap™ *II and Capnomac Ultima*™ *series* 201

Separate subroutines are then used to decode each data-string, and print the data to the screen. The alarm strings are temporarily displayed on the screen as and when they occur. Pressing <Q> will quit the program. An example of the screen when running the program is shown in Figure 13.3.

Program points

- Because all data-strings are terminated by ⟨CR⟩⟨LF⟩ it is convenient to access the serial port data using the LINE INPUT # statement, which allocates everything up to the ⟨CR⟩ character to a specified variable (see Chapter 5). For example, in the example program the input data-strings are placed in the variable dataline$ prior to decoding, using the following statement.

```
LINE INPUT #1, dataline$
```

However, this has the effect of now making each dataline$ (except the first) start with ⟨LF⟩ as shown below.

$$\underbrace{C03, 000, 012, \ldots, 420}_{\text{dataline\$}} \langle CR \rangle \underbrace{\langle LF \rangle C03, 000, 013, \ldots, 420}_{\text{dataline\$}} \langle CR \rangle \langle LF \rangle \ldots$$

The ⟨LF⟩ character now needs to be either removed, or allowed for when decoding the data-string. One way of doing this is to remove the ⟨LF⟩ character immediately following the LINE INPUT # statement, by preserving only that part of the data-string to the right of the ⟨LF⟩ character using the RIGHT$ statement in the following way.

```
LINE INPUT #1, dataline$
L% = LEN(dataline$)
dataline$ = RIGHT$(dataline$, L% - 1)
```

- It is useful to allow the data-string to be accessed by all the subroutines, and this is arranged using the COMMON SHARED dataline$ statement in the main module.
- It is convenient to be able to view the stored data while running the program. In this example the data can be viewed by pressing <V>. First the file is closed in order to write any outstanding data to the file; then a file viewing utility (SHOW.COM†) is used to view the file; finally the file is reopened so it can receive more data. The QuickBASIC code for this is as follows.

† SHOW.COM is marketed by Clockwork Software, Bidbury House, Havant, Hampshire, PO9 3JL, UK. Tel: +44–(0)1705–483217; Fax: +44–(0)1705–454233. See also Section 5.10.

```
    IF UCASE$(key$) = "V" THEN
        CLOSE #2
        REM use the SHOW utility to view file
        SHELL "show ultima.dat"
        OPEN "c:ultima.dat" FOR APPEND ACCESS READ WRITE AS #2
    END IF
```

  Further details on how to view files are given in Section 5.10.
- The time is printed to the data file (ultima.dat) at the beginning of each group of data. This is achieved using a two-character string (loop$) to which is added the letter A or B depending on which of the two loops is being executed at the time. Only if the end of loop$ consists of the combination AA will the time be printed to the file, following which the letter B is added to the end of loop$. The code used in the example program is as follows.

```
loop$ = RIGHT$(loop$ + "A", 2)
...
...
IF loop$ = "AA" THEN PRINT #2, TIME$
loop$ = loop$ + "B"
```

- While the program is designed to be used with the Capnomac Ultima™ it can be used to collect the data-strings from any Datex monitor. However, under these circumstances, the particular screen position to which the various data-strings are printed will have to be adjusted accordingly—see the SELECT CASE routine towards the end of the main module.

Example program

```
REM [ultima.bas]
REM program to access data from the Capnomac Ultima
REM
DECLARE SUB getdata ()
DECLARE SUB getB00data ()
DECLARE SUB getU01data ()
DECLARE SUB getU03data ()
COMMON SHARED dataline$
REM white text / blue background
```

```
REM COLOR 15, 1
CLS
OPEN "COM1:1200,N,8,1,CS,DS,CD" FOR INPUT AS #1
OPEN "c:ultima.dat" FOR OUTPUT AS #2
PRINT #2, "SAVING CAPNOMAC ULTIMA DATA", DATE$
LOCATE 1
PRINT "Program to access data from the Capnomac Ultima"
LOCATE 2
PRINT "All data saved to file <ultima.dat>"
LOCATE 3
PRINT "Press <Q> to QUIT;   <V> to view stored data"
LOCATE 2, 59
PRINT "waiting for data"
DO
    timezero = TIMER
    REM add slight delay to stop buffer emptying
    SLEEP 1
    DO
        REM add A to the loop$ and save last two characters
        loop$ = RIGHT$(loop$ + "A", 2)
        REM update screen clock
        LOCATE 1, 59: PRINT TIME$
        IF TIMER > timezero + 2 THEN
            LOCATE 2, 59
            PRINT "waiting for data" + SPACE$(1) + "(" +
LTRIM$(STR$(INT(TIMER - timezero))) + ")"
        END IF
        REM detect <Q> keypress to quit program
        key$ = INKEY$
        IF UCASE$(key$) = "Q" THEN
            CLOSE
            END
        END IF
        REM view the stored data by pressing <V>
        IF UCASE$(key$) = "V" THEN
            REM write all data in the buffer to file
            CLOSE #2
            REM use SHOW.COM to view the datafile
            SHELL "show ultima.dat"
            REM re-open the file without losing data
```

```
            OPEN "c:ultima.dat" FOR APPEND ACCESS READ WRITE
AS #2
            LOCATE 2, 59
            PRINT "waiting for data"
        END IF
        REM overwrite the *
        LOCATE 1, 73: PRINT SPACE$(1)
        REM loop if no data in buffer
    LOOP WHILE LOC(1) <= 1
    REM print current time to file on first loop
    IF loop$ = "AA" THEN PRINT #2, TIME$
    loop$ = loop$ + "B"
    REM indicate when data is being received
    LOCATE 1, 73: PRINT "*"
    LOCATE 2, 59: PRINT SPACE$(22)
    REM input one data-string from serial port buffer
    LINE INPUT #1, dataline$
    REM remove the initial LF character when present
    IF LEFT$(dataline$, 1) = CHR$(1Ø) THEN
        L% = LEN(dataline$)
        dataline$ = RIGHT$(dataline$, L% - 1)
    END IF
    REM read the initial string code
    code$ = LEFT$(dataline$, 3)
    SELECT CASE code$
        CASE "BØØ"
            PRINT #2, dataline$
            LOCATE 5: PRINT dataline$
            CALL getBØØdata
        CASE "UØ1"
            PRINT #2, dataline$
            LOCATE 6: PRINT dataline$
            CALL getUØ1data
        CASE "UØ3"
            PRINT #2, dataline$
            LOCATE 7: PRINT dataline$
            CALL getUØ3data
        CASE "CØØ"
            LOCATE 9: PRINT dataline$
            PRINT #2, dataline$
```

```
        CASE "C01"
            LOCATE 5: PRINT dataline$
            PRINT #2, dataline$
        CASE "C02"
            LOCATE 9: PRINT dataline$
            PRINT #2, dataline$
        CASE "C03"
            LOCATE 9: PRINT dataline$
            PRINT #2, dataline$
        CASE "C04"
            LOCATE 23: PRINT dataline$
            PRINT #2, dataline$
    END SELECT
    REM identify alarm strings (second character = 9)
    IF MID$(code$, 2, 1) = "9" THEN
        alarm$ = dataline$
        PRINT #2, dataline$
        REM overwrite last alarm string with blanks
        LOCATE 8: PRINT SPACE$(40)
        LOCATE 8: PRINT "ALARM: "; alarm$
    END IF
LOOP
END


SUB getB00data
    REM decoding the Ultima B00 data-string
    REM 16 groups of data
    REM group 2
    a$ = MID$(dataline$, 5, 3)
    hour$ = RIGHT$("0" + LTRIM$(STR$(VAL(a$))), 2)
    REM group 3
    a$ = MID$(dataline$, 9, 3)
    min$ = RIGHT$("0" + LTRIM$(STR$(VAL(a$))), 2)
    REM group 4
    etco2$ = MID$(dataline$, 13, 3)
    REM determine the Integer part
    I$ = RIGHT$("0" + LTRIM$(STR$(VAL(LEFT$(etco2$, 2)))), 2)
    REM determine the Decimal part
    D$ = LTRIM$(STR$(VAL(RIGHT$(etco2$, 1))))
```

```
            etco2$ = I$ + "." + D$
            REM groups 5-9 not used by this program
            REM group 10
            etaa$ = MID$(dataline$, 37, 3)
            I$ = LTRIM$(STR$(VAL(LEFT$(etaa$, 1))))
            D$ = RIGHT$("Ø" + LTRIM$(STR$(VAL(RIGHT$(etaa$, 2)))), 2)
            etaa$ = I$ + "." + D$
            REM group 11
            fiaa$ = MID$(dataline$, 41, 3)
            I$ = LTRIM$(STR$(VAL(LEFT$(fiaa$, 1))))
            D$ = RIGHT$("Ø" + LTRIM$(STR$(VAL(RIGHT$(fiaa$, 2)))), 2)
            fiaa$ = I$ + "." + D$
            REM group 12
            a$ = MID$(dataline$, 45, 3)
            AA$ = a$
            IF a$ = SPACE$(3) THEN AA$ = "NO AGENT    "
            IF a$ = "HAL" THEN AA$ = "HALOTHANE   "
            IF a$ = "ENF" THEN AA$ = "ENFLURANE   "
            IF a$ = "ISO" THEN AA$ = "ISOFLURANE  "
            IF a$ = "DES" THEN AA$ = "DESFLURANE  "
            IF a$ = "SEV" THEN AA$ = "SEVOFLURANE"
            REM group 13
            a$ = MID$(dataline$, 49, 3)
            rr$ = RIGHT$("Ø" + LTRIM$(STR$(VAL(a$))), 2)
            REM group 14
            gaspressure$ = MID$(dataline$, 53, 3)
            REM group 15
            rec.output$ = MID$(dataline$, 57, 3)
            REM group 16
            bØØstatus$ = MID$(dataline$, 61, 3)
            REM
            LOCATE 10, 2: PRINT "Time     = "; hour$ + ":" + min$ + " hrs"
            LOCATE 15, 2: PRINT "EtCO2 = "; etco2$ + " %"
            LOCATE 16, 2: PRINT "Agent = "; AA$
            LOCATE 17, 2: PRINT "Insp agent  = "; fiaa$ + " %"
            LOCATE 18, 2: PRINT "Exp agent   = "; etaa$ + " %"
            LOCATE 10, 40: PRINT "Resp rate = "; rr$ + " /min"
            LOCATE 20, 2: PRINT "BØØ status = "; bØØstatus$
        END SUB
```

```
SUB getU01data
    REM decoding the Ultima U01 data-string
    REM 20 groups of data
    REM
    REM group 3
    eto2$ = MID$(dataline$, 9, 3)
    REM determine the Integer part
    I$ = RIGHT$("0" + LTRIM$(STR$(VAL(LEFT$(eto2$, 2)))), 2)
    REM determine the Decimal part
    D$ = LTRIM$(STR$(VAL(RIGHT$(eto2$, 1))))
    eto2$ = I$ + "." + D$
    REM group 4
    fio2$ = MID$(dataline$, 13, 3)
    I$ = RIGHT$("0" + LTRIM$(STR$(VAL(LEFT$(fio2$, 2)))), 2)
    D$ = LTRIM$(STR$(VAL(RIGHT$(fio2$, 1))))
    fio2$ = I$ + "." + D$
    REM groups 5-14 not used by this program
    REM group 15
    a$ = MID$(dataline$, 57, 3)
    heart.rate$ = RIGHT$("00" + LTRIM$(STR$(VAL(a$))), 3)
    REM group 16
    a$ = MID$(dataline$, 61, 3)
    sat$ = RIGHT$("00" + LTRIM$(STR$(VAL(a$))), 3)
    REM groups 17-19 not used by this program
    REM group 20
    u01status$ = MID$(dataline$, 77, 3)
    REM
    LOCATE 13, 2: PRINT "EtO2 = "; eto2$ + " %"
    LOCATE 12, 2: PRINT "FiO2 = "; fio2$ + " %"
    LOCATE 11, 2: PRINT "HR = "; heart.rate$; " /min"
    LOCATE 14, 2: PRINT "Sat = "; sat$; " %"
    LOCATE 21, 2: PRINT "U01 status = "; u01status$
END SUB


SUB getU03data
    REM decoding the Ultima U03 data-string
    REM 20 groups of data
    REM group 2
```

```
expmv$ = MID$(dataline$, 5, 3)
Iexpmv$ = LEFT$(expmv$, 2)
Dexpmv$ = RIGHT$(expmv$, 1)
REM group 3
inspmv$ = MID$(dataline$, 9, 3)
Iinspmv$ = LEFT$(inspmv$, 2)
Dinspmv$ = RIGHT$(inspmv$, 1)
REM group 4 (exp TV (high - Litres))
a$ = MID$(dataline$, 13, 3)
Iexptv$ = LTRIM$(STR$(VAL(a$)))
REM group 5 (exp TV (low-mls))
Dexptv$ = MID$(dataline$, 17, 3)
REM group 6 (insp TV high (L))
a$ = MID$(dataline$, 21, 3)
REM determine the Integer value
Iinsptv$ = LTRIM$(STR$(VAL(a$)))
REM group 7 (insp TV low-mls)
Dinsptv$ = MID$(dataline$, 25, 3)
REM group 8 (V1.0 (%))
a$ = MID$(dataline$, 29, 3)
V1$ = RIGHT$("00" + a$, 2)
REM group 9 (compliance)
a$ = MID$(dataline$, 33, 3)
compliance = VAL(a$)
REM group 10 (peak airway pressure)
peakpressure% = VAL(MID$(dataline$, 37, 3))
REM group 11 (plateau airway pressure)
plateaupressure% = VAL(MID$(dataline$, 41, 3))
REM group 12 (PEEP)
peep% = VAL(MID$(dataline$, 45, 3))
REM group 13 (I:E ratio)
ie.ratio$ = MID$(dataline$, 49, 3)
Iie.ratio$ = MID$(ie.ratio$, 2, 1)
Die.ratio$ = RIGHT$(ie.ratio$, 1)
REM groups 14 - 18 not used by this program
REM group 19 (units status)
a$ = MID$(dataline$, 73, 3)
units$ = RIGHT$(a$, 2)
REM determine which units are being used
REM k is a factor used to scale the units correctly
```

```
        IF units$ = "ØØ" THEN
            pressureunits$ = "cms H2O"
            complianceunits$ = "mls/cm H2O"
            k = 1
        END IF
        IF units$ = "Ø1" THEN
            pressureunits$ = "kPa"
            complianceunits$ = "mls/kPa"
            k = 1Ø
        END IF
        IF units$ = "1Ø" THEN
            pressureunits$ = "mm Hg"
            complianceunits$ = "mls/mm Hg"
            k = 1
        END IF
    REM group 2Ø (status)
    uØ3status$ = MID$(dataline$, 77, 3)
    REM
    LOCATE 11, 4Ø
    PRINT "Insp TV = "; Iinsptv$ + "." + Dinsptv$ + " L"
    LOCATE 12, 4Ø
    PRINT "Exp TV  = "; Iexptv$ + "." + Dexptv$ + " L"
    LOCATE 13, 4Ø
    PRINT "Insp MV = "; Iinspmv$ + "." + Dinspmv$ + " L"
    LOCATE 14, 4Ø
    PRINT "Exp MV  = "; Iexpmv$ + "." + Dexpmv$ + " L"
    LOCATE 15, 4Ø
    PRINT "Compliance = "; RIGHT$("ØØ" + LTRIM$(STR$(
compliance / k)), 2) + SPACE$(1) + complianceunits$
    LOCATE 16, 4Ø
    PRINT "V(1.Ø) = "; V1$ + " %"
    LOCATE 17, 4Ø
    PRINT "Peak pressure = "; RIGHT$("ØØ" + LTRIM$(STR$(
peakpressure% * k)), 2) + SPACE$(1) + pressureunits$
    LOCATE 18, 4Ø
    PRINT "Plat. pressure = "; RIGHT$("ØØ" + LTRIM$(STR$(
plateaupressure% * k)), 2) + SPACE$(1) + pressureunits$
    LOCATE 19, 4Ø
    PRINT "PEEP = "; RIGHT$("ØØ" + LTRIM$(STR$(peep% * k)),
2) + SPACE$(1) + pressureunits$
```

```
    LOCATE 20, 40
    PRINT "I:E ratio = "; 1; ":" + SPACE$(1) + Iie.ratio$
+ "." + Die.ratio$
    LOCATE 22, 2: PRINT "U03 status = "; u03status$
END SUB
```

14
The Graseby 3400 syringe pump

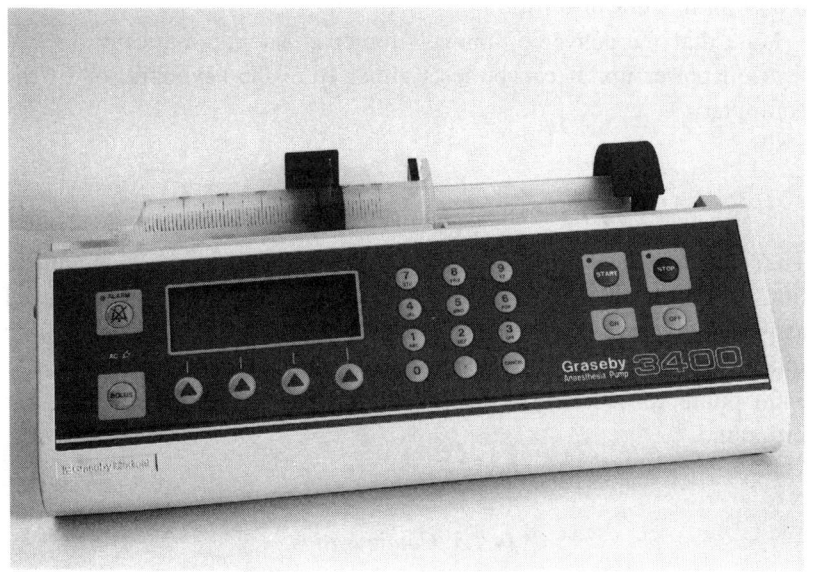

14.1 Introduction

The Graseby 3400 syringe pump† caters for a wide range of syringes (5–60 ml), and can deliver maintenance flow rates in the range 0.1–400 ml/hr in steps of 0.1 ml/hr. It has a bolus facility which allows flow rates up to 1200 ml/hr. When disconnected from the mains supply the pump will operate for more than 10 hours on internal rechargeable batteries.

The pump can be operated manually using touch-keys on the front panel, and all information regarding the pump's activity is shown on a liquid-crystal display (LCD). The 3400 pump can also be computer driven via the serial port, using a maximum bit-rate of 9600 bps. For

---

† Graseby Medical Limited, Colonial Way, Watford, Hertfordshire, WD2 4GL, UK. Tel: +44–(0)1923–246434. Fax: +44–(0)1923–231595.

safety, the <STOP> key on the front panel will override computer-based instructions.

The electrical safety classification of the Graseby 3400 syringe pump is Type CF.†

14.1.1 Volume infused

The pump keeps a running total of the delivered volume, and this is maintained when the pump is stopped and restarted. The range is 0–999 ml in steps of 0.1 ml.

Note that the delivered volume counter is *not* automatically reset to zero on power up. It can be reset either from the keyboard, or by the computer.

14.1.2 Communications software version

That part of the pump's software which implements serial communications (**Protocol** software) is currently at version 2.0. This value is returned as part of the reply message to the 'check pump status' and 'check pump rate' commands. This allows computer programs written to drive the 3400 pump to check that the Protocol version is appropriate for the program.

14.1.3 Configuration

The Graseby 3400 must be initially configured for bit-rate, syringe type, language, and maximum prescribable flow-rate via the **Configuration** mode‡, which is accessed as follows.

(1) First stop the pump by pressing the <STOP> key.
(2) Simultaneously press the second triangular key from the right *and* the <BOLUS> key until the graphics window displays CONFIGURATION?
(3) Now release the two touch-keys, and quickly (within 2 seconds) press the <START> key. The graphics window will now display the Configuration menu, starting with the syringe type.

† See Chapter 7 for further details.
‡ Note that the 'bolus' rate is set separately—see Section 14.1.4 on maximum infusion rates.

Table 14.1. *Graseby 3400 configuration options.*

Option	Comments
Syringe type	A wide range of syringes can be used – see pump manual for full listing.
Bit-rate	300, 600, 1200, 2400, 4800, 9600.
Language	English, German, French, Italian, Dutch.
LCD contrast	1–20
Maximum rate	0.1–1200 mls/hr

Table 14.2. *Graseby 3400 maximum infusion rates.*

Syringe size (ml)	Maximum rate (ml/hr)
50–60	1200.0
30–35	600.0
20	400.0
10	200.0
5	100.0

(4) Step through the menu (use the <NEXT> key) and set the options (use the <CHANGE> key) as required. Pressing the <STOP> key will exit the menu and return the pump to its normal operating mode.

The options accessed via the Configuration mode are shown in Table 14.1.

14.1.4 Maximum infusion rates

The maximum prescribable infusion rate can be set within the range 0.1–1200 ml/hr by accessing the Configuration mode. However, the maximum infusion rate for both maintenance and bolus infusions does vary with syringe size as shown in Table 14.2. Rates above 400 ml/hr cannot be set from the front panel except in Bolus mode.

Changing the bolus rate. The bolus rate is changed by first pressing the <BOLUS> key and then pressing the <CHANGE> key. The new bolus rate can then be entered from the numeric keypad. After the new rate has been entered, then press the <BOLUS> key to complete the change.

Table 14.3. *Graseby 3400 serial port.*

Pin No.	Name	Comments
1	—	Not connected
2	RxD	Receives data
3	TxD	Transmits data
4	—	Not connected
5	GND	Signal ground
6	DSR	Active handshake-out, i.e. the pump holds this pin HIGH (positive) only when it is ready to receive data. This pin should therefore be wired to the PC's CTS pin
7	RTS	Always held HIGH by the pump when it is powered up
8	CTS	This line must be held HIGH to enable the pump to output data to the computer
9	—	Not connected

14.1.5 Start-up time

The time taken for the pump to achieve the set infusion rate after the syringe is first loaded is known as the **start-up** time. This varies with both infusion rate and syringe size; the slower the infusion rate the longer the start-up time, with large syringes being worse than small ones in this respect.

Typical start-up times for a 50 ml syringe (i.e. immediately following loading the syringe) are as follows: 3 mins for a flow rate of 5 ml/hr, and 15 mins for a flow rate of 1 ml/hr.

14.2 Serial port

A male 9-pin D-type serial port is located on the rear panel of the pump. The pins used for communication are shown in Table 14.3. Only six pins are used for communications; the remaining pins are not connected internally.

The Graseby 3400 serial port requires a minimum input voltage (± 6 volts). This means that some portable PCs with low-voltage serial ports may be unable to drive the Graseby 3400.

Table 14.4. *Graseby 3400 protocol.*

Bit rate	300, 600, 1200, 2400, 4800, 9600
Data bits	8
Parity	None
Stop bits	1

14.2.1 Protocol options

With the exception of the bit-rate, which can be varied between 300 and 9600 bps, the protocol options are fixed as shown in Table 14.4. The bit-rate is set on the pump by entering the Configuration mode, and stepping through the bit-rate options (see Section 14.1.3).

14.2.2 Cable connections

Figure 14.1 indicates a convenient wiring configuration for interfacing to a PC.

- **RTS** The pump maintains its RTS line HIGH (positive) when it is powered up. This pin is probably best wired to the PC's DSR line since the PC requires its DSR line to be held HIGH in order for it to be able to read an incoming byte (see Section 4.5.3). A communications fault (i.e. pump power failure or serial port disconnection) can then be detected by the PC by monitoring the status of its own DSR line. If this is not HIGH then a fault exists.
- **DSR** The pump's DSR line is the active output handshaking line (control line), and is set HIGH (positive) only when the pump is ready to receive data. This pin should therefore be wired to the PC's CTS line, since the PC checks that its own CTS line is being held HIGH before outputting data (see Section 4.5.2).
- **CTS** The pump's CTS line must be held HIGH (positive) by the PC in order for the pump to be able to output data. Since QuickBASIC automatically sets the computer's RTS and DTR lines HIGH on executing the OPEN COM statement† (unless the RS option is used), the pump's CTS can be wired to either RTS or DTR at the PC.

† See Chapter 5 and Appendix 6 for details of the OPEN COM statement.

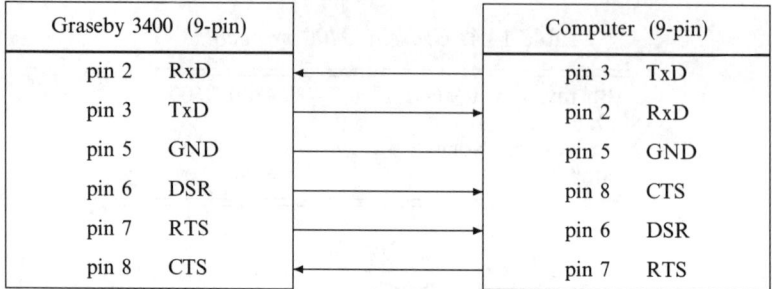

Fig. 14.1. Wiring diagram for the Graseby 3400.

14.3 Commands and replies

There are a number of **commands** available for communicating with the pump, each generating a **reply**. Commands either instruct the pump (e.g. stop the pump), or request data (e.g. send total volume infused). Replies return status information, and also indicate when the command syntax is incorrect.

The 3400 pump uses a two-character hexadecimal checksum (i.e. an 8-bit checksum) for both commands and replies; this is described more fully in Section 14.3.4 below.

14.3.1 Command string structure

Command messages are transmitted by the computer, and require the command and parameter (where appropriate) to be enclosed within angle brackets, followed by the two-character hexadecimal checksum and ⟨CR⟩ as follows.

$$\underbrace{\langle<\rangle \overbrace{\langle\text{command}\rangle\langle\text{parameter}\rangle}^{\textit{command message}} \langle>\rangle\langle\text{checksum}\rangle\langle\text{CR}\rangle}_{\textit{command string}}$$

The components of the command string are detailed below.

<   The 'start of command' character (ASCII 60).
command   A four-character command-code (capital letters only).
parameter   A variable length decimal number. Note that the command parameter (when applicable) is the infusion rate ×10 since this avoids the use of decimal points. For

The Graseby 3400 syringe pump 217

Table 14.5. *Graseby 3400 command messages.*

Meaning	Command	Parameter	Example string
Start pump	STRT	—	<STRT>C7⟨CR⟩
Stop pump	STOP	—	<STOP>C0⟨CR⟩
Change rate	CHGR	0–12000	<CHGR145>38⟨CR⟩
Get pump-rate	GETR	—	<GETR>AC⟨CR⟩
Get volume infused	TOTL	—	<TOTL>BD⟨CR⟩
Reset volume infused	ZTOT	—	<ZTOT>CB⟨CR⟩
Check pump	CHCK	—	<CHCK>93⟨CR⟩
Check pump-rate	CHKR	0–12000	<CHKR1200>65⟨CR⟩

example, the command string <CHGR145>38⟨CR⟩ tells the pump to change rate to 14.5 ml/hr.

> The 'end of command' character (ASCII 62).

checksum A two-character hexadecimal checksum.

⟨CR⟩ The packet terminating character. The Graseby 3400 command message format specifies that the message must be terminated with a ⟨CR⟩. However, care must be taken not to inadvertently send *two* ⟨CR⟩'s to the pump, since this is easily done if a ⟨CR⟩ is included in the string to be transmitted using the PRINT# statement *without* a following semicolon to suppress the ⟨CR⟩ which is otherwise routinely added by the PRINT# statement (see Section 5.3.1).

If two ⟨CR⟩'s are included in a command string received by the pump, it will therefore return two reply messages, thinking that two command messages were sent. The second reply message will therefore be <SXIVLD>54⟨CR⟩⟨LF⟩ indicating a syntax error (see Table 14.6).

For convenience, examples of the various commands and parameters together with the full command string, are listed in Table 14.5.

14.3.2 Reply string structure

Reply messages are transmitted by the pump in response to a command message. The reply string consists of an initial acknowledge-code (OK, SX, or CE), followed by the original command (STRT, STOP, etc.), an optional status code (STBY, INFS, or ALRM), an optional parameter, checksum, and

Table 14.6. *Graseby 3400 acknowledge and status codes.*

	Code	Meaning
ACK-codes	OK	The command has been actioned and/or the reply is valid.
	SX	The string contained a syntax error. The command was not actioned.
	CE	The message contained a command error. The general format was correct, but either a parameter was out of range, or the pump was not in the correct state to be able to action the command. The command was not actioned.
Status codes	STBY	The pump is stopped and is in standby mode.
	INFS	The pump is infusing.
	ALRM	The pump is in an alarm state. Note that alarms can only be cleared from the front panel; in addition, the 'occlusion' alarm state can only be cleared by first opening the syringe 'plunger clamp'. Alarms are accompanied by a message displayed in the pump's LCD window.
	IVLD	The command message was invalid.

$\langle CR \rangle \langle LF \rangle$. The acknowledge and status codes are shown in Table 14.6. The general structure of the reply string is as follows.

$$\underbrace{\langle < \rangle \overbrace{\langle \text{ACK-code} \rangle \langle \text{command} \rangle \langle \text{status} \rangle \langle \text{parameter} \rangle}^{\text{reply message}} \langle > \rangle \langle \text{checksum} \rangle \langle CR \rangle \langle LF \rangle}_{\text{reply string}}$$

An important feature of the Graseby 3400 reply message format is the inclusion of the initiating command, which is extremely valuable from a programing point of view.

14.3.3 The commands

The eight commands which are used to control the pump are now described in detail. Note that the Graseby 3400 protocol requires all commands to be in uppercase letters. Table 14.7 summarises the command and reply strings.

The Graseby 3400 syringe pump 219

- **Start pump**   The command to start the pump is STRT. It takes no parameter as the infusion rate is set using a separate command (see below). If the infusion rate is zero, then the pump will reply with OKSTRTSTBY.
  Command: STRT
  Example replies: OKSTRTINFS   OKSTRTSTBY

- **Stop pump**   The command to stop the pump is STOP. The normal reply has STBY status
  Command: STOP
  Example reply: OKSTOPSTBY

- **Change rate**   The command to change the infusion rate is CHGR followed by the 'rate' parameter (1–12000). Note that the rate parameter is the *true* rate ×10; i.e. a rate parameter of 155 corresponds to a *true* rate of 15.5 ml/hr. If the pump is stopped and in standby mode when a 'change rate' command is received, then the pump will remain stopped, change its rate setting, and then reply using the status code STBY. If the 'change rate' command is used while the pump is infusing, the pump will sound a 'beep' to indicate that the rate has changed.†
  Example command: CHGR145
  Example replies: OKCHGR145   OKCHGRSTBY145

- **Get pump rate**   The command for getting the current infusion rate is GETR. It returns a rate parameter in the range 1–12000 corresponding to a true value in the range 0.1–1200 ml/hr.
  Command: GETR
  Example reply: OKGETRINFS145

- **Get volume infused**   The command for getting the total volume infused is TOTL. It returns a volume parameter in the range 0–9999 corresponding to a true value in the range 0–999.9 ml.
  Command: TOTL
  Example reply: OKTOTLINFS543

- **Reset volume-infused counter**   The command to reset the volume-infused counter to zero is ZTOT. Note that this command will *only* work if the pump is stopped. If the pump is infusing when it receives the command, then it replies using the error code CE (see Table 14.6).
  Command: ZTOT
  Example replies: OKZTOTSTBY   CEZTOTINFS

† Recent software versions allow the beep to be disabled.

Table 14.7. *Examples of command and reply strings.*

Command string	Reply string
<STRT>C7⟨CR⟩	<OKSTRTINFS>91⟨CR⟩⟨LF⟩
<STOP>C0⟨CR⟩	<OKSTOPSTBY>9C⟨CR⟩⟨LF⟩
<CHGR145>38⟨CR⟩	<OKCHGR145>02⟨CR⟩⟨LF⟩
<GETR>AC⟨CR⟩	<OKGETRINFS145>10⟨CR⟩⟨LF⟩
<TOTL>BD⟨CR⟩	<OKTOTLINFS211>1B⟨CR⟩⟨LF⟩
<ZTOT>CB⟨CR⟩	<CEZTOTINFS>83⟨CR⟩⟨LF⟩
<CHCK>C3⟨CR⟩	<OKCHCKINFSV2.0>43⟨CR⟩⟨LF⟩
<CHKR1200>65⟨CR⟩	<OKCHKRINFSV2.0>52⟨CR⟩⟨LF⟩

- **Check pump status** The command for getting the pump's current status is CHCK. The pump returns the status parameter, together with the version number of the Protocol software which implements the serial communications (currently V2.0).
  Command: CHCK
  Example reply: OKCHCKINFSV2.0   OKCHCKALRMV2.0

- **Check pump-rate** The command for checking the current infusion rate is CHKR. The rate parameter is the *expected* infusion rate, and must be in the range 1–12000, i.e. corresponding to a true value in the range 0.1–1200 ml/hr. The pump returns the status parameter together with the version number of the Protocol software which implements the serial communications (currently V2.0). *This command must be sent to the pump at least every 3 seconds in order to sustain a continuous infusion.* If the infusion rates do not correspond, the pump replies with the CE error code. If the correct command is not sent within 3 seconds, then the pump enters an alarm state and stops infusing.
  Example command: CHKR443
  Example replies: OKCHKRINFSV2.0   CECHKRV2.0

14.3.4 The checksum

The checksum used by the Graseby 3400 pump is an 8-bit Σ-checksum† (i.e. *modulo*256), expressed in hexadecimal notation (i.e. two characters), and is used for both command and reply messages. The Graseby

† See Section 3.4.1 for details of this particular checksum.

The Graseby 3400 syringe pump 221

3400 checksum includes the start-of-message symbol < (ASCII 60), the command-code, the parameter (when used), and the end-of-message symbol > (ASCII 62).

Note that the Graseby 3400 checksum is always expressed as two hexadecimal characters, even when the decimal checksum is less than 16. For example, a reply checksum of 14 is expressed by the pump as 0E. However, the QuickBASIC HEX$(14) will return only E. When checking the reply to see whether the message agrees with the returned checksum, it is important therefore that the program adds one leading zero when determining hexadecimal checksums for values less than 16 (see Section 3.4).

14.4 Example interactive program

When writing programs for the Graseby 3400 pump, it is useful to first make an interactive utility program for testing the various commands and showing the replies and checksums. An example of such a program is shown below, and indicates how to send command messages interactively from the keyboard, collect the reply and save it to a log file.

The following example QuickBASIC 4.5 program prompts the operator for a command, and sends it to the pump on pressing <ENTER>. The program then displays both the command and reply messages, and also prints all messages to a log file (log3400.dat) in the same directory (opened as #2). Pressing <Q> exits from the program.

The screen appears as shown in Figure 14.2.

```
enter a command for the pump    STOP

buffer emptied OK
sending message         <STOP>C0
reply =                 <OKSTOPSTBY>9C

press any key to continue (<Q> to quit)
```

Fig. 14.2. An example of the screen when using the interactive program **grasebya.bas**.

Program points

- Check that both the program and syringe pump are configured for the same bit rate.
- In the subroutine SEND there is no ⟨CR⟩ in the string to be sent to the pump (s$ = CHR$(60) + UCASE$(s$) + CHR$(62)) since the final ⟨CR⟩ is added by the PRINT# statement.
- Since all Graseby 3400 commands must be in uppercase, the subroutine SEND does the conversion automatically. Lowercase letters can therefore be entered from the keyboard.
- Note that the SLEEP statement is followed by z$ = INKEY$. This is to remedy a QuickBASIC 'bug' whereby the keyboard buffer fails to be cleared following SLEEP (see Microsoft, 1989e).

Example program

```
REM [grasebya.bas]
REM interactive program for Graseby 3400 syringe pump
DECLARE SUB emptybuffer ()
DECLARE SUB send (s$)
DECLARE SUB getreply ()
DECLARE FUNCTION checksum% (c$)
CLEAR
OPEN "COM1:9600,N,8,1,CS,DS" FOR RANDOM ACCESS READ WRITE
                                                         AS #1
OPEN "c:log3400.dat" FOR OUTPUT AS #2
DO
    CLS
    LOCATE 5, 5
    INPUT "enter a command for the pump "; pumpCOMMAND$
    PRINT
    IF UCASE$(pumpCOMMAND$) = "Q" THEN
        CLOSE #1, #2
        END
    END IF
    CALL send(pumpCOMMAND$)
    CALL getreply
    PRINT "press any key to continue (<Q> to quit)"
    SLEEP : z$ = INKEY$ : IF z$ = "Q" THEN END
```

```
LOOP
END



FUNCTION checksum% (c$)
    REM generates an 8-bit checksum
    sum% = 0
    FOR J = 1 TO LEN(c$)
        sum% = sum% + ASC(MID$(c$, J, 1))
    NEXT J
    checksum% = sum% MOD 256
END FUNCTION


SUB emptybuffer
    REM empties the receive buffer
    DO WHILE NOT EOF(1)
        buff$ = INPUT$(LOC(1), #1)
    LOOP
    PRINT "Buffer empty"
END SUB


SUB getreply
    a$ = ""
    LF$ = CHR$(10)
    starttime = TIMER :REM set timer for time-out
    DO
        DO
            a$ = a$ + INPUT$(LOC(1), #1)
            L% = INSTR(1, a$, LF$): REM looking for LF
            IF TIMER > starttime + 3 THEN END
        LOOP UNTIL L% > 0
        reply$ = MID$(a$, 1, L%)
        PRINT "reply = ", , reply$
        PRINT #2, "reply = ", reply$
        a$ = RIGHT$(a$, LEN(a$) - L%)
    LOOP UNTIL LEN(a$) = 0
END SUB
```

```
SUB send (s$)
    CALL emptybuffer
    s$ = CHR$(60) + UCASE$(s$) + CHR$(62)
    checksumhex$ = HEX$(checksum%(s$))
    PRINT #1, s$ + checksumhex$
    PRINT #2, s$ + checksumhex$
    PRINT "sending message ", s$ + checksumhex$
END SUB
```

14.5 Programming a continuous infusion

When controlling the pump during a continuous infusion, the pump's keyboard is locked out with the exception of the <STOP> key. This is a safety feature which allows the pump to be taken over manually, if necessary, by first stopping the pump and then adjusting the infusion rate.

14.5.1 Pump time-out

In order for the computer to sustain a continuous infusion, it is necessary to send a correct 'check rate' command (CHGR...) at least once every 3 seconds. Failing to do so results in the pump generating a *time-out* error causing an alarm state, and the pump stops. This is indicated by the message COMMS FAILURE in the pump's LCD window. An example of the check-rate command and reply is shown in Table 14.7.

14.5.2 Programing considerations

Since the version of the pump's Protocol software which implements the serial communications may be upgraded from time to time, it is important that the program detects the Protocol version used by the pump, and aborts if this is different from the expected version.

The program should also detect and respond appropriately to 'alarm' and 'standby' states as and when they occur, allowing the operator to either adjust the pump and continue with the infusion, or quit the program. Communication failures should also be detected (e.g. power failure, accidental switch off, or serial cable disconnection).

After sending a command, the reply relating to the command should always be collected and analysed before sending another command. In

The Graseby 3400 syringe pump 225

addition, the linking of replies to their initiating commands is facilitated by emptying the receive buffer immediately before sending a command. Note that Graseby's inclusion in replies of the initiating command is very useful for linking replies to their commands.

On receipt of a reply, its message should be checked against the returned checksum. If the reply indicates that either the syntax was invalid, or that the checksum was incorrect, then the error-handler should be called (the subroutine PUMPERROR in the example program below). Alternatively, the reply can be ignored, and the initiating command transmitted again.

For accurate control, the timing of infusion-rate changes is best related to delivered volume as measured by the pump itself rather than to the computer's time clock. Similarly, program variables are best chosen so that they indicate the units, e.g. rate.mlhr as a variable for the rate in ml/hr etc.

The program should also incorporate some system for checking that all calculations are performed correctly, in order to serve as a check against program corruption, and duplication of variables against PC RAM corruption.

14.5.3 Example program for a continuous infusion.

The following example QuickBASIC 4.5 program illustrates a method of driving the Graseby 3400 pump to help maintain anaesthesia using the intravenous anaesthetic drug Propofol. The example program delivers the infusion rates given in Table 14.8, which are those described by Roberts *et al.* (1988) to supplement fentanyl and nitrous oxide anaesthesia. Note that the example program does *not* incorporate a system for checking calculations of rate, volume etc.

The infusion rate can be changed within the range 1–12 (mg/kg)/hr (1, 2, 3...) at any time by pressing the <ESCAPE> key and then selecting an infusion rate by pressing one of the computer's 12 <FUNCTION> keys. The information regarding the progress of the infusion is given on the screen as shown in Figure 14.3.

Program points

- The program uses the subroutine RUNPUMP to drive the pump and sustain a continuous infusion, as well as for checking the pump rate and delivered volume, and writing data to the screen. Any problems are

```
Serial Coms data logged to file c:coms-log.dat     <Q> to quit
Time 15:04:02                                <ESC> to change rate
Elapsed time = 00:01:15

    weight = 76 kg
    drug = PROPOFOL 10 mg/ml
    infusion mode = STEP1 [dose rate 10 mg/kg/hr]
                        [duration 10 mins]
    status = INFUSING
    pump rate = 76 mls/hr
    volume delivered = 1.6 mls
    target volume = 12.66 mls

serial port activity 720
```

Fig. 14.3. An example of the screen while running the continuous infusion program **grasebyb.bas**. In this example the program has been running for 1 min 15 seconds, and is in the STEP1 phase, with 1.6 mls having been delivered. STEP2 will start when the target volume of 12.66 mls has been delivered.

Table 14.8. *Graseby 3400 regimen used in the example program for a continuous intravenous infusion using Propofol. The computer controlled infusion is started immediately following induction of anaesthesia.*

Step 1	10 (mg/kg)/hr for 10 mins
Step 2	8 (mg/kg)/hr for 10 mins
Step 3 (maintenance)	6 (mg/kg)/hr

directed to the error-handler subroutine PUMPERROR. The two infusion steps at rates 10 and 8 (mg/kg)/hr are controlled by the subroutine STEPPUMP. The maintenance infusion at 6 (mg/kg)/hr is controlled by the subroutine MAINTENANCE. The subroutine FUNCTIONKEY allows the infusion rate to be changed (in the range 1–12 (mg/kg)/hr) by pressing one of the 12 <FUNCTION> keys. The remaining subroutines send the command, get the reply, and empty the buffer.

- The parameters of the infusion regimen (infusion rates and times) are specified at the end of the main module in the following statements.

    ```
    CALL steppump(10, 10): REM (rate mg/kg/hr, time mins)
    CALL steppump(8, 10): REM (rate mg/kg/hr, time mins)
    CALL maintenance(6): REM (rate mg/kg/hr)
    ```

- The infusion rate is altered by using the <ESCAPE> and <FUNCTION>

- keys as described above. The scan codes for the various keys are given in Appendix 3. A note on trapping keys is given in Section 5.14.
- A bolus infusion of the drug (Propofol) can be given at any time using the front panel, by first stopping the pump. Following the bolus the program is restarted by pressing <C>, as indicated on the screen.
- The fastest bit rate (9600 bps) is used in view of the pump's time-out being only 3 seconds.
- If the serial connections are not those indicated in Figure 14.1 then changes may need to be made to the options in the OPEN COM statement.
- The example program uses COM1. If another COM port is used then appropriate changes will need to be made to the OPEN COM statement, and to the address used by the modem status register (see Section 4.4.5) in the program's DSR function.
- The value indicating serial port activity is incremented each time the subroutine SEND is called.
- Note that the variable replytimezero in the subroutine GETREPLY is used to implement a 2-second time-out for the reply wait time. The construction used is described in Section 5.12, and is also used in the **grasebya.bas** program.
- The program allows for two concentrations of Propofol, namely 10 mg/ml and 20 mg/ml.
- Enabling the Serial Coms log is particularly useful when debugging. The log (saved in the file c:coms-log.dat) records the details of every communication, and is therefore too detailed for general use. Note that the Serial Coms log accumulates at the rate of approximately 3 Mb per hour! An extract of the log is shown in Figure 14.4.
- A convenient way of viewing the Coms log file is to use one of the file viewing utilities (e.g. VIEW.EXE; see Section 5.10), and include the following routine at the end of the SHUTDOWN subroutine, between the CLOSE and the END statements.

```
IF log$ = "on" THEN
   PRINT : PRINT
   PRINT "inspect coms log file?  Y/N"
   SLEEP: key$ = INKEY$
   IF UCASE$(key$) = "Y" THEN SHELL "view c:coms-log.dat"
END IF
```

- It is important to check the acknowledge codes in the replies from the pump for the CE and SX codes (see Table 14.6). For example if the program is started while the pump is already running, then the pump will not respond to commands to change the rate. However, this problem is easily detected since under these circumstances the pump returns the CE acknowledge code in response to both the CHGR and CHKR commands.

Note that in order to avoid trapping the CE code directly from the GETREPLY subroutine, the program sets the variable ackerror$ and uses this to call the PUMPERROR subroutine from the RUNPUMP subroutine.

Example program†

```
REM [grasebyb.bas]
REM anaesthesia program for Graseby 3400 pump
REM (protocol version 2.0)
REM drug PROPOFOL (10 mg/ml or 20 mg/ml)
REM using Roberts et al. (1988) regimen
REM 10mg/kg/hr (10 mins), 8mg/kg/hr (10mins),
REM and then maintained at 6mg/kg/hr.
DECLARE FUNCTION checksumhex$ (c$)
DECLARE FUNCTION elapsedtime$ (seconds)
DECLARE FUNCTION DSR$ ()
DECLARE SUB pumperror ()
DECLARE SUB shutdown ()
DECLARE SUB maintenance (r.mgkghr)
DECLARE SUB steppump (r.mgkghr, td.mins)
DECLARE SUB runpump ()
DECLARE SUB getreply ()
DECLARE SUB setup ()
DECLARE SUB send (s$)
DECLARE SUB emptybuffer ()
DECLARE SUB functionkey ()
COMMON SHARED fullreply$, pumpstatus$, status$, mode$, p
COMMON SHARED weight.kg, conc.mgml, stepcount, log$
COMMON SHARED rate.mgkghr, rate.mlhr, targetvolume, volume
COMMON SHARED targettime.secs, timezero, timedelay.mins
COMMON SHARED ackcode$, ackerror$
CLEAR
```

† WARNING – The programs contained in this book are examples only. Anyone intending to make use of them for a specific purpose needs to bear in mind the author and publisher's disclaimer as detailed on p. xix.

```
REM check if pump is powered up by looking at DSR status
DO WHILE DSR$ = "low"
    CLS
    LOCATE 5
    PRINT "PUMP SWITCHED OFF / SERIAL CABLE FAULT"
    PRINT "press a key when ready / <Q> to quit"
    SLEEP: key$ = INKEY$: IF UCASE$(key$) = "Q" THEN END
LOOP
CLS
LOCATE 1, 2: PRINT "opening the port"
REM delay in case pump was off and key pressed too early
SLEEP 1
OPEN "COM1: 9600,N,8,1,CS,DS" FOR RANDOM ACCESS READ
                                            WRITE AS #1
REM check protocol version
CALL send("CHCK"): CALL getreply
version$ = MID$(fullreply$, 12, 4)
LOCATE , 2: PRINT "Protocol version  = "; version$
IF version$ <> "V2.0" THEN
    CLS
    PRINT "SOFTWARE VERSION ERROR"
    PRINT "pump version = "; version$
    END
END IF
REM log facility
logloop:
LOCATE 5, 2
PRINT "enable Serial Comms LOG facility? (Y/N)"
SLEEP: key$ = INKEY$
SELECT CASE UCASE$(key$)
    CASE "Y"
        log$ = "on"
        OPEN "c:coms-log.dat" FOR OUTPUT AS #2
        PRINT #2, "port open OK", DATE$, TIME$
    CASE ELSE
        log$ = "off"
END SELECT
propofolconcloop:
CLS
LOCATE 5, 30: PRINT "PROPOFOL CONCENTRATION"
```

```
          LOCATE 10, 2: INPUT "Enter PROPOFOL concentration (10 mg/ml
                                            or 20 mg/ml)"; conc.mgml
     SELECT CASE conc.mgml
          CASE 10, 20
               LOCATE 10, 2: PRINT "PROPOFOL concentration =";
                              conc.mgml; " mg/ml"; SPACE$(30)
               LOCATE 12, 2: PRINT "is this correct?   (Y/N)
                                                        <Q> to quit"
               SLEEP: key$ = INKEY$
               SELECT CASE UCASE$(key$)
                    CASE "Y"
                    CASE "Q"
                         CLOSE
                         END
                    CASE ELSE
                         CLS
                         GOTO propofolconcloop
               END SELECT
          CASE ELSE
               CLS
               GOTO propofolconcloop
     END SELECT
     weightloop:
     CLS
     LOCATE 5, 35: PRINT "WEIGHT"
     LOCATE 10, 2: INPUT "Enter weight in Kg"; weight.kg
     LOCATE 10, 2: PRINT "weight="; weight.kg; " kg"; SPACE$(30)
     LOCATE 12, 2: PRINT "is this correct?   (Y/N)   <Q> to quit"
     SLEEP: key$ = INKEY$
     SELECT CASE UCASE$(key$)
          CASE "Y"
               IF weight.kg = 0 THEN
                    LOCATE 8, 2: PRINT "weight = 0 ERROR"
                    LOCATE 12, 2: PRINT SPACE$(30)
                    GOTO weightloop
               END IF
          CASE "Q"
               CLOSE
               END
          CASE ELSE
```

```
            CLS
            GOTO weightloop
END SELECT
CLS
LOCATE 2, 5: PRINT "weight = "; weight.kg; "kg"
LOCATE 4, 5: PRINT "PROPOFOL concentration = "; conc.mgml;
                                                  "mg/ml"
LOCATE 10, 5: PRINT "press <S> to start pump (press <Q>
                                                  to quit)"
DO WHILE key$ <> "Q" OR key$ <> "S"
    key$ = UCASE$(INKEY$)
    IF key$ = "Q" THEN
        CLOSE
        END
    END IF
    IF key$ = "S" THEN EXIT DO
LOOP
CLS
CALL setup
CALL steppump(10, 10): REM (rate mg/kg/hr, time mins)
CALL steppump(8, 10): REM (rate mg/kg/hr, time mins)
CALL maintenance(6): REM (rate mg/kg/hr)
END

FUNCTION checksumhex$ (c$)
    REM generates a two character hex 8-bit checksum
    sum% = 0
    FOR J = 1 TO LEN(c$)
        sum% = sum% + ASC(MID$(c$, J, 1))
    NEXT J
    checksum% = sum% MOD 256
    checksumhex$ = RIGHT$("0" + HEX$(checksum%), 2)
END FUNCTION

FUNCTION DSR$
    REM using computer's DSR to detect status of pump's RTS
    REM computer's DSR is controlled by MSR bit-5
    REM using COM1
    msrcom1% = &H3FE: msrcom2% = &H2FE
    reg% = msrcom1%
```

```
    IF (INP(reg%) AND 2 ^ 5) = 2 ^ 5 THEN
        DSR$ = "high"
        ELSE
        DSR$ = "low"
    END IF
    REM IF (INP(reg%) AND 2 ^ 5) = 0 THEN DSR$ = "low"
END FUNCTION

FUNCTION elapsedtime$ (seconds)
    min% = INT(seconds / 60) MOD 60
    hour% = INT(seconds / 3600) MOD 24
    sec% = INT(seconds) MOD 60
    hour$ = RIGHT$("0" + LTRIM$(STR$(hour%)), 2)
    min$ = RIGHT$("0" + LTRIM$(STR$(min%)), 2)
    sec$ = RIGHT$("0" + LTRIM$(STR$(sec%)), 2)
    elapsedtime$ = hour$ + ":" + min$ + ":" + sec$
END FUNCTION

SUB emptybuffer
    DO WHILE NOT EOF(1)
        buff$ = INPUT$(LOC(1), #1)
    LOOP
    IF log$ = "on" THEN PRINT #2, "Buffer emptied OK"
END SUB

SUB functionkey
    IF log$ = "on" THEN
        PRINT #2, "Calling functionkey to change rate"
    END IF
    REM set rate to zero
    CALL send("CHGR0"): CALL getreply
    REM stop pump
    CALL send("STOP"): CALL getreply
    CLS
    LOCATE 4, 5: PRINT "Pumped stopped"
    LOCATE 5, 5: PRINT "Last rate"; rate.mgkghr; "mg/kg/hr"
    LOCATE 7, 5
    PRINT "To change DOSE rate:- press FUNCTION key F(n)
to get N mg/kg/hr."
    BEEP
```

```
SLEEP: key$ = INKEY$
SELECT CASE key$
    CASE CHR$(0) + CHR$(59)
        rate.mgkghr = 1
    CASE CHR$(0) + CHR$(60)
        rate.mgkghr = 2
    CASE CHR$(0) + CHR$(61)
        rate.mgkghr = 3
    CASE CHR$(0) + CHR$(62)
        rate.mgkghr = 4
    CASE CHR$(0) + CHR$(63)
        rate.mgkghr = 5
    CASE CHR$(0) + CHR$(64)
        rate.mgkghr = 6
    CASE CHR$(0) + CHR$(65)
        rate.mgkghr = 7
    CASE CHR$(0) + CHR$(66)
        rate.mgkghr = 8
    CASE CHR$(0) + CHR$(67)
        rate.mgkghr = 9
    CASE CHR$(0) + CHR$(68)
        rate.mgkghr = 10
    CASE CHR$(0) + CHR$(133)
        rate.mgkghr = 11
    CASE CHR$(0) + CHR$(134)
        rate.mgkghr = 12
    CASE ELSE
END SELECT
rate.mlhr = rate.mgkghr * weight.kg / conc.mgml
CALL send("CHGR" + LTRIM$(STR$(rate.mlhr * 10)))
CALL getreply
CALL send("STRT"): CALL getreply
CLS
LOCATE 1, 54: PRINT "press <Q> to quit"
LOCATE 2, 54: PRINT "press <ESC> to change rate"
END SUB

SUB getreply
    a$ = ""
    replytimezero = TIMER
```

```
    LF$ = CHR$(10)
    cr$ = CHR$(13)
    DO
        DO
            a$ = a$ + INPUT$(LOC(1), #1)
            L% = INSTR(1, a$, LF$): REM looking for LF
            IF TIMER > replytimezero + 2 THEN
                status$ = "COMMUNICATION ERROR"
                IF log$ = "on" THEN PRINT #2, "no reply
from pump error"
                LOCATE 12, 20: PRINT SPACE$(50)
                LOCATE 12, 20
                PRINT "status = "; "COMMUNICATION ERROR"
                LOCATE 20, 5
                PRINT "No reply from pump"
                PRINT "? communication error"
                CALL pumperror
                GOTO endreply
            END IF
        LOOP UNTIL L% > 0
        fullreply$ = MID$(a$, 1, L%)
        IF log$ = "on" THEN PRINT #2, "reply = ",
fullreply$, TIME$
        REM check the checksum
        fullreplycksum$ = MID$(fullreply$, LEN(fullreply$)
- 3, 2)
        reply$ = LEFT$(fullreply$, (LEN(fullreply$) - 4))
        replycksum$ = checksumhex$(reply$)
        IF replycksum$ <> fullreplycksum$ THEN
            LOCATE 12, 34
            PRINT "REPLY-CHECKSUM ERROR    "; fullreply$
            LOCATE 13, 54
            PRINT "calculated cksum = "; replycksum$
            CALL pumperror
        END IF
        REM determine the ACK code
        ackcode$ = MID$(fullreply$, 2, 2)
        IF ackcode$ = "CE" OR ackcode$ = "SX" THEN
ackerror$ = ackcode$
        a$ = RIGHT$(a$, LEN(a$) - L%)
```

```
        LOOP UNTIL LEN(a$) = 0
endreply:
END SUB

SUB maintenance (r.mgkghr)
    mode$ = "maintenance"
    IF log$ = "on" THEN PRINT #2, "start of maintenance"
    rate.mgkghr = r.mgkghr
    rate.mlhr = rate.mgkghr * weight.kg / conc.mgml
    CALL send("CHGR" + LTRIM$(STR$(rate.mlhr * 10)))
    CALL getreply
    CALL runpump
END SUB

SUB pumperror
    IF log$ = "on" THEN PRINT #2, "pumpstatus$ = ALRM or
STBY "
    BEEP: BEEP
    IF ackerror$ = "CE" OR ackerror$ = "SX" THEN
        ackerror$ = ""
        LOCATE 22: PRINT " ACKnowledge code error (CE, SX)
********** "
        LOCATE 23: PRINT SPACE$(30)
        LOCATE 23: PRINT " pump NOT being controlled by
computer"
        LOCATE 24
        PRINT " STOP pump: press <C> to continue /
<Q> to QUIT              "
    ELSE
        LOCATE 22: PRINT " ALARM / STANDBY condition
**************** "
        LOCATE 23: PRINT SPACE$(30)
        LOCATE 23: PRINT " pump stopped"
        LOCATE 24
        PRINT " reset pump: press <C> to continue /
<Q> to QUIT              "
    END IF
alarmloop:
    PRINT
    SLEEP: key$ = INKEY$
```

```
    SELECT CASE UCASE$(key$)
        CASE "Q"

            IF status$ = "COMMUNICATION ERROR" THEN
                CLOSE
                CLS
                END
            END IF
            CALL shutdown
        CASE "C"
            CLS
            LOCATE 1, 54: PRINT "Press <Q> to quit"
            IF log$ = "on" THEN
                PRINT #2, "C-key pressed"
                LOCATE 1, 2
                PRINT "Serial Comms Data logged to file
c:coms-log.dat"
                ELSE
                LOCATE 1, 2
                PRINT "Serial Comms data NOT being logged"
            END IF
            LOCATE 3, 2: PRINT "starting pump"
            CALL send("STRT"): CALL getreply
            CALL send("CHGR" + LTRIM$(STR$(rate.mlhr * 10)))
            CALL getreply
        CASE ELSE
            LOCATE 24, 55: PRINT "INVALID KEY - <C> or <Q>"
            GOTO alarmloop
    END SELECT
END SUB

SUB runpump
    IF log$ = "on" THEN
        LOCATE 1, 2
        PRINT "Serial Comms Data logged to file
c:coms-log.dat"
        PRINT #2, "start of runpump"
        ELSE
        LOCATE 1, 2: PRINT "Serial Comms data NOT being
logged"
```

The Graseby 3400 syringe pump

```
    END IF
    REM start of loop
    DO
        LOCATE 1, 54: PRINT "Press <Q> to quit"
        LOCATE 2, 54: PRINT "Press <ESC> to change rate"
        key$ = INKEY$
        IF UCASE$(key$) = "Q" THEN CALL shutdown
        IF key$ = CHR$(27) THEN CALL functionkey
        CALL send("CHKR" + LTRIM$(STR$(rate.mlhr * 10)))
        CALL getreply
        CALL send("TOTL")
        CALL getreply
        REM: determine no of chars up to the > char
        la% = INSTR(1, fullreply$, CHR$(62))
        REM <OKTOTLINFS276>8Ecrlf
        pumpstatus$ = MID$(fullreply$, 8, 4)
        IF pumpstatus$ = "ALRM" THEN status$ =
"** ALARM **"
        IF pumpstatus$ = "STBY" THEN status$ =
"** STANDBY **"
        IF pumpstatus$ = "INFS" THEN status$ = "INFUSING"
        v$ = MID$(fullreply$, 12, la% - 1)
        volume = VAL(v$) / 10
        REM print data to screen
        LOCATE 2, 2: PRINT "Time "; TIME$
        LOCATE 3, 2
        PRINT "Elapsed time = "; elapsedtime$(TIMER
- timezero)
        LOCATE 23, 2: PRINT "Serial port activity"; p
        LOCATE 6, 20: PRINT "Weight ="; weight.kg; " kg"
        LOCATE 8, 20: PRINT "Drug = PROPOFOL"; conc.mgml;
"mg/ml"
        SELECT CASE mode$
            CASE "step1", "step2"
                LOCATE 10, 20: PRINT SPACE$(57)
                LOCATE 10, 20
                PRINT "Infusion mode = "; UCASE$(mode$);
"  [dose rate "; rate.mgkghr; " mg/kg/hr]"
                LOCATE 11, 20: PRINT SPACE$(57)
                LOCATE 11, 43: PRINT "[duration = ";
```

```
        timedelay.mins; "mins]"
                    LOCATE 18, 20: PRINT SPACE$(57)
                    LOCATE 18, 20: PRINT "Target volume = ";
(INT(targetvolume * 100) / 100); "mls"
                CASE "maintenance"
                    LOCATE 10, 20: PRINT SPACE$(57)
                    LOCATE 10, 20
                    PRINT "Infusion mode = "; UCASE$(mode$);
"  [dose rate "; rate.mgkghr; " mg/kg/hr]"
                    LOCATE 11, 20: PRINT SPACE$(57)
                    LOCATE 18, 20: PRINT SPACE$(57)
            END SELECT
            LOCATE 12, 20: PRINT SPACE$(54)
            LOCATE 12, 20: PRINT "Status = "; status$
            LOCATE 14, 20: PRINT SPACE$(54)
            LOCATE 14, 20: PRINT "Pump rate ="; rate.mlhr;
"mls/hr"
            LOCATE 16, 20: PRINT SPACE$(54)
            LOCATE 16, 20: PRINT "Volume delivered ="; volume;
"mls"
            REM monitor status code to see if pump infusing
            SELECT CASE pumpstatus$
                CASE "ALRM", "STBY"
                    CALL pumperror
            END SELECT
            REM check the ACK code
            IF ackerror$ = "CE" OR ackerror$ = "SX" THEN
CALL pumperror
            REM check whether volume delivered has reached
targetvolume
            SELECT CASE mode$
                CASE "induction", "step1", "step2"
                    IF volume >= targetvolume THEN EXIT DO
            END SELECT
        LOOP
END SUB

SUB send (s$)
    CALL emptybuffer
    s$ = CHR$(60) + s$ + CHR$(62)
```

```
        p = p + 1
        PRINT #1, s$ + checksumhex(s$)
        IF log$ = "on" THEN PRINT #2, s$ + checksumhex(s$),
TIME$
END SUB

SUB setup
        mode$ = "step1"
        REM set the delivered volume counter to zero
        CALL send("ZTOT"): CALL getreply
        REM set pump rate to zero
        CALL send("CHGR0"): CALL getreply
        REM start the pump
        CALL send("STRT"): CALL getreply
        timezero = TIMER
        CALL runpump
END SUB

SUB shutdown
        CLS
        LOCATE 10, 20
        PRINT "Session terminated   (<Q> pressed)"
        CALL send("CHGR0"): CALL getreply: REM set rate to zero
        CALL send("STOP"): CALL getreply: REM stop pump
        IF log$ = "on" THEN PRINT #2, "shutdown routine called"
        CLOSE : REM close all ports
        END
END SUB

SUB steppump (r.mgkghr, td.mins)
        IF stepcount = 2 THEN mode$ = "step2"
        rate.mgkghr = r.mgkghr
        timedelay.mins = td.mins
        initialvolume = volume
        stepvolume = rate.mgkghr * weight.kg * timedelay.mins
/ conc.mgml / 60
        targetvolume = initialvolume + stepvolume
        rate.mlhr = rate.mgkghr * weight.kg / conc.mgml
        stepcount = 2
        CALL send("CHGR" + LTRIM$(STR$(rate.mlhr * 10)))
```

```
       CALL getreply
       CALL runpump
END SUB
```

A copy of the beginning of the Coms log for the above example program is shown in Figure 14.4.

```
port open OK   07-29-1993 17:49:19
Buffer emptied OK
<ZTOT>CB        17:49:26
reply =         <OKZTOTSTBY>A7
                17:49:26
Buffer emptied OK
<CHGR0>CE       17:49:26
reply =         <OKCHGRSTBY0>AA
                17:49:26
Buffer emptied OK
<STRT>C7        17:49:26
reply =         <OKSTRTINFS>91
                17:49:26
start of runpump
Buffer emptied OK
<CHKR12000>95 17:49:26
reply =         <OKCHKRINFSV2.0>52
                17:49:26
Buffer emptied OK
<TOTL>BD        17:49:26
reply =         <OKTOTLINFS0>B7
                17:49:26
Buffer emptied OK
<CHKR12000>95 17:49:26
reply =         <OKCHKRINFSV2.0>52
                17:49:26
Buffer emptied OK
<TOTL>BD        17:49:26
reply =         <OKTOTLINFS0>B7
                17:49:26
Buffer emptied OK
<CHKR12000>95 17:49:26
reply =         <OKCHKRINFSV2.0>52
                17:49:27
Buffer emptied OK
<TOTL>BD        17:49:27
reply =         <OKTOTLINFS0>B7
                17:49:27
```

Fig. 14.4. Extract of the Serial Coms Log (c:coms-log.dat) during the beginning of the example continuous infusion program **grasebyb.bas**.

15

The Ohmeda 9000 syringe pump

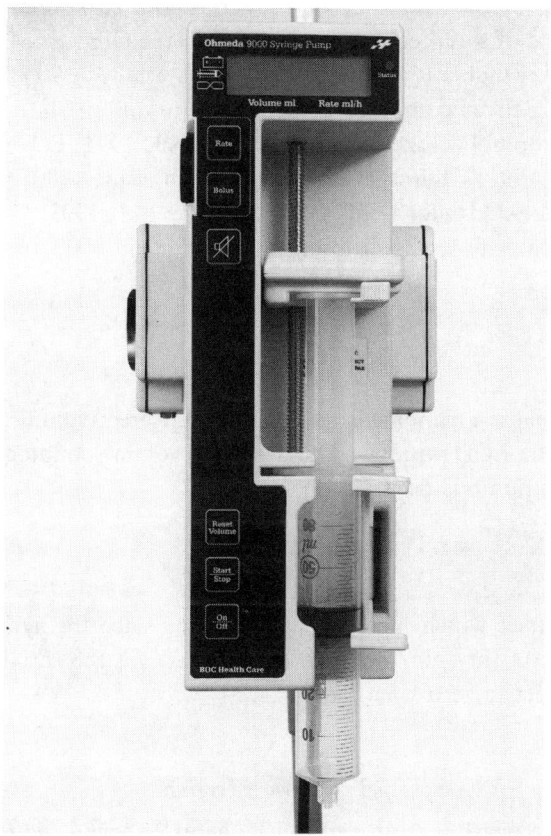

15.1 Introduction

The Ohmeda 9000 syringe pump† consists of two primary components; the syringe pump itself, and the supporting Power Interface Backbar (PIB).

The syringe pump is completely portable, and when disconnected from the backbar will operate for up to 8 hours on internal batteries under

---

† Ohmeda Anaesthesia Systems, Station Road, Steeton, West Yorkshire, BD20 6RB, UK. Tel: +44–(0)1535–656016. Fax: +44–(0)1535–653690.

typical operating conditions. The pump caters for a range of syringe size (10–60 ml), and can deliver maintenance flow rates in the range 0.1–200 ml/hr. The pump has a bolus facility which can deliver rates up to 1200 ml/hr. All information regarding the pump's activity is shown on a liquid-crystal display (LCD).

The pump can be operated either manually using touch-keys on the front panel, or by the computer via the serial port. A pamphlet covering various aspects of serial communications with the Ohmeda 9000 syringe pump is also available (Sainsbury, 1993). The Ohmeda 9000 pump has been used to deliver computer controlled infusions of the intravenous anaesthetic propofol (Stokes *et al.*, 1990; Peacock, 1991; D'Hulster *et al.*, 1991; Kenny, 1991; Church *et al.*, 1991; Marsh *et al.*, 1990; Kenny and White, 1990, 1992; Taylor *et al.*, 1993; Skipsey *et al.*, 1993).

The electrical safety classification of the Ohmeda 9000 syringe pump is Type BF.†

15.1.1 Volume infused

The pump keeps a running total of the delivered volume, which is displayed in the LCD window. The delivered volume counter is reset to zero when the pump is powered on.

15.1.2 Clock

An internal clock which indicates *elapsed* time since the syringe pump was switched on (hr/min/sec), can be accessed via the serial interface, and can be reset to zero when necessary.

15.1.3 Software version

The pump's software version can not be accessed using the touch-keys. However, there have been no software revisions, and therefore all pumps will respond in the same way to a given program.

15.1.4 Backbar

The Ohmeda 9000 is normally supplied with a single Power Interface Backbar (PIB), which incorporates an AC supply lead and a battery charger. The optional RS-232 version of the syringe pump has an

† See Chapter 7 for further details.

Table 15.1. *Ohmeda 9000 bolus rates.*

Syringe size ml	Maximum ml/hr	Median ml/hr	Minimum ml/hr
50–60	1200	600	300
20–49	450	350	300
10–19	300	220	180

optically isolated serial interface on the backbar, and a three-metre interface cable. A three-position PIB is also available which allows up to three pumps to be run simultaneously.

15.1.5 Bolus rates

Three bolus rates are available for a given syringe size, as shown in Table 15.1. The maximum bolus rate is 1200 ml/hr for the 50–60 ml syringe size.

15.1.6 Syringe configuration

Although the Ohmeda 9000 pump will automatically detect the syringe size, the pump must be initially configured for syringe manufacturer by selecting one of the three options from the syringe menu. The menu is accessed by switching the pump on while pressing the <ALARM MUTE> key.†

15.1.7 Start-up time

The time taken for the pump to achieve the set infusion rate after the syringe has been loaded is known as the **start-up** time, and is generally longer the bigger the syringe. For example when the pump is primed using the bolus facility, the time taken to achieve a set infusion rate of 2 ml/hr using a Becton Dickinson 50 ml syringe is less than three minutes.

15.1.8 Communication modes

The Ohmeda 9000 has two communication modes; **Local mode** and **Remote mode**. When in Local mode, the pump's data-logging facility can

† See the Operation and Maintenance manual for details.

be used to save a record of the pump status, by connecting the pump to either a printer or a computer via the serial interface.

- **Local mode** When the pump is first switched on, it powers up in Local mode with the data-logging facility *enabled*. The pump can also operate in Local mode with the data-logging facility *disabled*, but this can only be done by interfacing the pump to a computer.
- **Remote mode** The pump can be made to operate in Remote mode (a 'slave' mode) by interfacing it to a computer, and sending the appropriate commands to the pump via the serial interface. Under these circumstances, the pump becomes completely controlled by the computer, and the pump's touch-keys are then locked out except for the <MUTE> key and the <START/STOP> key. However, there is a built-in safety feature associated with the Remote mode, such that if the pump's <START/STOP> key is pressed while the pump is in Remote mode, the pump will automatically exit and return to Local mode with the data-logging facility *disabled* and the delivery rate set to *zero*.

15.2 Serial port

A female 9-pin D-type serial interface port is located on the backbar. The serial interface is optically isolated from the pump, and the backbar must be powered on in order for the interface to be operational. The serial interface will accept voltages in the range ± 5 to ± 15 volts.

The pins used for communication are shown in Table 15.2. Pins 1, 4, 6, 9 are not connected internally.

- **RxD** This pin must be held LOW (negative) for data to be output. A printer, if attached, must therefore maintain this pin LOW. If a computer is used, then this pin must be connected to the computer's Transmit pin (TxD) since the computer holds this pin LOW unless it is transmitting data.
- **Pin-7** This pin is used as a power input to drive the pump's TxD line, and is therefore effectively an Output Enable pin, since it must be held HIGH (positive) by the computer (or printer) to enable both data output (TxD) and RTS (see below). Pin-7 requires to be held ≥ 5 volts for adequate operation.

This unusual arrangement is to eliminate the requirement for a separate fully isolated secondary winding on the transformer, and allows the pump's serial interface to take power from the host computer to drive the pump's TxD line. This is achieved using a spare output control line

Table 15.2. *Ohmeda 9000 serial port.*

Pin No.	Name	Comments
1	—	
2	TxD	Transmits data
3	RxD	Receives data
4	—	
5	GND	Signal ground
6	—	
7	POWER	Must be held HIGH (positive)
8	RTS	Goes HIGH (positive) when pump is both powered on by the backbar *and* switched on, providing that pin-7 is also held HIGH
9	—	

Table 15.3. *Ohmeda 9000 protocol.*

Bit rate	1200
Data bits	7
Parity	Odd
Stop bits	1

from the computer (e.g. RTS or DTR) to charge a capacitor through a diode to provide the negative supply of the pump's TxD line.†

- **RTS** This pin goes HIGH (positive) only when the backbar is powered on *and* the pump is switched on *and* pin-7 is held HIGH. This pin can therefore be used to indicate whether all the conditions for serial interfacing have been met.

15.2.1 Protocol options

The single backbar for the Ohmeda 9000 pump has a fixed protocol as shown in Table 15.3.

A three-position backbar is also available, and allows up to three syringe pumps to be used at once. Each pump position uses the same Data, Parity, and Stop bits, but uses different bit rates for each pump (i.e. either 300, 600, 1200 bps).

† Martyn Gray, Ohmeda; personal communication.

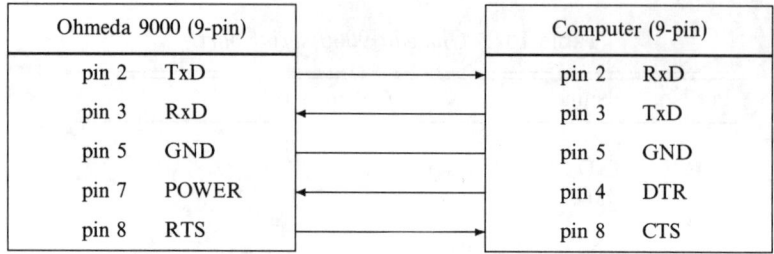

Fig. 15.1. Suggested pin connections for the Ohmeda 9000.

15.2.2 Cable connections

Figure 15.1 shows the necessary connections to a PC having a 9-pin RS-232 connector. Since the pump requires its pin-7 to be held HIGH (positive) this can be done by wiring it to either the computer's RTS or DTR pins, since these are automatically set HIGH by QuickBASIC on opening the COM port. Furthermore, the PC requires its DSR to be held HIGH in order to read incoming data, and this is best achieved by either (a) joining the computer's DSR pin back to its own DTR, or (b) disabling the computer's DSR checking by using the DS option in the QuickBASIC OPEN COM statement (see Section 5.2.3).

The pump's RTS can be monitored by wiring it to any of the computer's remaining input control lines (e.g. DCD, CTS or RI) and then programming the computer to check whether this line is HIGH before proceeding with the program.

The suggested wiring configuration shown in Figure 15.1 makes use of the computer's CTS to monitor the pump's RTS (pin-8). This configuration therefore maintains the computer's CTS HIGH when the pump is operational. Programs using this wiring configuration will therefore need to use the DS option in the OPEN COM statement in order to disable the computer's DSR checking routine since the computer's DSR is not being held HIGH.

15.3 Commands and replies

There are a number of **commands** available for communicating with the pump, each generating a **reply**. Note that the pump does not recognise lower-case letters in commands.

Commands either instruct the pump (e.g. stop the pump), or request data (e.g. return the total volume infused). Replies return status information, and also indicate whether the command syntax was acted upon. If the checksum facility is enabled, then all commands and replies are accompanied with a checksum. Three categories of commands are available, as follows.

- General commands, which can be used in both Local and Remote modes.
- Commands which can *only* be used in Remote mode.
- Commands which can *only* be used when the data-logging facility is enabled.

15.3.1 Command format

All commands consist of the control character ⟨ESC⟩ followed by the code SP, a command-code, a space ␣ or checksum depending on whether the checksum facility has been enabled or not, and terminated by ⟨CR⟩ as follows.

⟨ESC⟩SP⟨command-code⟩␣⟨CR⟩
⟨ESC⟩SP⟨command-code⟩⟨checksum⟩⟨CR⟩

All command-codes are listed in Table 15.4.

15.3.2 Reply format

Replies have a similar structure to commands with the exception that replies are prefixed with a colon : as follows.

:SP⟨reply-code⟩␣⟨CR⟩
:SP⟨reply-code⟩⟨checksum⟩⟨CR⟩

The pump responds to a command with either :SPY, or :SPN, or with the requested data :SP⟨data⟩, depending on whether the pump has recognised the command as being valid or not under the circumstances. For example, in response to a command to enter the Remote mode while the pump is running, the pump will reply with :SPN, and the command will not be executed. This is because Remote mode can *only* be entered while the pump is stopped.

When the checksum is enabled, the negative and affirmative replies for the Ohmeda 9000 are :SPYi and :SPNt respectively. Table 15.4 shows all the command-codes and their affirmative replies.

Table 15.4. *Local and Remote mode command-codes.*
§ *the S and CV codes only work if the pump is stopped.* ¶ *indicates commands only available in Remote mode.* ␣ *indicates a space.* † *mm indicates the manufacturer; ss indicates syringe size.*

Meaning	Command	Reply
Enable checksum	E	:SPYi
Disable checksum	D	:SPY␣
Return bolus rates	?B	:SPB1200.0␣0600.0␣0300.0␣
Return elapsed time	?C	:SPChhmmss␣
Return motor current	?I	:SPiii␣
Return infusion rate	?R	:SPRrrrr.r␣
Return status	?S	:SPSsss␣
Return syringe type †	?T	:SPTmm␣ss␣
Return delivered volume	?V	:SPVvvvv.v␣
Return compressed data	?	:SP␣hhmmss␣rrrr.r␣vvvv.v␣sss␣␣
		(time) (rate) (volume) (status)
Enable Printer format	P	:SPY␣
Enable Compressed format	Q	:SPY␣
Enter Remote mode §	S	:SPY␣(disables data-logger)
¶ Start pump at rate rrr.r	CRrrr.r	:SPY␣
¶ Stop pump	CS	:SPY␣
¶ Reset volume counter §	CV	:SPY␣
¶ Reset elapsed time counter	CC	:SPY␣
¶ Start pump at bolus rate 1=1200, 2=600, 3=300	CBn (n=1,2,3)	:SPY␣
¶ Exit Remote mode	L	:SPY␣(disables data-logger)
¶ Exit Remote mode	X	:SPY␣(enables data-logger)

15.3.3 Status codes

The three-letter status code (sss) given in the replies to the command-codes ? (return compressed data) and ?S (return status data) is an integer encoded number for which the codings for the first, second, and third numbers are shown in Table 15.5.

15.4 The checksum

Although the checksum facility can be used in both Local and Remote modes, its use is particularly recommended when the pump is operated in Remote mode. When the checksum facility is enabled, a checksum is

Table 15.5. *Ohmeda 9000 status codes.*

First number	Second number	Third number
1. (Local mode) OK	0. No syringe fitted	0. No alarm
2. (Local mode) alert	1. Syringe fitted and pump stopped	1. Communication failure
3. (Local mode) alarm	2. Infusing	2. Syringe empty
4. (Remote mode) OK	3. Bolus mode	3. Syringe clamp has moved
5. (Remote mode) alert		4. Occlusion
6. (Remote mode) alarm		5. Flat battery
		6. Near end of syringe
		7. Low battery

sent following all command strings (i.e. following both Command and Reply codes).

The Ohmeda 9000 uses a checksum known as a **two's complement** 7-bit checksum (TC-checksum—see Section 3.4.2 for details). An example program to determine this checksum is given in Section 5.15.

15.4.1 Command checksum (*TC-checksum*)

The pump's checksum includes the ⟨ESC⟩ character, the SP code and the command-code as follows.

$$\underbrace{\langle\text{ESC}\rangle\text{SP}\langle\text{command-code}\rangle}_{checksum}\langle\text{checksum}\rangle\langle\text{CR}\rangle$$

The Ohmeda's 7-bit two's complement checksum is calculated as follows.†

$$\text{checksum} = 128 - (\text{string}) modulo 128$$

In the example interactive program given below for testing Local and Remote mode commands, a function called TWOSCHECKSUM is used to calculate the checksum using the above formula.

† See Section 3.4.2 for details.

15.4.2 Reply checksum

When the checksum is *enabled*, the Reply format is either an acknowledgment, e.g. :SPYi or :SBNt, or :SP followed by the requested data and checksum as shown below.

:SPYi
:SPNt
:SP⟨data⟩⟨checksum⟩

Owing to a minor error in the pump's software, all replies are prefixed with a colon : instead of the usual ⟨ESC⟩ control character.† However, the pump actually calculates the reply checksum as if replies were prefixed by ⟨ESC⟩ as intended.

Since the difference between the ASCII values of ⟨ESC⟩ (ASCII 27) and the colon (ASCII 58) is 31, the reply checksum is calculated as follows, where the term 'string' refers to the sum of the ASCII values of the three characters :SP and the reply-code.

$$(\text{string} + \text{checksum}) modulo\, 128 = 31$$

$$\text{checksum} = 128 - (\text{string}) modulo\, 128 + 31$$

For example, when the checksum facility is enabled, the affirmative reply is :SPYi. The appropriate checksum is the letter i (ASCII 105) since the sum of the ASCII values of the string :SPY is 310, as follows.

$$\binom{:}{58} + \binom{S}{83} + \binom{P}{80} + \binom{Y}{89} = 310$$

i.e. $\text{checksum} = 128 - (310) modulo\, 128 + 31 = 105$

15.4.3 Enabling the checksum facility

This is achieved using the E code. This code is sent as follows

⟨ESC⟩SPE␣⟨CR⟩

Since the checksum facility is *enabled* by this command, the reply includes a checksum, and is :SPYi.

† Martyn Gray, Ohmeda; personal communication.

15.4.4 Disabling the checksum facility

This is achieved by using the D code followed by the appropriate checksum. In this case, the checksum is the tilde (~), which has the ASCII value 126. The command will therefore be sent as follows:

⟨ESC⟩SPD~⟨CR⟩

Since the checksum facility is *disabled* by this command, the pump gives :SPY as the reply.

15.5 Data-logging

When the pump's data-logging facility is enabled, the pump automatically outputs a status log every 5 minutes, and also whenever the status of the pump is changed (e.g. whenever the various touch-keys on the front panel are pressed). The actual time of sending each data-log is at 5, 10, 15 ... minutes according to the pump's internal *elapsed-time* clock.

15.5.1 Enabling the data-logging facility

Although the pump has no command for specifically enabling data-logging, the data-logging facility can be enabled in one of three ways; these are as follows.

- Switch the pump off and then on again. The pump automatically powers up in Local mode with the data-logging facility enabled.
- If already in Local mode with the data-logger disabled, then enter Remote mode (using the S code), and then return to Local mode with data-logging enabled by using the X code (see Table 15.4).
- If already in Remote mode, then exit using the X code which will also enable data-logging (see Table 15.4).

In order to enable data output, not only must the pump's Receive pin (RxD) be maintained LOW (negative), but also the pump's pin-7 must be maintained HIGH. Satisfying both these conditions will enable the Log data to be output via the pump's Transmit pin (TxD). If a printer is used to record the Log data directly, then the interface cable must maintain these pins appropriately.

15.5.2 Data format

Two commands are available to determine the format of the Log data. The Printer format is enabled using the P code, and the Compressed format is enabled using the Q code (see Table 15.4). Note that these two commands will only work providing the data-logging facility is enabled.

Since the ASCII code for ⟨ESC⟩ is 27, and that for a space (⊔) is 32, the Log data format can be set by the program using the following lines of QuickBASIC, where in this example the sequence of codes for enabling the Printer format is placed in a string called printerformat$.

```
compressedformat$ =  CHR$(27) + "SP" + "Q" + CHR$(32)
printerformat$ =  CHR$(27) + "SP" + "P" + CHR$(32)
PRINT #1, printerformat$
```

Note that the terminal ⟨CR⟩ is added automatically by the PRINT statement.

Printer format. This is the default format for the Log data, which is automatically enabled when the pump is powered on. Printer format results in the following output format (spaces are shown here as the ⊔ symbol).

⟨LF⟩⟨CR⟩
Time⊔hh:mm:ss⟨LF⟩⟨CR⟩
⊔⊔⊔⊔⊔⟨status message⟩⟨LF⟩⟨CR⟩
⊔⊔⊔⊔⊔Rate⊔⊔⊔⊔⊔⊔⊔⊔⊔nnnn.n⊔ml/hr⟨LF⟩⟨CR⟩
⊔⊔⊔⊔⊔Total⊔volume⊔nnnn.n⊔ml⟨LF⟩⟨CR⟩

Note that the time indicated in the Printer format is the time *elapsed* since the pump was powered up. Regarding the status message, a number of messages are possible; the full list of status messages being as follows.

- Infusing with ...
- Bolus infusion
- Bolus volume ...
- Pumped stopped
- ** Near end of syringe **
- ** SYRINGE EMPTY **

Compressed data format. This format for Log data is enabled using the Q code (see Table 15.4) providing that the data-logging facility is already enabled.

The Compressed data format gives *elapsed* time (hhmmss), rate (rrrr.r), total volume (vvvv.v), and status (sss). The Compressed data format together with an example is as follows (spaces are shown here as the ␣ symbol).

hhmmss␣rrrr.r␣vvvv.v␣sss␣␣⟨LF⟩⟨CR⟩
013025␣0040.0␣0012.0␣120␣␣⟨LF⟩⟨CR⟩

15.5.3 Program to save Log data

An example QuickBASIC 4.5 program which will access the Ohmeda 9000 Log data and save it to a file (log9000.dat) is given below. The program prompts the operator to select the required data format (Printer or Compressed), and then captures the Log data transmitted whenever the pump's soft keys are pressed, as well as the pump's regular 5-minute Log data output. Pressing <Q> will quit the program.

Program points

- The backbar must be powered on.
- Before running the program first switch the pump off and then on again, to make sure the pump is in Local mode with the data-logging facility enabled.
- The program assumes that the pump is attached to serial port 1 (COM1) using the wiring configuration shown in Figure 15.1. Since this configuration does not hold the computer's DSR HIGH, the DS option must be used in the OPEN COM statement in order to disable the computer's DSR checking (see Chapter 5). The CS option should be used if the computer's CTS is not wired to the pump's RTS.
- Note that the last two characters of each Log data output using the Printer format are ⟨LF⟩⟨CR⟩. This means that a program to save the Log data must inspect the data-strings up to the ⟨CR⟩ character, and then discard the ⟨LF⟩⟨CR⟩ pair. In view of this the following two lines appear in the loop which reads the software buffer a$.

```
L% = INSTR(1, a$, CHR$(13))
data$ = MID$(a$, 1, L% - 2)
```

Example program

```
REM [log9000.bas]
CLEAR
CLS : LOCATE 7
PRINT "A data-logging program for the Ohmeda 9000 pump"
OPEN "COM1:1200,0,7,1,CS,DS" FOR RANDOM ACCESS READ WRITE
                                                               AS #1
OPEN "c:logdata.dat" FOR OUTPUT AS #2
PRINT #2, "Log data from Ohmeda 9000 pump", TIME$, DATE$
PRINT
PRINT "communications open OK (press <Q> to quit)"
PRINT
PRINT "Select data format: <P> (printer)"
PRINT "                    <C> (compressed)"
PRINT
SLEEP: KEY$ = INKEY$
SELECT CASE UCASE$(KEY$)
    CASE "P"
        PRINT #1, CHR$(27) + "SP" + "P" + CHR$(32)
        PRINT "Printer format enabled"
    CASE "C"
        PRINT #1, CHR$(27) + "SP" + "Q" + CHR$(32)
        PRINT "Compressed format enabled"
END SELECT
PRINT "waiting for data"
DO
    DO
        a$ = a$ + INPUT$(LOC(1), #1)
        L% = INSTR(1, a$, CHR$(13))
        KEY$ = INKEY$
        IF UCASE$(KEY$) = "Q" THEN
            CLOSE #1, #2
            END
        END IF
    LOOP UNTIL L% > 0
    data$ = MID$(a$, 1, L% - 2)
    PRINT data$
    PRINT #2, data$
    a$ = RIGHT$(a$, LEN(a$) - L%)
```

LOOP
END

Log data (Printer format). An example of the Log data using the default Printer format is shown below.

```
Time 00:15:40
     Infusing with BD 50
     Rate          0087.0 ml/hr
     Total volume 0023.4 ml

Time 00:15:47
     Bolus infusion
     Rate          1200.0 ml/hr
     Total volume 0024.0 ml

Time 00:16:05
     Bolus volume 0005.9 ml
     Rate          0087.0 ml/hr
     Total volume 0029.8 ml

Time 00:16:20
     Pump stopped
     Rate          0087.0 ml/hr
     Total volume 0030.0 ml

Time 00:17:30
     ** Near end of syringe **
     Rate          0087.0 ml/hr
     Total volume 0035.0 ml

Time 00:18:14
     ** SYRINGE EMPTY **
     Alarm condition
     Rate          0087.0 ml/hr
     Total volume 0038.3 ml
```

Log data (Compressed format). An example of the Log data using the default Compressed format is shown below.

```
001540  0087.0  0023.4  120
```

```
001547 1200.0 0024.0 130
001605 0087.0 0029.8 120
001620 0087.0 0030.0 110
001730 0087.0 0035.0 226
001814 0087.0 0038.8 322
```

15.6 Local mode

When in Local mode, data can be accessed by the computer using a number of commands, either with or without the optional checksum facility.

When the pump is first switched on it powers up in Local mode with the data-logging facility enabled. However, although command-codes can be used with the data-logging facility enabled this is not advisable, as a request for specific data from the keyboard could then coincide with a stream of Log data from the pump, and cause confusion. It is best, therefore, to initially disable the data-logging facility on entering Local mode when intending to send command-codes from the computer.

15.6.1 Disabling the data-logging facility

Unfortunately there is no command which directly disables the data-logging facility. However, the data-logging facility can be disabled *indirectly* by first entering Remote mode (using the S code) for which data-logging is automatically disabled, and then returning to Local mode using the L code (see Table 15.4). Note that leaving Remote mode using the X code will *enable* data-logging on return to Local mode.

15.6.2 Local mode options

The possible options which can be taken when operating in Local mode are listed below, together with the relevant command-codes. A full list of all command-codes is given in Table 15.4.

- Use the computer for data-logging purposes
- Disable the data-logging facility
- Enable data-logging (code X)
- Enter Remote mode (code S)
- Enable the checksum facility (code E)
- Disable the checksum facility (code D)

The Ohmeda 9000 syringe pump 257

- Enable Compressed format data-logging mode (code Q)
- Enable Printer format data-logging mode (code P)
- Request data (use command-codes with data-logging disabled)
  - Bolus rates (code ?B)
  - Elapsed time (code ?C)
  - Motor current (code ?I)
  - Infusion rate (code ?R)
  - Status (code ?S)
  - Syringe type (code ?T)
  - Total volume delivered (code ?V)
  - Compressed data (code ?)

15.7 Remote mode

Remote mode (a 'slave' mode) is entered from Local mode. This is achieved by first stopping the pump using the <START/STOP> key on the front panel, and then using the S code. The reply :SPY indicates that Remote mode has been entered successfully.

Once in Remote mode data-logging is automatically disabled, and a 10 second time-out comes into operation unless either the set infusion rate is zero, or the pump has been stopped (using the code CS). Unless the pump receives a correct command at least every 10 seconds, the pump will alarm and cease to function.

15.7.1 Remote mode options

Once in Remote mode the possible options are given below. A full list of commands is given in Table 15.4.

- Request data
- Send Remote mode pump commands
- Exit Remote mode (code X, code L)
- Enable the checksum facility (code E)
- Disable the checksum facility (code D)

15.7.2 To exit Remote mode

Two codes can be used to exit Remote mode and return to the Local mode. These are the X code and the L code. These have different effects on the data-logging facility within the subsequent Local mode as follows.

258   *Chapter 15*

- **L code**   This exits from Remote mode under all conditions. The pump rate is automatically set to zero, and the pump enters Local mode with the data-logging facility *disabled*.
- **X code**   This command will only exit from Remote mode providing the pump is first stopped (using the code CS). The pump enters Local mode with the data-logging facility *enabled*.

15.8 Interactive program for Local/Remote mode

When writing programs for the pump it is useful to first make an interactive utility program for testing the various commands and showing the replies and checksums. An example of such a program is shown below, and indicates how to send commands interactively from the keyboard. The program shows both the current mode (Local or Remote) and the current checksum status (on or off) on the screen. If the checksum facility is enabled, the program will automatically supply the checksum; i.e. in this case enter *only* the command-code.

For example, Figure 15.2 shows the screen following keying in the command-code ? while in Local mode with the data-logger disabled and with the checksum enabled. The 'key' entry shows that the entered code is ?. The 'command' entry shows that the full command (including the checksum) sent to the pump was ←SP♥, where the symbol ← is the graphic representation of the control character ⟨ESC⟩. The symbol ♥ is the graphic representation of the control character ⟨ETX⟩, whose value (ASCII 3) is the value of the checksum.† (see Appendix 1 for details of the ASCII code).

The 'reply' entry shows that in this case there is an undocumented space‡ between the end of the reply and the reply checksum (¶). This point illustrates the value of experimenting with an interactive program to check the command and reply syntax.

Note that all the command-codes are listed in Table 15.4.

Program points

- Before running the program switch the pump off and then on again, to make sure the pump is in Local mode with data-logger enabled.

† Note that in cases where PCs represent the control characters using the ^ notation, the symbols ←SP♥ will appear as ^[SP^C.

‡ This space is not documented in the pump's 'operation and maintenance' manual.

The Ohmeda 9000 syringe pump 259

```
checksum status = ON  mode = LOCAL + Log OFF

enter pump command-code (enter <q> to quit)
use CAPITAL letters and a SPACE if necessary

Enter <CODE><ENTER>

key = ?

command =←SP?♥
reply = :SP 010542 0017.5 0003.4 110 ¶
```

Fig. 15.2. The screen when using the example interactive program for Local/Remote mode **lr9000.bas**.

- The program uses the subroutine GETREPLY to collect the reply, and a function TWOSCHECKSUM to calculate the checksum.
- Both DSR and CTS checking by the computer are disabled using the CS and DS options in the OPEN COM statement.
- Entering <q> will quit the program. The capital letter Q cannot be used as Q is one of the Ohmeda 9000 command-codes.
- Occasionally strange effects are seen when either the command or reply is printed to the screen; e.g. characters being overwritten etc. These effects occur whenever the checksum equals the ASCII value of a control character which moves the cursor to a new position (see Appendix 1 for details of the ASCII code).
  This is because the function TWOSCHECKSUM uses the variable twoschecksum$ which is defined as the character having the same ASCII value as the checksum, in the following line.

  twoschecksum$ = CHR$(128 - sum% MOD 128)

  This effect can be avoided by printing the checksum as its decimal or hexadecimal value; for example, using the following line.

  twoschecksum% = 128 - sum% MOD 128

- The characters ⟨ESC⟩, ⟨CR⟩ and ⟨SPACE⟩ are redefined near the beginning of the program as ESC$, CR$, and SPAC$ respectively in order to make the program more readable.

  ESC$ = CHR$(27)
  SPAC$ = CHR$(32)
  CR$ = CHR$(13)

Note that SPAC$ is used for ⟨SPACE⟩, since SPACE$ is a reserved keyword in QuickBASIC.

- The program can be enhanced considerably by including the subroutine FULLCODE given in Section 5.6, and the following line in the subroutine GETREPLY.

```
PRINT "fullcode = "; fullcode(a$)
```

This then adds an additional line under the 'reply', which indicates all the spaces and ⟨CR⟩ characters.

Example program

```
REM [lr9000.bas]
DECLARE SUB fullcode (r$)
REM Ohmeda 9000 pump
REM interactive LOCAL/REMOTE mode program
DECLARE SUB getreply ()
DECLARE FUNCTION twochecksum$ (c$)
COMMON SHARED reply$
CLEAR
ESC$ = CHR$(27): SPAC$ = CHR$(32): CR$ = CHR$(13)
tilde$ = CHR$(126)
OPEN "COM1:1200,0,7,1,CS,DS" FOR RANDOM ACCESS READ WRITE
                                                        AS #1
CLS : LOCATE 7
PRINT "communications open OK"
start:
REM  get pump status to see whether pump is stopped
PRINT "Checking  pump status"
PRINT #1, ESC$ + "SP" + "?S" + SPAC$
CALL getreply
IF MID$(reply$, 6, 1) = "1" THEN
    REM disable data logging facility
    PRINT "Entering REMOTE mode"
    PRINT #1, ESC$ + "SP" + "S" + SPAC$
    CALL getreply
    PRINT "Returning to LOCAL mode with data-logger disabled"
    PRINT #1, ESC$ + "SPL" + SPAC$
    CALL getreply
```

```
ELSE
    BEEP
    PRINT "pump is running"
    PRINT "stop pump, and then press ENTER"
    SLEEP: x$ = INKEY$
    GOTO start
END IF
PRINT "get status again to check mode"
PRINT #1, ESC$ + "SP" + "?S" + SPAC$
CALL getreply
SELECT CASE MID$(reply$, 5, 1)
    CASE "1", "2", "3"
        mode$ = "LOCAL + Log ON"
    CASE "4", "5", "6"
        mode$ = "REMOTE"
END SELECT
cksum$ = "OFF"
SLEEP 1
DO
    CLS
    LOCATE 2
    pump$ = ""
    PRINT STRING$(50, "*")
    PRINT "checksum status = "; cksum$, " mode = "; mode$
    PRINT
    PRINT "enter pump command code (enter <q> to quit)"
    PRINT "use CAPITAL leters and  a SPACE if necessary"
    PRINT
    IF cksum$ = "ON" THEN
        PRINT "Enter  < CODE >< ENTER >"
    ELSE
        PRINT SPACE$(30)
        LOCATE 8: PRINT "Enter  < CODE >< SPACE>< ENTER >"
    END IF
    PRINT
    DO
        DO: key$ = INKEY$: LOOP UNTIL key$ <> ""
        SELECT CASE key$
            CASE CR$
                EXIT DO
```

```
                CASE "q"
                    REM return pump to LOCAL mode
                    REM with data-logger disabled
                    IF cksum$ = "ON" THEN
                        PRINT #1, ESC$ + "SPD" + tilde$
                        CALL getreply
                    END IF
                    IF mode$ = "REMOTE" THEN
                        PRINT #1, ESC$ + "SPX" + SPAC$
                        CALL getreply
                    END IF
                    CLOSE #1, #2
                    END
                CASE SPAC$
                    k$ = "SPACE"
                CASE ELSE
                    k$ = key$
            END SELECT
            PRINT "key = "; k$
            pump$ = pump$ + key$
    LOOP
    PRINT
    IF cksum$ = "ON" THEN
        pump$ = pump$ + twoschecksum$(pump$)
    END IF
    E$ = "E" + SPAC$
    S$ = "S" + SPAC$
    L$ = "L" + SPAC$
    x$ = "X" + SPAC$
    Yi$ = ":SPYi"
    Y$ = ":SPY" + SPAC$
    SELECT CASE cksum$
        CASE "OFF"
            PRINT "command = "; ESC$ + "SP" + pump$
            PRINT #1, ESC$ + "SP" + pump$
            CALL getreply
            IF pump$ = E$ AND reply$ = Yi$ THEN cksum$ = "ON"
            IF pump$ = S$ AND reply$ = Y$ THEN mode$ = "REMOTE"
```

```
            IF pump$ = L$ AND reply$ = Y$ THEN mode$ =
"LOCAL + Log OFF"
            IF pump$ = x$ AND reply$ = Y$ THEN mode$ =
"LOCAL + Log ON"
        CASE "ON"
            PRINT "command = "; ESC$ + "SP" + pump$
            PRINT #1, ESC$ + "SP" + pump$
            CALL getreply
            IF pump$ = "D" + tilde$ AND reply$ = Y$ THEN
cksum$ = "OFF"
            IF pump$ = "So" AND reply$ = Yi$ THEN mode$ =
"REMOTE"
            IF pump$ = "Lv" AND reply$ = Yi$ THEN mode$ =
"LOCAL + Log OFF"
            IF pump$ = "Xj" AND reply$ = Yi$ THEN mode$ =
"LOCAL + Log ON"
    END SELECT
    PRINT STRING$(57, "*")
    LOCATE 23
    PRINT "press a key to continue"
    SLEEP: z$ = INKEY$
LOOP
END


SUB fullcode (r$)
SHARED code$
code$ = ""
FOR j = 1 TO LEN(r$)
    ch$ = MID$(r$, j, 1)
    IF ASC(ch$) < 33 THEN
        char$ = "<" + LTRIM$(STR$(ASC(ch$))) + ">"
        IF ch$ = CHR$(13) THEN char$ = "<CR>"
        IF ch$ = CHR$(10) THEN char$ = "<LF>"
        IF ch$ = CHR$(32) THEN char$ = "<SPACE>"
        IF ch$ = CHR$(27) THEN char$ = "<ESC>"
        IF ch$ = CHR$(7) THEN char$ = "<BEL>"
    ELSE
        char$ = ch$
    END IF
```

```
            code$ = code$ + char$
    NEXT j
    PRINT "fullcode = "; code$
    REM PRINT #2, "fullcode = "; code$
END SUB



SUB getreply
    a$ = ""
    CR$ = CHR$(13)
    DO
        DO
            a$ = a$ + INPUT$(LOC(1), #1)
            L% = INSTR(1, a$, CR$)
        LOOP UNTIL L% > 0
        reply$ = MID$(a$, 1, L% - 1)
        PRINT "reply = "; reply$
        CALL fullcode(a$)
        a$ = RIGHT$(a$, LEN(a$) - L%)
        REM LOOP UNTIL EOF(1)
    LOOP UNTIL LEN(a$) = 0
END SUB



FUNCTION twoschecksum$ (c$)
    k$ = CHR$(27) + "SP" + c$
    sum% = 0
    FOR j = 1 TO LEN(k$)
        sum% = sum% + ASC(MID$(k$, j, 1))
    NEXT j
    twoschecksum$ = CHR$(128 - sum% MOD 128)
END FUNCTION
```

15.9 Programming a continuous infusion

When controlling the Ohmeda 9000 pump during a continuous infusion, all the pump's touch-keys are locked out with the exception of the <START/STOP> key. This is a safety feature which allows the pump to be taken over manually, if necessary, by first stopping the pump and then adjusting the infusion rate.

15.9.1 Pump time-out

In order for the computer to sustain a continuous infusion, it is necessary to send at least one valid command every 10 seconds. Failing to do so results in the pump generating a time-out error causing an alarm state, and the pump stops.

15.9.2 Programming considerations

The program should detect and respond appropriately to 'alarm' states as and when they occur, allowing the operator to either adjust the pump and continue with the infusion, or quit the program. Communication failures should also be detected (e.g. power failure, accidental switch off, or serial cable disconnection). This can be done by monitoring the status of the pump's RTS line.

After sending a command, the reply relating to the command should always be collected and analysed before sending another command. In addition, the linking of replies to their initiating commands can be facilitated by emptying the receive buffer immediately before sending a command.

On receipt of a reply, its message should be checked against the returned checksum. If the reply does not agree with the checksum then an error-handler should be called to alert the operator, and stop the pump if necessary. Alternatively, the reply can be ignored, and the initiating command transmitted again.

For accurate control, the timing of infusion rate changes is best related to delivered volume as measured by the pump itself rather than to the computer's time clock. Similarly, program variables are best chosen so that they indicate the units, e.g. `rate.mlhr` as a variable for the rate in ml/hr etc.

The program should also incorporate some system for checking that all calculations are performed correctly, in order to serve as a check against program corruption.

Note that in the example program given below many of the above suggestions are not implemented.† This is because the program described in this book is simply to illustrate methods of programming the syringe pump; the author is not trying to give a complete and safe program ready for real-life applications.

---

† Many of these aspects are incorporated into the example continuous infusion program for the Graseby 3400 syringe pump described in Chapter 14.

15.9.3 Example program for continuous infusion

The following example QuickBASIC 4.5 program illustrates a method of driving the Ohmeda 9000 pump to deliver a continuous infusion with variable flow rates.

For example, the pump could be used to induce anaesthesia, and then maintain a given plasma concentration of an intravenous anaesthetic agent, by varying the flow rate according to an algorithm based on various patient parameters, e.g. weight, age, height etc.

The example program given below starts by checking the pump status code to see whether the conditions necessary for entering the Remote mode are met (i.e. pump must be stopped etc.). The program then enters the Remote mode, and resets the pump's elapsed-time and delivered-volume counters to zero. It then instructs the pump to deliver the bolus flow rates 1200, 600, 300 ml/hr for 10, 20, and 30 seconds respectively. Following this, the flow rate is decreased to 50 ml/hr. The pump status data is updated on the computer every 2 seconds, and gives the time, elapsed time, pump rate, and volume delivered. Pressing <Q> will quit the program at any stage.

The program comprises of the main module (terminated by the END statement), and seven short subroutines, namely EMPTYBUFFER (flushes the input buffer), SEND (sends the control codes), SECONDS (generates a time delay of S seconds), REPLY (gets the reply from the input buffer), GETDATA (gets and processes the data from the input buffer), and RATE (allows a specific infusion rate to be set).

Program points

- The COMMON SHARED data$ statement allows both the main module and the SECONDS subroutine to use the data$ generated by the REPLY subroutine.
- Note the use of the CALL emptybuffer statement at the beginning of the SEND subroutine, so that only the required reply will be read from the input buffer. This is important here because when the pump is first switched on, it enters Local mode with the data-logger enabled, and so unwanted data may accumulate in the input buffer when the pumped is stopped manually using the touch-keys before running the program.
- Note the use of the LTRIM$ function in the RATE subroutine, where it is used to remove the space reserved for the sign immediately in front of the rate number.

- Once the pump rate is less than 100 ml/hr, it is then necessary to insert a leading zero immediately following the CR code, in order to adhere to the CRnnn.n format. For example, the command to set a rate of 73 ml/hr must be sent as CR073.0. If a rate of less than 10 ml/hr was wanted, then two leading zeros would be needed after the CR code (see Chapter 5 for details of using the LTRIM$ function). The 0.1 is added on to the rate as a simple way of making sure that the rate always has one decimal place.

Example program

```
REM [ci-9000.bas]
REM OHMEDA 9000 pump
DECLARE SUB emptybuffer ()
DECLARE SUB send (s$)
DECLARE SUB seconds (s%)
DECLARE SUB reply ()
DECLARE SUB getdata ()
DECLARE SUB rate (r.mlhr)
COMMON SHARED data$
OPEN "COM1:1200,0,7,1,CS,DS,OP10000" FOR RANDOM ACCESS
                                         READ WRITE AS #1
OPEN "c:datafile" FOR OUTPUT AS #2
CLS : LOCATE 7
checkstatus:
data$ = ""
PRINT "pump must be STOPPED in order to access remote mode"
PRINT "press a key to continue (or <Q> to quit)"
DO: key$ = INKEY$: LOOP UNTIL key$ <> ""
IF UCASE$(key$) = "Q" THEN
    CLOSE
    END
END IF
CALL send("?S"): REM get status
PRINT
PRINT "pump status = "; data$
IF VAL(MID$(data$, 6, 1)) <> 1 THEN
    PRINT "The pump is still running"
    GOTO checkstatus
```

```
END IF
PRINT "REMOTE mode entered OK"
CALL send("S"): BEEP
CALL send("CV"): PRINT "resetting the volume"
CALL send("CC"): PRINT "resetting the time"
REM **** start of infusion routine ****
PRINT
PRINT "start fast bolus rate for 10 secs"
CALL send("CB1"): BEEP: REM CB1=1200 ml/hr
CALL seconds(10): REM wait 20 seconds
PRINT "start medium bolus rate for 20 secs"
CALL send("CB2"): BEEP: REM CB2 = 600 ml/hr
CALL seconds(20)
PRINT "start slow bolus rate for 30 secs"
CALL send("CB3"): BEEP: REM CB3 = 300 ml/hr
CALL seconds(30)
PRINT "final rate of 50 ml/hr for 10 secs"
CALL rate(50)
CALL seconds(10): BEEP
PRINT "end of infusion"
REM  exit Remote mode and shut pump down
CALL send("L")
CLOSE #1, #2
END



SUB emptybuffer
    REM this flushes the input buffer
    DO WHILE NOT EOF(1)
        buff$ = INPUT$(LOC(1), #1)
    LOOP
END SUB



SUB getdata
    CALL send("?"): REM gets data in compressed format
    et$ = MID$(data$, 5, 6): REM elapsed time
    eth$ = LEFT$(et$, 2): REM hrs
    etm$ = MID$(et$, 3, 2): REM mins
    ets$ = RIGHT$(et$, 2): REM secs
```

```
    R$ = MID$(data$, 12, 6): REM pump rate
    V$ = MID$(data$, 19, 6): REM volume delivered
    PRINT "Time = "; TIME$; " "; "Elapsedtime = "; eth$;
":"; etm$; ":"; ets$; " "; "Rate = "; R$; " "; "Volume
= "; V$; "mls"
    PRINT #2, "Time = "; TIME$; " "; "Elapsedtime = ";
eth$; ":"; etm$; ":"; ets$; " "; "Rate = "; R$; " ";
"Volume = "; V$; "mls"
END SUB



SUB rate (r.mlhr)
    REM max rate = 999.9, min rate = 0.1
    REM make number have 1 decimal place
    r.mlhr = (INT(r.mlhr * 10)) / 10
    r.mlhr = r.mlhr + .1
    REM make number have nnn.n format
    R$ = RIGHT$("000" + LTRIM$(STR$(r.mlhr)), 5)
    CALL send("CR" + R$)
END SUB



SUB reply
    REM gets the reply
    a$ = ""
    DO
        DO
            a$ = a$ + INPUT$(LOC(1), #1)
            L% = INSTR(1, a$, CHR$(13))
        LOOP UNTIL L% > 0
        data$ = MID$(a$, 1, L% - 1)
        a$ = RIGHT$(a$, LEN(a$) - L%)
    LOOP UNTIL LEN(a$) = 0
END SUB



SUB seconds (s%)
    REM this causes a delay of S seconds
    timenow = TIMER
    k$ = ""
```

```
        DO
            SLEEP 2
            CALL getdata
            REM include a Quit routine while pump is running
            k$ = INKEY$
            IF k$ = "q" THEN
                  CALL send("L")
                  CLOSE #1, #2
                  END
            END IF
        LOOP UNTIL TIMER >= timenow + s%
END SUB


SUB send (s$)
      REM this sends the control codes
      CALL emptybuffer
      se$ = CHR$(27) + "SP" + s$ + CHR$(32)
      PRINT #1, se$
      CALL reply
END SUB
```

An extract of the log data saved to the disk when running the above example program for controlling a continuous infusion is shown in Figure 15.3.

```
Time = 19:37:47   Elapsedtime = 00:00:21   Rate = 0600.0   Volume = 0005.4mls
Time = 19:37:49   Elapsedtime = 00:00:23   Rate = 0600.0   Volume = 0005.7mls
Time = 19:37:52   Elapsedtime = 00:00:25   Rate = 0600.0   Volume = 0006.1mls
Time = 19:37:54   Elapsedtime = 00:00:27   Rate = 0600.0   Volume = 0006.5mls
Time = 19:37:56   Elapsedtime = 00:00:30   Rate = 0600.0   Volume = 0006.9mls
Time = 19:37:59   Elapsedtime = 00:00:32   Rate = 0600.0   Volume = 0007.3mls
Time = 19:38:01   Elapsedtime = 00:00:35   Rate = 0300.0   Volume = 0007.5mls
Time = 19:38:03   Elapsedtime = 00:00:37   Rate = 0300.0   Volume = 0007.7mls
Time = 19:38:06   Elapsedtime = 00:00:39   Rate = 0300.0   Volume = 0007.9mls
Time = 19:38:08   Elapsedtime = 00:00:42   Rate = 0300.0   Volume = 0008.1mls
Time = 19:38:10   Elapsedtime = 00:00:44   Rate = 0300.0   Volume = 0008.3mls
Time = 19:38:12   Elapsedtime = 00:00:46   Rate = 0300.0   Volume = 0008.5mls
Time = 19:38:15   Elapsedtime = 00:00:48   Rate = 0300.0   Volume = 0008.7mls
Time = 19:38:17   Elapsedtime = 00:00:51   Rate = 0300.0   Volume = 0008.8mls
Time = 19:38:19   Elapsedtime = 00:00:53   Rate = 0300.0   Volume = 0009.0mls
Time = 19:38:21   Elapsedtime = 00:00:55   Rate = 0300.0   Volume = 0009.2mls
Time = 19:38:24   Elapsedtime = 00:00:58   Rate = 0300.0   Volume = 0009.4mls
Time = 19:38:26   Elapsedtime = 00:01:00   Rate = 0300.0   Volume = 0009.6mls
Time = 19:38:28   Elapsedtime = 00:01:02   Rate = 0300.0   Volume = 0009.8mls
Time = 19:38:31   Elapsedtime = 00:01:04   Rate = 0300.0   Volume = 0010.0mls
Time = 19:38:33   Elapsedtime = 00:01:07   Rate = 0050.0   Volume = 0010.0mls
Time = 19:38:35   Elapsedtime = 00:01:09   Rate = 0050.0   Volume = 0010.1mls
Time = 19:38:38   Elapsedtime = 00:01:11   Rate = 0050.0   Volume = 0010.1mls
Time = 19:38:40   Elapsedtime = 00:01:14   Rate = 0050.0   Volume = 0010.1mls
Time = 19:38:42   Elapsedtime = 00:01:16   Rate = 0050.0   Volume = 0010.2mls
```

Fig. 15.3. An extract of the Log data generated by the continuous infusion program **ci-9000.bas**. The Log data is saved in the file datafile.

16

The Vitalograph Compact II spirometer

by
F. Jahan

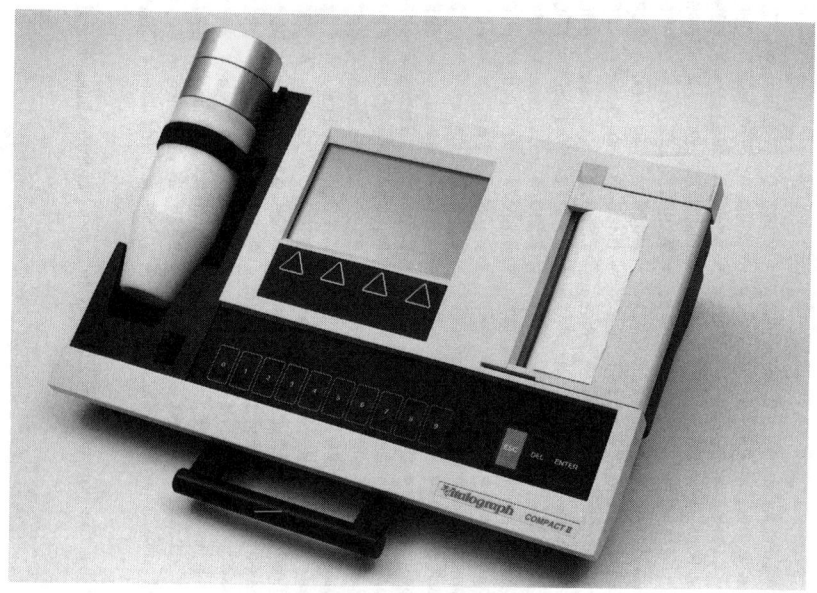

16.1 Introduction

The Vitalograph† Compact II is a portable mains powered spirometer which measures inspiratory and expiratory air flow parameters. All results can be printed out on the spirometer's inbuilt printer, which also displays the data graphically.

The Compact II has a 9-pin serial port, and is compatible with both the Epson FX-80 and FX-85 printers via the Epson 8148 Serial Interface card. Full details regarding switch settings are given in the User Manual.

The Compact II spirometer complies with the recommendations of the American Thoracic Society (1987), and its performance has been reviewed by Roget & Shield (1986), and Nelson et al. (1990). The

† Vitalograph Limited, Maids Moreton House, Buckingham, MK18 1SW, UK.
  Tel: +44–(0)1280–822811. Fax: +44–(0)1280–823302.

Table 16.1. *Vitalograph Compact II serial port.*

Pin No.	Name	Comments
1	+5 volts	50 mA max
2	TTL input	Factory use only
3	TxD	Transmits data (± 13 volts)
4	−15 volts	
5		Not connected
6	+15 volts	
7	GND	Signal ground
8		Not connected
9	RTS	Must be held HIGH (positive) to enable data output.

electrical safety classification of the Vitalograph Compact II flowhead and tubing is Type BF.†

16.1.1 Software version

The latest software at the time of writing is 66.345 version 5 (introduced in 1993), and is available in a number of different languages.

The software version number is the last digit of the **Software reference number**, which is which displayed at the bottom right-hand corner of the **Set-up** menu screen. An example is as follows.

SOFTWARE REF. : 66.045/5

The Software reference number is also printed at the end of any data output on Compact II's inbuilt printer.

16.2 Serial port

A 9-pin D-type female serial port is located at the rear of the spirometer. The pins used for communication are shown in Table 16.1.

16.2.1 Protocol

The Compact II has a fixed protocol as shown in Table 16.2.

† See Chapter 7 for further details.

Table 16.2. *Vitalograph Compact II protocol.*

Bit rate	4800
Data bits	8
Parity	None
Stop bits	1

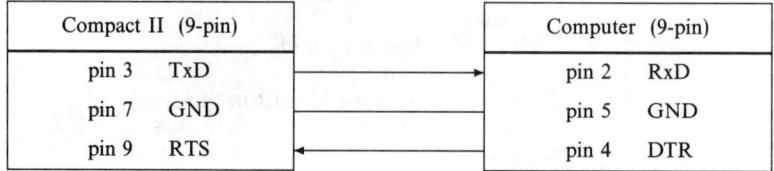

Fig. 16.1. Vitalograph Compact II wiring configuration.

16.2.2 *Cable connections*

Figure 16.1 indicates a suitable wiring configuration for interfacing to a PC.

- **RTS** This is the spirometer's handshake line, and must be held HIGH (positive) in order to *enable* data output. If during data transmission the PC suddenly pulls the Compact II's RTS LOW, then data output will cease until its RTS is held HIGH again. Note that the Compact II has no time-out on this line, so if the RTS is not returned HIGH then data output will cease indefinitely.

In practice, the Compact II's RTS can be wired to either of the PC's output control lines (DTR or RTS), since QuickBASIC automatically sets both of these lines HIGH on opening the serial port.†

If RTS is *not* held HIGH when selecting the key options EXTERNAL PRINT (Serial Mode 1)‡ or TRANSMIT RESULTS (Serial Mode 3) in order to initiate data transmission via the Compact II's serial port, then the following screen message is displayed.

> ENSURE EXTERNAL DEVICE IS CONNECTED AND
> ON-LINE; THEN RESELECT FROM MAIN MENU

† See Section 5.16 for details regarding control of the PC's DTR and RTS.
‡ See Table 16.3 for details of the Serial Modes.

The Vitalograph Compact II spirometer

Table 16.3. *External (serial) communications menu.*

Serial Mode	Description
1	Printout without graphs—best Test
2	Printout with graphs—best Test
3	Results only—best Test
4	Results only—last Test
5	Results and Flow data—last Test

If RTS is *not* held HIGH when data is to be transmitted automatically (Serial Modes 4 and 5), the Compact II temporarily displays the following screen message.

> NO CONNECTION FOR DATA TRANSMISSION

When data is being transmitted via the serial port, this is indicated by the following screen message

> DATA BEING TRANSMITTED

16.3 Communication Modes

The Vitalograph Compact II has five serial communication modes, which are accessed via the **External Communications** menu (see Table 16.3), which itself is accessed via the **Set-up** menu. The options which can be selected from the External Communications menu will be referred to throughout this Chapter as the **Serial Modes**.

Of the five Serial modes, *only* Serial Mode 2 (Printout with graphs—best Test) is unsuitable for use with a PC, since this Serial mode is specifically for use with an Epson printer (FX-80; FX-85). The Serial communication modes are now described in turn.

- **Serial Mode 1 (Printout without graphs—best Test).** This mode outputs the data in table form, and is designed for use with an Epson printer. However, since the few additional control characters which are transmitted when using this mode are easily removed, this mode can be used with PCs without difficulty. Serial data transmission is initiated by pressing the EXTERNAL PRINT soft key (option 0; main menu).
- **Serial Mode 2 (Printout with graphs—best Test).** This mode is designed for use with an Epson printer, and is *not* suitable for PCs.

- **Serial Mode 3 (Results only—best Test).** This mode outputs the best Test results in a compressed form (i.e. a list of values only). The data is output in the following order: Message number (1 value), Patient Reference data (4 values), the best Pre results (25 values), the best Post results if Post tests have been made (25 values), Predicted values (25 values). All data fields are transmitted; those parameters not selected from the parameter list (option 2; Set-up menu) are filled with zeros. Serial data transmission is initiated by pressing the TRANSMIT RESULTS soft key (option 0; main menu).
- **Serial Mode 4 (Results only—last Test).** This mode outputs the data from the last test (Pre or Post) in compressed form (i.e. a list of values only). The data is output in the following order: Message number (1 value), Patient Reference data (4 values), the last Test (Pre or Post; 25 values), Predicted values (25 values). All data fields are transmitted; those parameters not selected from the parameter list (option 2; Set-up menu) are filled with zeros. Serial data transmission is initiated automatically following each Test, providing the Compact II's RTS is held HIGH.
- **Serial Mode 5 (Results and Flow Data—last Test).** This mode is essentially the same as the previous mode, except that the measured Flow data is also transmitted. The data is output in the following order: Message number (1 value), Patient Reference data (4 values), the last Test (Pre or Post; 25 values), Predicted values (25 values), number of Flow data points (1 value), Flow data (maximum 2001 values). Serial data transmission is initiated automatically following each Test, providing the Compact II's RTS is held HIGH.

16.4 Data format

The Compact II spirometer outputs data via the serial port in either a Table or List format depending on the Serial Mode being used. These are now described in turn.

16.4.1 Table format (Serial Mode 1)

When the Compact II is in Serial Mode 1 (Printout without graphs; see Table 16.3), the serial data is formatted in the form of a convenient table of results which, when printed out, can then be put into the patient's notes (see Figure 16.2). The table format is the same as that printed out using the Compact II's own internal printer.

Table 16.4. *Message number coding. The * indicates that with these modes the serial data is transmitted automatically.*

Serial mode	Results	Message number	Total No. of values
1	Printout without graphs	—	—
2	Printout with graphs	—	—
3	Best test (Pre)	01	55
	Best test (Pre + Post)	03	80
4 *	Last test (Pre)	00	55
	Last test (Post)	02	55
5 *	Last test (Pre + Flow)	04	2057
	Best test (Post + Flow)	06	2057

16.4.2 List format (Serial Modes 3, 4, 5)

When the Compact II is in one of the Serial Modes 3, 4, 5 (see Table 16.3) the output data is in the form of a long list of all of the values of the various measured parameters.

The number of values transmitted via the serial port can vary between 55 and 2057, depending on the particular Serial Mode (3, 4, or 5) and the tests which have been done (Pre, Post, or both)—see Table 16.4.

The list of results consists of a number of component sets of data which are transmitted in a strict sequence, the order being as follows.

(1) Message number
(2) Patient reference data
(3) Test data—Pre results (last or best)
(4) Test data—Post results (last or best)
(5) Predicted data
(6) Flow data

Message number. The Message number (00–06)† is always the first value to be transmitted, and is the key to processing the data since it indicates how the data is formatted (see Table 16.4).

The Message number is always transmitted as two digits (e.g. 04) and

† Note that Message number 05 is not allocated at present.

is terminated with a ⟨CR⟩. An example of the format is as follows.

04⟨CR⟩

Patient reference data. This data is always transmitted, and immediately follows the Message number. The Patient Reference data consists of the following 4 data items in this order; reference number (up to a total of 15 digits), age (years; 2 digits), height (cm or inches; 3 digits), sex (M, F; 1 character).

Note that if the number field for the reference number is not filled, then the remaining positions are filled with spaces. Regarding the height, a three-figure value is regarded as being in centimetres, and a two-figure value is regarded as being in inches.

As an example, the Patient Reference data for a male (ref no. 1993001) of age 35 years and height 180 cm is output in the following format.

1993001⎵⎵⎵⎵⎵⎵⎵⎵⟨CR⟩
35⟨CR⟩
180⟨CR⟩
M⟨CR⟩

Test data. The Test data-set refers to a set of 25 measured parameters transmitted in a fixed order (see Table 16.5). Where a particular parameter is not measured (i.e. not selected from the parameter list†) the number field will be filled with zeros.

Either one or two groups of Test data will be transmitted depending on the Serial Mode and the tests performed. For example, two Test data groups will be transmitted *if* Serial Mode 3 has been selected (i.e. best test—Pre and Post results Mode; see Table 16.4) *and* both Pre and Post tests have been performed. When two sets of Test data are transmitted they are sent consecutively, with the Pre results immediately followed by the Post results.

Predicted data. The Predicted data-set consists of the predicted values of the same 25 parameters, and in the same order, as the Test data (see Table 16.5). The Predicted data set is *always* transmitted, and immediately follows the Test data.

Flow data. Flow data is only associated with Serial Mode 5. Under these circumstances, a large number of flow values (max 2001) are transmitted

† The parameter list is accessed by selecting option 2 from the Set-up menu.

Table 16.5. *Test data. Note that the same data set is used for Pre, Post, and Predicted data.*

Order	Format	Parameter	Units
1	nn.nn⟨CR⟩	VC	L
2	nn.nn⟨CR⟩	IVC	L
3	nn.nn⟨CR⟩	FVC	L
4	nn.nn⟨CR⟩	$FEV_{0.5}$	L
5	-nnn⟨CR⟩	$FEV_{0.5}/FVC$	ratio
6	nn.nn⟨CR⟩	FEV_1	L
7	-nnn⟨CR⟩	FEV_1/VC	ratio
8	-nnn⟨CR⟩	FEV_1/IVC	ratio
9	-nnn⟨CR⟩	FEV_1/FVC	ratio
10	nn.nn⟨CR⟩	FEV_3	L
11	-nnn⟨CR⟩	FEV_3/FVC	ratio
12	nnnn⟨CR⟩	PEF	L/min
13	nn.nn⟨CR⟩	$FEF_{0.2-1.2}$	L/sec
14	nn.nn⟨CR⟩	$FEF_{25\%-75\%}$	L/sec
15	nn.nn⟨CR⟩	FMFT	sec
16	nn.nn⟨CR⟩	$FEF_{75\%-85\%}$	L/sec
17	nn.nn⟨CR⟩	$FEF_{25\%}$	L/sec
18	nn.nn⟨CR⟩	$FEF_{50\%}$	L/sec
19	nn.nn⟨CR⟩	$FEF_{75\%}$	L/sec
20	nn.nn⟨CR⟩	PIF	L/sec
21	nn.nn⟨CR⟩	$FIF_{75\%}$	L/sec
22	nn.nn⟨CR⟩	$FIF_{50\%}$	L/sec
23	nn.nn⟨CR⟩	$FIF_{25\%}$	L/sec
24	nnnn⟨CR⟩	MVV_{IND}	L/min
25	nnnn⟨CR⟩	MVV_f	L/min

immediately following the Predicted data. Each value is terminated by ⟨CR⟩.

The first item of the Flow data-set is a value giving the number of Flow data items which are being transmitted. All subsequent Flow values are in litres/min and represent the flow rate measured at 10 ms intervals over a period of 20 seconds. Flow sampling stops when the flow is less than 20 ml/sec for a period of 30 seconds.

Each Flow value consists of four digits prefixed by a sign which indicates whether the flow is inspiratory (−) or expiratory (+).

An example of the first few items of a Flow data-set is as follows, where the first value represents the total number of Flow values to be transmitted. The + sign indicates that the measured flow rate was *expiratory*.

2001⟨CR⟩
+0010⟨CR⟩
+0015⟨CR⟩
+0032⟨CR⟩
+0063⟨CR⟩
+0082⟨CR⟩
+0105⟨CR⟩
...
...

16.5 Serial Mode 1 (printout without graphs)

This Serial mode (see Table 16.3) transmits a formatted tabular printout of results via the serial port (see Figure 16.2).

Once this mode has been selected and the spirometry tests performed, transmitting the data via the serial port is initiated by pressing the EXTERNAL PRINT key (option 0; main menu), and then selecting one of the two parameter selection keys (SELECTED or SCREENING). Note that the Compact II's RTS must be held HIGH before the parameter selection key is pressed, in order to enable data output.

16.5.1 Program for accessing the data

An example QuickBASIC 4.5 program to access the Serial Mode 1 data is given below. However, this mode was originally intended for data transfer straight to an Epson printer, and therefore the data contains a number of additional control characters which are used to control the printer. Generally when intercepting data destined for printers, all the control characters except ⟨LF⟩ and ⟨CR⟩ will need to be removed by the program, in order to reveal the required data which can then be processed by the PC.

One way of making all the control characters 'visible' is to use the FULLCODE subroutine described in Section 5.6, which prints all the control characters in anglebrackets ⟨ ⟩. Where the letter codes are not given, the example subroutine FULLCODE gives the ASCII decimal value, e.g. ⟨9⟩.

In this particular case, all the additional control characters are found to be located in two areas of the data, namely towards the beginning and near the end. For example, the first 87 characters of the data stream which gave rise to Figure 16.2 are as follows. A space is indicated by the ⊔ symbol.

The Vitalograph Compact II spirometer

⟨LF⟩⟨LF⟩⟨CR⟩⟨14⟩␣␣␣␣␣␣␣␣␣␣␣VITALOGRAPH␣COMPACT␣II⟨LF⟩⟨CR⟩
⟨14⟩␣␣␣␣␣␣␣␣␣␣␣- -⟨LF⟩⟨CR⟩⟨ESC⟩⟨1⟩⟨20⟩DAT
E␣␣␣␣:

The last 104 characters of the data stream are as follows.

-4⟨LF⟩⟨CR⟩FEF75-85%␣1.32␣␣␣2.08␣157␣␣␣1.53␣116␣␣␣-26⟨LF⟩⟨CR⟩⟨LF⟩
⟨LF⟩⟨CR⟩⟨ESC⟩A⟨8⟩⟨ESC⟩A⟨12⟩⟨9⟩⟨9⟩⟨9⟩⟨9⟩⟨9⟩PHYSICIAN␣␣_ _ _ _ _
_ ⟨LF⟩⟨CR⟩⟨12⟩

Thus the Serial Mode 1 data output starts with two ⟨LF⟩ characters, and ends with the second of two Formfeed characters (ASCII 12). Note also that the data includes two '⟨ESC⟩A' sequences which also need to be removed.

```
         VITALOGRAPH COMPACT II
         ----------------------
DATE    : 19-07-93

NAME    : _____
REF.NO. : 1
AGE     : 35
SEX     : MALE
HEIGHT  : 180 CM
NORMALS : ECCS 1983

PRE  : 2 TESTS -36.4%
POST : 2 TESTS -20.7%
VALUES AT B.T.P.S.:-

A.T.S. BEST.     PRE          POST         CHANGE
       PRED     MEAS    %    MEAS    %       %
VC      5.35    -.--   --    -.--   --      --
FVC     5.10    4.57   90    4.76   93       4
FEV1    4.24    3.83   90    3.82   90       0
FEV1/VC%  81     --    --     --    --      --
FEV1/FVC% 83    84      1    80     -3      -3
PEF      582   329     57   359     62       9
FEF25-75% 4.69  3.81   81   3.66    78      -4
FEF75-85% 1.32  2.08  157   1.53   116     -26

PHYSICIAN _____
```

Fig. 16.2. An example of the Table format output by the example program for the 'Printout without graphs' option (Serial Mode 1) **vital-1.bas**.

Program points

- The example program uses COM1. If a different serial port is used, then appropriate changes will have to be made to the OPEN COM statement.
- The example program collects the data, and then removes all the control characters except for ⟨CR⟩, ⟨LF⟩, and spaces.
- Note that once the unwanted control characters have been removed, and the new 'clean' string (f$) passed back to a$ (a$=f$), the statement L% = INSTR(1,a$,cr$) has to be used a second time as the number of characters in the string may now be less than before.
- Since the final character of the data is not ⟨CR⟩, the program uses a convenient way of combining the removal of the two additional 'A' characters and terminating, by detecting the string AAPHYSICIAN, replacing it with PHYSICIAN and the signature line, and then quitting the loop.
- The data is saved in the file printout.dat which can then be printed out to give the results in the format shown in Figure 16.2.

Example program

```
REM [vital-1.bas]
REM Vitalograph Compact II
REM program for PRINTOUT WITHOUT GRAPHS
CLS
PRINT "Vitalograph Compact II spirometer: Serial Mode 1"
PRINT "opening the port"
OPEN "COM1:4800,N,8,1,CS,DS" FOR INPUT AS #1
OPEN "printout.dat" FOR OUTPUT AS #2
PRINT "waiting for data from spirometer"
PRINT "press <Q> to quit"
PRINT "press EXTERNAL PRINT key (0) from main menu"
cr$ = CHR$(13): REM   carriage return CR
a$ = ""
DO
    DO
        REM collect the data up to the next CR character
        a$ = a$ + INPUT$(LOC(1), #1)
        L% = INSTR(1, a$, cr$)
        key$ = INKEY$
```

```
            IF UCASE$(key$) = "Q" THEN
                CLOSE #1, #2
                END
            END IF
        LOOP UNTIL L% > 0
        REM remove all unwanted control characters
        f$ = ""
        FOR j = 1 TO LEN(a$)
            char$ = MID$(a$, j, 1)
            IF ASC(char$) >= 32 OR ASC(char$) = 13 OR
ASC(char$)= 10 THEN f$ = f$ + char$
        NEXT j
        a$ = f$
        REM remove LF and CR characters prior to printing
        L% = INSTR(1, a$, cr$)
        data$ = MID$(a$, 1, L% - 2)
        REM remove the two AA characters from last line
        IF LEFT$(data$, 11) = "AAPHYSICIAN" THEN
            PRINT
            PRINT "PHYSICIAN _____"
            PRINT #2, "PHYSICIAN _____"
            EXIT DO
        END IF
        PRINT data$
        PRINT #2, data$: REM print data to a file
        a$ = RIGHT$(a$, LEN(a$) - L%)
LOOP
CLOSE #1, #2
BEEP
END
```

An example of the output of the above example program is shown in Figure 16.2.

16.6 Serial Modes 3, 4, 5 (results and flow data)

When using these Modes from the External Communications menu (accessed from the Set-up menu) the data is transmitted via the serial port either completely automatically (immediately after the Compact II displays the results on the screen—Modes 4, 5), or in response to pressing the TRANSMIT RESULTS key† (Mode 3).

The number of data values transmitted depends on both the Serial Mode selected and the particular tests performed (Pre, Post, or both). With Serial Mode 5 the Flow data is also transmitted (see Table 16.4). Note that the key to processing the data is the Message number.

16.6.1 Program to access the Results and Flow data

An example QuickBASIC 4.5 program which accesses all the Results and Flow data is given below. Three subroutines are used.

Note that the complete data-set is saved in the file `alldata.dat`. The program also saves the Results and Flow data in separate files, namely `results.dat` and `flowdata.dat` respectively. All three data files can then be inspected by pressing the appropriate key from an option menu.

Program points

- The example program uses `COM1` in the `OPEN COM` statement.
- The Receive buffer is increased from the default 512 bytes to 3000 bytes using the `RB3000` option in the `OPEN COM` statement.
- The program's main module looks at data-line 56 when using Serial Mode 5 (Message number 4, 6) in order to read the total number of Flow data items to be transmitted (`flowno`), by setting the variable `finalno` initially to 56 for these Modes. Once `flowno` has been read, `finalno` is then set to 56 + `flowno`.
- The Flow data is numbered using the counter `nflow` which is set to zero when line 56 is read.
- The subroutine FORMATRESULTS formats the Results data (see Figure 16.4), making use of the Message number, and saves the data in the file `results.dat`.
- The subroutine OPTIONS gives a list of options which print the three data files to the screen by calling the subroutine READFILE. However, it is often much more convenient to use a commercial file-viewer (e.g. SHOW.COM‡) to view the data files, and an example of how to do this is given in the OPTIONS subroutine. For example, if SHOW.COM

† Option 0; main menu.
‡ SHOW.COM is marketed by Clockwork Software, Bidbury House, Havant, Hampshire, PO9 3JL, UK. Tel: +44–(0)1705–483217; Fax: +44–(0)1705–454233. See also Section 5.10.

were to be used to inspect the file results.dat in this case then the code would be as follows.

```
SHELL "show results.dat"
CLS
CALL options
```

- The subroutine READFILE prints the chosen file to the screen, and scrolls the file when the keyboard SPACE-bar is pressed. Note that the statement IF LOF(1) < 100 ... is there to take into account the number of characters which are always written to the beginning of this file. Note that if a commercial file-viewer is used (see Section 5.10) then the subroutine READFILE is not necessary.

Example program

```
REM [vital345.bas]
REM Vitalograph compact II serial MODES 3, 4, 5
DECLARE SUB formatresults ()
DECLARE SUB options ()
DECLARE SUB readfile (filename$)
DIM SHARED matrix(25, 3)
DIM SHARED label$(25)
COMMON SHARED messagenumber, reference, age, height, sex$
CLS
PRINT " Vitalograph Compact II. Serial Modes 3,4,5"
PRINT " opening the serial port"
OPEN "COM1: 4800,N,8,1,CS,DS,RB3000" FOR INPUT AS #1
PRINT " port open OK - waiting for data"
PRINT " Press <Q> to quit"
OPEN "results.dat" FOR OUTPUT AS #2
PRINT #2, " RESULTS - press <SPACE> to view (<Q> to quit)"
OPEN "alldata.dat" FOR OUTPUT AS #3
PRINT #3, " ALL DATA - press <SPACE> to view (<Q> to quit)"
cr$ = CHR$(13)
DO
    DO
        REM input the data one line at a time
        a$ = a$ + INPUT$(LOC(1), #1)
        L% = INSTR(1, a$, cr$)
```

```
            key$ = INKEY$
            IF UCASE$(key$) = "Q" THEN
                CLOSE
                END
            END IF
        LOOP UNTIL L% > 0
        data$ = MID$(a$, 1, L% - 1)
        n = n + 1: nflow = nflow + 1
        PRINT n, data$: REM print all data to the screen
        PRINT #3, n, data$: REM print all data to file
        REM read the message number
        IF n = 1 THEN
            messagenumber = VAL(data$)
            SELECT CASE messagenumber
                CASE 0, 1, 2
                    finalno = 55
                CASE 3
                    finalno = 80
                CASE 4, 6
                    finalno = 56
            END SELECT
        END IF
        IF n = 2 THEN reference = VAL(data$)
        IF n = 3 THEN age = VAL(data$)
        IF n = 4 THEN height = VAL(data$)
        IF n = 5 THEN sex$ = data$
        IF n = 56 AND messagenumber = 4 OR n = 56
AND messagenumber = 6 THEN
            flowno = VAL(data$)
            finalno = 56 + flowno
            nflow = 0
            OPEN "flowdata.dat" FOR OUTPUT AS #4
            PRINT #4, " FLOW DATA - press <SPACE> to view data
(Q to quit)"
            PRINT #4, "Total No. of flow data items = "; flowno
            PRINT #4,
            PRINT #4, "Order", "Flow", "Time"
            PRINT #4, , "(L/min)", "(secs)"
        END IF
        IF flowno > 0 AND n > 56 THEN PRINT #4, nflow, data$,
```

```
(nflow) / 100
    IF n >= 6 AND n <= 30 THEN j = 1
    IF n >= 31 AND n <= 55 THEN j = 2
    IF n >= 56 AND n <= 80 THEN j = 3
    IF n >= 6 THEN I = (n - 5) MOD 25
    matrix(I, j) = VAL(data$)
    IF n = finalno THEN EXIT DO
    a$ = RIGHT$(a$, LEN(a$) - L%)
LOOP
REM print test results to a file formatted in columns
CALL formatresults
CLOSE
CALL options
END


SUB formatresults
    label$(1) = "VC (L)"
    label$(2) = "IVC (L)"
    label$(3) = "FVC (L)"
    label$(4) = "FEV 0.5 (L)"
    label$(5) = "FEV 0.5/FVC (ratio)"
    label$(6) = "FEV 1 (L)"
    label$(7) = "FEV 1/VC (ratio)"
    label$(8) = "FEV 1/IVC (ratio)"
    label$(9) = "FEV 1/FVC (ratio)"
    label$(10) = "FEV 3 (L)"
    label$(11) = "FEV 3/FVC (ratio)"
    label$(12) = "PEF (L/min)"
    label$(13) = "FEF 0.2-1.2 (L/sec)"
    label$(14) = "FMEF (L/sec)"
    label$(15) = "FMFT (sec)"
    label$(16) = "FEF 75%-85% (L/sec)"
    label$(17) = "FEF 25% (L/sec)"
    label$(18) = "FEF 50% (L/sec)"
    label$(19) = "FEF 75% (L/sec)"
    label$(20) = "PIF (L/sec)"
    label$(21) = "FIF 75% (L/sec)"
    label$(22) = "FIF 50% (L/sec)"
    label$(23) = "FIF 25% (L/sec)"
```

```
        label$(24) = "MVV IND (L/min)"
        label$(25) = "MVV DIR (L/min)"
        REM
        REM print the reference data to file
        PRINT #2, "Time = "; TIME$, "Date = "; DATE$
        PRINT #2, "Ref. No. = "; reference
        PRINT #2, "Age = "; age
        PRINT #2, "Height = "; height
        PRINT #2, "Sex = "; sex$
        PRINT #2,
        SELECT CASE messagenumber
            CASE 0, 1, 4
                SELECT CASE messagenumber
                    CASE 0, 4
                        IF messagenumber = 0 THEN serialmode = 4
                        IF messagenumber = 4 THEN serialmode = 5
                        bestlast$ = "Last"
                    CASE 1
                        serialmode = 3
                        bestlast$ = "Best"
                END SELECT
                PRINT #2, "Serial Mode = "; serialmode
                PRINT #2, bestlast$
                PRINT #2, "Pre Data", "Predicted", "Parameter
(units)"
                FOR I = 1 TO 25
                    PRINT #2, matrix(I, 1), matrix(I, 2),
label$(I)
                NEXT I
            CASE 2, 6
                IF messagenumber = 2 THEN
                    serialmode = 4
                    ELSE serialmode = 5
                END IF
                PRINT #2, "Serial Mode = "; serialmode
                PRINT #2, "Best"
                PRINT #2, "Post Data", "Predicted", "Parameter
(units)"
                FOR I = 1 TO 25
                    PRINT #2, matrix(I, 1), matrix(I, 2),
```

The Vitalograph Compact II spirometer

```
label$(I)
            NEXT I
        CASE 3
            PRINT #2, "Serial Mode = 3"
            PRINT #2, "Best", "Best"
            PRINT #2, "Pre Data", "Post Data", "Predicted",
"Parameter(units)"
            FOR I = 1 TO 25
                PRINT #2, matrix(I, 1), matrix(I, 2),
matrix(I, 3), label$(I)
            NEXT I
    END SELECT
END SUB


SUB options
    PRINT : PRINT : PRINT
    PRINT " SELECT OPTIONS"
    PRINT
    PRINT " view RESULTS data   :  press  <R>"
    PRINT " view FLOW data      :  press  <F>"
    PRINT " view ALL the data   :  press  <A>"
    PRINT
    PRINT " (press <Q> to quit)"
optionsline1:
    DO
        key$ = INKEY$
    LOOP WHILE key$ = ""
    SELECT CASE UCASE$(key$)
        CASE "R"
            CALL readfile("results.dat")
            REM example of using third-part viewer
            REM SHELL "show results.dat"
            REM CLS
            REM CALL options
        CASE "F"
            CALL readfile("flowdata.dat")
        CASE "A"
            CALL readfile("alldata.dat")
        CASE "Q"
```

```
            CLOSE
            END
        CASE ELSE
            GOTO optionsline1
    END SELECT
END SUB


SUB readfile (filename$)
    f$ = filename$
    CLS
    LOCATE 5, 5
    OPEN f$ FOR INPUT AS #1
    IF LOF(1) < 100 THEN
        PRINT "THERE IS NO DATA"
        CLOSE
        CALL options
    END IF
    REM print the first 5 lines of the file
    FOR j = 1 TO 5
        LINE INPUT #1, a$
        PRINT a$
    NEXT j
    REM print a line each time a key is pressed
    DO UNTIL EOF(1)
        LINE INPUT #1, a$
        PRINT a$
        DO
            key$ = INKEY$
        LOOP WHILE key$ = ""
        IF UCASE$(key$) = "Q" THEN EXIT DO
    LOOP
    CLOSE
    CLS
    CALL options
END SUB
```

Data file (`alldata.dat`*).* The complete data output by the Compact II is saved in the file `alldata.dat`, and an example of the format of this data is shown below, where the number on the left (added by the program) gives the order of the data. The first value is the Message number, which in this example is 03. The Patient Reference data starts at line 2, and the Pre results start at line 6 (see Table 16.5). Note that this example shows the initial part of the 'raw' data which generated the results shown in Figure 16.4.

```
ALL DATA - press <SPACE> to view data (<Q> to quit)
 1         03
 2         123
 3         44
 4         180
 5         M
 6         00.00
 7         00.00
 8         04.30
 9         02.11
10         +049
11         03.49
12         +000
13         +000
14         +081
...        ...
...        ...
...        ...
```

The following example is of part of the file `alldata.dat` when using Serial Mode 5 (gets Flow data), and shows the point where the Predicted data ends (line 55) and the Flow data begins (line 56). Note that the Flow data *always* starts at line 56; the first value being the number of Flow data values to follow (2001 in this example). All the Flow values are prefixed with a sign to indicate inspiration (−) or expiration (+).

```
...        ...
...        ...
51         03.28    [predicted FIF 75%]
52         04.86    [predicted FIF 50%]
53         04.10    [predicted FIF 25%]
54         0122     [predicted MVV IND]
```

55	0122	[predicted MVV f (End of Results)]
56	2001	[Number of flow data items to follow]
57	+0008	[Flow data begins here....]
58	+0013	
59	+0017	
60	+0018	
61	+0019	
62	+0020	
63	+0020	
64	+0021	
65	+0021	
66	+0023	
...	...	
...	...	
2057	+0001	

*Data file (*results.dat*).* The results are formatted and saved in the file results.dat which can then be printed out. An example of the format of the results using the above example program is shown in Figure 16.4.

*Data file (*flowdata.dat*).* The file flowdata.dat contains the Flow data (column 2), and the time (column 3). The following example is a typical extract from this file, and shows the beginning, region of maximum flow rate, and the region where the flow returns to zero.

```
FLOW DATA - press <SPACE> to view data (<Q> to quit)
Total No. of flow data items = 2001
```

Order	Flow (L/min)	Time (secs)
1	+0008	.01
2	+0010	.02
3	+0013	.03
4	+0014	.04
...	...	...
...	...	...
48	+0321	.48
49	+0323	.49
50	+0325	.5
51	+0325	.51
52	+0328	.52

53	+0322	.53
54	+0318	.54
...	...	...
...	...	...
298	+0011	2.98
299	+0009	2.99
300	+0006	3
301	+0003	3.01
302	+0001	3.02
303	−0000	3.03

The file `flowdata.dat` can now be exported into a graph plotting package if required. For example, Figure 16.3 shows the flow data plotted from a typical file, using the freeware package GNUPLOT.†

For most ordinary purposes the flow data output by the Compact II is adequate as it stands. However, if accurate *volume* data are required, then extensive further processing of the flow data is necessary (e.g. using back extrapolation) as described by the guidelines established by the American Thoracic Society (1987).

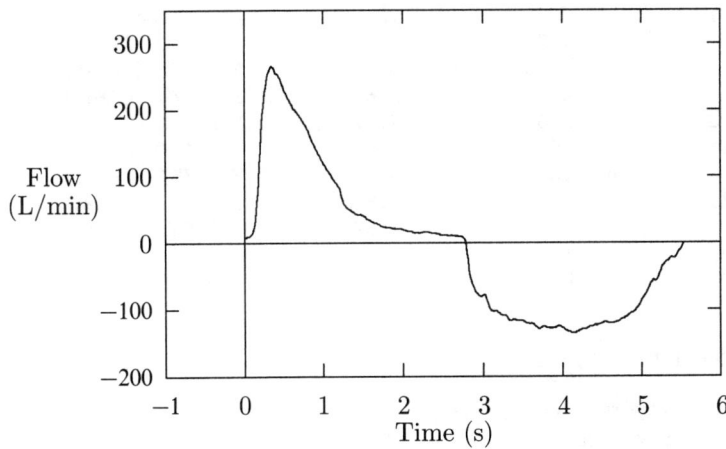

Fig. 16.3. Flow/volume data from file `flowdata.dat` plotted using the freeware package GNUPLOT.

† See Appendix 7 for details of GNUPLOT.

```
RESULTS - press <SPACE> to view data (<Q> to quit)

Time = 18:58:35              Date = 09-02-1993
Ref. No. = 123
Age = 44
Height = 180
Sex = M

Serial Mode = 3
Best         Best
Pre Data     Post Data    Predicted    Parameter(units)
0            0            4.79         VC (L)
0            0            4.79         IVC (L)
4.3          4.37         4.79         FVC (L)
2.11         2.43         3.17         FEV 0.5 (L)
49           56           66           FEV 0.5/FVC (ratio)
3.49         3.72         3.74         FEV 1 (L)
0            0            78           FEV 1/VC (ratio)
0            0            78           FEV 1/IVC (ratio)
81           85           77           FEV 1/FVC (ratio)
4.27         0            4.73         FEV 3 (L)
99           0            99           FEV 3/FVC (ratio)
268          383          592          PEF (L/min)
4.45         5.91         7.66         FEF 0.2-1.2 (L/sec)
3.52         3.9          3.87         FEF 25%-75% (L/sec)
.61          .56          .61          FMFT (sec)
1.79         1.82         1.12         FEF 75%-85% (L/sec)
4.44         4.93         8.08         FEF 25% (L/sec)
3.58         4.18         5.66         FEF 50% (L/sec)
2.3          2.55         2.71         FEF 75% (L/sec)
.01          .04          8.92         PIF (L/sec)
0            .02          4.55         FIF 75% (L/sec)
.01          .03          5.58         FIF 50% (L/sec)
0            .02          5.27         FIF 25% (L/sec)
131          139          141          MVV IND (L/min)
0            0            0            MVV f (L/min)


SELECT OPTIONS

view RESULTS data   :  press <R>
view FLOW data      :  press <F>
view ALL the data   :  press <A>
(press <Q> to quit)
```

Fig. 16.4. Example of the Results data as viewed on the screen.

17

The Ohmeda 7800 ventilator

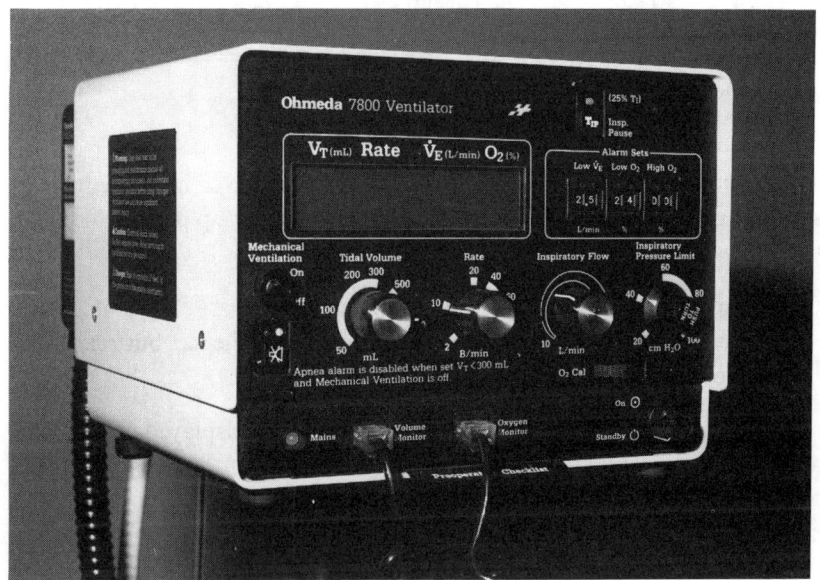

17.1 Introduction

The Ohmeda 7800† is a time-cycled ventilator designed for use in anaesthesia. Information regarding the ventilator's activity is shown on a liquid-crystal display. More detailed information, both digital (parameter values and alarm settings) and analog (pressure and oxygen concentration), is available via the serial port.

The electrical safety classification of the Ohmeda 7800 ventilator is Type BF.‡

---

† Ohmeda Anesthesia Systems, Ohmeda Drive, P.O. Box 7550, Madison, Wisconsin 53707, USA. Tel: +1–608–2211551. Fax: +1–608–2229147.
‡ See Chapter 7 for further details.

Table 17.1. *Ohmeda 7800 serial port.*

Pin No.	Format	Name	Comments
2	RS-232	TxD	Transmits data.
3	RS-232	RxD	Receives data.
7	RS-232	GND	Signal ground.
18	Analog	Oxygen (ground)	
19	Analog	Oxygen (shield)	
20	Analog	Oxygen (signal)	0 to 100% (0–1 volt)
23	Analog	Pressure (signal)	-20 to 120 cm H_2O (0–1 volt)
24	Analog	Pressure (shield)	
25	Analog	Pressure (ground)	

17.1.1 Software version

The version of the ventilator's software (4.xx) is displayed in the ventilator **set-up page** shown in the liquid-crystal display. The set-up page is accessed as follows.

(1) Switch the 'mechanical ventilation' switch off.
(2) Press and continue to hold down the 'alarm silence' button.
(3) Now press the 'inspiration pause' button.

This results in the following set-up page being displayed, which indicates the ventilator (7800), software version (4.xx), driving gas (/O, oxygen), language (English), and operating height above sea level (300 m).

```
7800 REV 4.xx /O
ENGLISH  300 M
```

17.2 Serial port

A 25-pin female D-type serial port is located on the rear panel of the ventilator. The communications interface provides for both digital (serial) and analog data, as shown in Table 17.1. Note that the 7800 requires a minimum signal of ± 5 volts to drive its RxD line (pin-3).

17.2.1 Protocol options

The serial protocol is shown in Table 17.2. The bit-rate is fixed at 1200 bps.

Table 17.2. *Ohmeda 7800 serial protocol.*

Bit rate	1200
Data bits	7
Parity	Odd
Stop bits	1

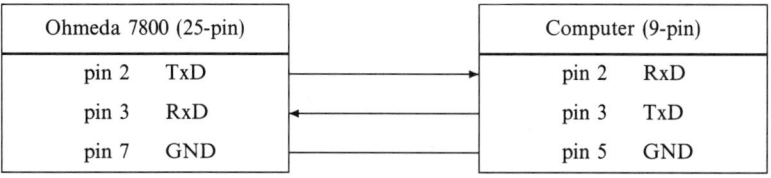

Fig. 17.1. Ohmeda 7800 wiring diagram.

17.2.2 Cable connections

Figure 17.1 indicates the wiring configuration for interfacing to a PC.

17.3 Communication modes

The Ohmeda 7800 has two operating modes, namely **Auto-output** mode and **Slave** mode. Data can be output in either mode, and consists of the **Measured data** (values of the measured parameters) and the **Status data** (values of the parameters set on the ventilator, and a number of status bytes). Note that the Status data output using the Compressed format is more comprehensive than that output using the Printer format (see Section 17.5).

17.3.1 Auto-output mode

This is the default mode for the ventilator immediately following power-on. In this mode the ventilator outputs digital data automatically via the serial port, either every 10 seconds or following each breath, whichever is the most frequent. Data can be output in either Printer format or Compressed format, although immediately following power-on data is output in Printer format (the default format). Note that when the Compressed format is used in Auto-output mode, an 'alarms silenced' string (:VTR) is transmitted by the ventilator whenever the button for silencing the alarms is pressed.

Table 17.3. *Ohmeda 7800 ventilator command codes and checksums.*

Code	Meaning	Checksum	
X	Auto-output mode	99	c
S	Slave mode	104	h
P	Printer format data mode	107	k
Q	Compressed format data mode	106	j
E	Enable checksum mode	—	—
D	Disable checksum mode	117	u
CS	Silence alarms	37	%
?	Request data	124	¦

17.3.2 Slave mode

The 7800 can be switched to Slave mode by sending the command-code S (see Table 17.3) from the computer. When in Slave mode data is *only* output in response to a 'send data' command (command-code ?). Data can be output in either Printer format or Compressed format.

Note that when in Slave mode the value returned for the *maximum pressure* is that at the moment the ventilator receives the 'send data' command. The *maximum pressure* returned in Slave mode therefore varies considerably depending on the exact moment in the respiratory cycle that the ventilator receives the command. In view of this the *maximum pressure* is best obtained from data output while in Auto-output mode, since this data relates to the last complete respiratory cycle.

17.4 Commands and replies

There are eight **commands** available for communicating with the ventilator, each generating a **reply**. A command consists of a command-code prefixed by the capital letters VT as follows.

⟨VT⟩⟨command-code⟩

Note that none of the commands can alter ventilator function, although one command is available for silencing alarms. All other commands simply influence the way data can be accessed via the serial port.

The command-codes and their meaning are shown in Table 17.3.

17.4.1 Command string structure

Commands are transmitted by the computer within a command string which must adhere to the format shown below. Note that when the checksum mode is *enabled*, a checksum replaces the space ␣ in the command string.

⟨ESC⟩VT⟨command-code⟩␣⟨CR⟩
⟨ESC⟩VT⟨command-code⟩⟨checksum⟩⟨CR⟩

When sending commands using QuickBASIC, care must be taken not to inadvertently send *two* ⟨CR⟩ characters to the ventilator. This is easily done if a ⟨CR⟩ is included in the command string to be transmitted using a PRINT# statement *without* a following semicolon.†

For example, the QuickBASIC statement to send a command to switch the ventilator to Slave mode (command-code S) via a COM port designated as #1 would be as follows since ⟨ESC⟩ is ASCII 27, and a space ␣ is ASCII 32.

PRINT #1, CHR$(27) + "VTS" + CHR$(32)

Note that the final ⟨CR⟩ is *not* included here, since there is no semicolon following the PRINT# statement.

17.4.2 Reply string structure

All reply strings from the Ohmeda 7800 have one of the two formats shown below, depending on whether data is returned or not. When the checksum mode is *enabled*, ⟨checksum⟩ replaces the space ␣.

:VT⟨reply-code⟩␣⟨CR⟩
:VT⟨reply-code⟩⟨data⟩␣⟨CR⟩

Unless data is returned (in response to the command-code ?) the reply is in the form of an acknowledgment. In response to a command to change Mode (e.g. change to Slave mode) this is either affirmative (:VTY), or negative (:VTN). In response to a command to silence alarms, this is either affirmative (:VTR), or negative (:VTN).

Following a command to send data (command-code ?), the Ohmeda 7800 outputs *two* data-strings; the first one being the Measured data (reply-code D), and the second one being the Status data (reply-code Q) as follows.

† In QuickBASIC the semicolon suppresses the ⟨CR⟩⟨LF⟩ pair which is otherwise added—see Section 5.3.1.

:VTD⟨data⟩␣⟨CR⟩
:VTQ⟨data⟩␣⟨CR⟩

Note that both the data-set *and* the format of the data will depend on the current data format mode of the ventilator (either Printer format or Compressed format). These two data formats are detailed in the next Section.

17.5 Data formats

The Ohmeda 7800 ventilator outputs data in one of two formats as follows. Note that there are no time-stamps associated with either of the data formats.

- Printer format (enabled using the command-code P)
- Compressed format (enabled using the command-code Q)

Data can be output in either format in both Auto-output and Slave mode. The command-codes to switch formats are shown in Table 17.3. Note that the data-set which is output when using the Compressed format is much more comprehensive than that output using the Printer format. The Printer format data-set is included in the Compressed data-set. These two data formats are now described in detail.

17.5.1 Printer format data mode

When the Ohmeda 7800 outputs data in Printer format, both the Measured and Status data are displayed on a single line in columns, with leading zeros suppressed, as shown in Figure 17.2. An explanatory header, preceded by six blank lines, is printed after every 59 outputs. Details of the header codes are shown in Table 17.4.

17.5.2 Compressed format data mode

When the Compressed format is used data is output in the form of *three* data-strings; a Measured data-string, a Status data-string, and an 'alarm silenced' data-string. These are now described in turn.

Measured data. The Compressed format Measured data-string is distinguished by the reply-code D, and is made up of 30 bytes including the ⟨CR⟩. If the checksum mode has been enabled, then a checksum

⟨CR⟩⟨LF⟩
⟨CR⟩⟨LF⟩
⟨CR⟩⟨LF⟩
⟨CR⟩⟨LF⟩
⟨CR⟩⟨LF⟩
⟨CR⟩⟨LF⟩
S␣MEAS␣␣TV␣␣␣␣VE␣␣␣RR␣␣O2␣MAX␣␣PT␣MIN␣␣SET␣␣VT␣␣RR␣␣IF␣␣␣␣␣I:E␣␣␣PL␣␣LVE␣LO␣HO␣MV␣I P⟨CR⟩⟨LF⟩
n␣␣␣␣␣␣nnnn␣n.nn␣␣nnn␣n n n␣nnn␣␣nnn␣␣␣␣␣nnnn␣nnn␣nnn␣1:nnn . n␣nnn␣n . n␣nn nn␣␣␣n␣␣␣n⟨CR⟩⟨LF⟩

S MEAS	TV	VE	RR	O2	MAX	PT	MIN	SET	VT	RR	IF	I:E	PL	LVE	LO	HO	MV	IP
	502	5.04	10	39	28	0	2		570	10	12	1: 1.1	46	1.5	25	0	1	0
	499	5.08	10	39	28	0	2		570	10	12	1: 1.1	46	1.5	25	0	1	0
	499	5.08	10	39	28	0	2		570	10	12	1: 1.1	46	1.5	25	0	0	0
	506	5.03	10	39	27	0	2		570	10	12	1: 1.1	46	1.5	25	0	1	0
	515	5.04	10	39	28	0	3		570	10	12	1: 1.1	46	1.5	25	0	1	0
	521	5.09	10	39	28	0	3		570	10	12	1: 1.1	46	1.5	25	0	1	0
	508	5.06	10	39	27	0	2		570	10	12	1: 1.1	46	1.5	25	0	1	0
	502	5.04	10	39	28	0	2		570	10	12	1: 1.1	46	1.5	25	0	1	0

Fig. 17.2. Ohmeda 7800 Printer Format: details of header and data strings, and a typical example of data output. The symbol ␣ indicates a space.

Table 17.4. *Printer format.*

Heading	Format	Description	Units
S	n	measured sigh breath status	1=on, 0=off
TV	nnnn	measured tidal volume	mL
VE	nn.nn	measured minute volume	L
RR	nnn	measured respiratory rate	breaths/min
O_2	nnn	measured oxygen concentration	%
PK	nnn	measured maximum pressure	cm H_2O
PT	nnn	measured plateau pressure	cm H_2O
EE	nnn	measured minimum pressure	cm H_2O
VT	nnnn	set tidal volume	mL
RR	nnn	set respiratory rate	breaths/min
IF	nnn	set inspiratory flow	L/min
I:E	1:nnn.n	set I:E ratio	—
PL	nnn	set peak pressure alarm limit	cm H_2O
LVE	n.n	set low minute volume alarm limit	L
LO	nn	set low oxygen conc. alarm limit	%
HO	nn	set high oxygen conc. alarm limit	% (0=100%)
MV	n	mechanical ventilation status	1=on, 0=off
IP	n	inspiratory pause status	1=on, 0=off

replaces the space ␣ shown in the format below. Details of the Measured data-string are shown in Table 17.5.

:VTDaaaabbbbdddeeefffggghhhs␣⟨CR⟩

A single status byte is returned with the Measured data-string. The byte is bit-encoded (see Table 17.5), and is expressed as the ASCII character having the same decimal value as the byte.

For example, suppose the status byte is the character A (ASCII 65), as shown in the example below. The binary equivalent of 65 is 01000001b, and therefore bit-0 = 1 and bit-6 = 1. Since Table 17.5 indicates that bit-6 (D6) is always 1, it follows that the status byte A indicates that the data relates to a new breath.

A typical example of a Measured data-string output in Compressed format is as follows.

:VTD053000636012033020010001A

There are only 29 characters in the string, and so the last character (A)

Table 17.5. *Compressed format: details of Measured data-string. Each entry is zero filled and right justified (i.e. 95 for aaaa = 0095). Bits set (1) in the status byte (s) indicate that the condition is active. X = not used (set to 0).*

Code	Description	Units
aaaa	measured tidal volume	mL
bbbb	measured minute volume	L×100
ddd	measured respiratory rate	breaths/min
eee	measured oxygen concentration	% (0–100)
fff	measured maximum pressure	cm H_2O
ggg	measured plateau pressure	cm H_2O
hhh	measured minimum pressure	cm H_2O
s	measured data status byte	—
	Status byte	
bit-0	0 = 10 sec data; 1 = newbreath data	
bit-1	0 = normal breath; 1 = sigh	
bit-2	X	
bit-3	X	
bit-4	X	
bit-5	X	
bit-6	1	
bit-7	0	

must be the status byte which is followed by a space, i.e. the checksum mode is not enabled. Comparing the data-string with Table 17.5 shows that the above data-string represents the following data.

Measured tidal volume	530 ml
Measured minute volume	6.36 L
Measured respiratory rate	12 breaths/min
Measured oxygen concentration	33%
Measured maximum pressure	20 cm H_2O
Measured plateau pressure	10 cm H_2O
Measured minimum pressure	1 cm H_2O
Status byte	A ≡ ASCII 65 ≡ 01000001b

Status data. The Compressed format Status data-string is distinguished by the reply-code Q, and is made up of 37 bytes including the ⟨CR⟩. If the checksum mode has been enabled, then a checksum replaces the space ⊔. The Status string includes six status bytes (s_1-s_6), as shown in the format below.

:VTQaaaabbbdddeeeefffgghhiijjs$_1$s$_2$s$_3$s$_4$s$_5$s$_6$⊔⟨CR⟩

Details of the Status data-string are shown in Table 17.6. Details of the six status bytes are shown in Table 17.7.

A typical example of a Status data-string output in Compressed format is as follows.

:VTQ04400100190033050251525000@@@@@H

In this example there are only 35 characters in the string, and so there must be a space following the last character, i.e. the checksum mode is not enabled. Comparing the data-string with Table 17.6 shows that the above data-string represents the following data.

Set tidal volume	440 ml
Set respiratory rate	10 breaths/min
Set inspiratory flow	19 L/min
Set I:E ratio	1:3.3
Set peak pressure alarm	50 cm H_2O
Set sustained pressure alarm	25 cm H_2O
Set low minute volume alarm	15 L/min
Set low oxygen alarm limit	25%
Set high oxygen alarm limit	100%
Status bytes	byte 1 = @ ≡ ASCII 64 ≡ 01000000b
	byte 2 = @ ≡ ASCII 64 ≡ 01000000b
	byte 3 = @ ≡ ASCII 64 ≡ 01000000b
	byte 4 = @ ≡ ASCII 64 ≡ 01000000b
	byte 5 = @ ≡ ASCII 64 ≡ 01000000b
	byte 6 = H ≡ ASCII 74 ≡ 01001000b

Comparing the status bytes with Table 17.7 shows that only the sixth status byte has an additional bit set (bit-3), which indicates that the ventilator is switched on.

17.6 The checksum

The Ohmeda 7800 checksum is a **two's complement** 7-bit checksum (see Section 3.4.2). For commands, the checksum includes the ⟨ESC⟩ control character but not the ⟨CR⟩ as follows.

Table 17.6. *Compressed format: details of Status data-string.* Each entry is zero filled and right justified (i.e. 95 in aaaa = 0095). Bits set (1) in status bytes s_1-s_6 indicate that the condition is active.

Code	Description	Units
aaaa	Set tidal volume	mL
bbb	Set respiratory rate	breaths/min
ddd	Set inspiratory flow	L/min
eeee	Set I:E ratio	1:eee.e (not rounded)
fff	Set peak pressure alarm limit	cm H_2O
gg	Set sustained pressure alarm limit	cm H_2O
hh	Set low minute volume alarm limit	L×10
ii	Set low oxygen conc. alarm limit	%
jj	Set high oxygen conc. alarm limit	%
$s_1 s_2 s_3 s_4 s_5 s_6$	status bytes	—

$$\underbrace{\langle\text{ESC}\rangle\text{VT}\langle\text{command-code}\rangle}_{checksum}\langle\text{checksum}\rangle\langle\text{CR}\rangle$$

For replies, the checksum includes the characters :VT but not the ⟨CR⟩. For example, consider the command message VT? (send data). The full command string together with the ASCII values is shown below.

⟨ESC⟩⟨V T ?⟩⟨checksum⟩⟨CR⟩
 27   86 84 63

Since the sum of the ASCII characters is 260, the checksum is therefore given by

$$\text{checksum} = 128 - 260(modulo\,128)$$
$$= 128 - 4$$
$$= 124$$
$$\text{checksum (ASCII character)} = |$$

The string to be sent is therefore ⟨ESC⟩⟨VT?⟩⟨|⟩⟨CR⟩. This would be sent using QuickBASIC via a serial port designated as #1 as

PRINT #1, CHR$(27) + "VT?" + CHR$(124)

A QuickBASIC 4.5 routine to determine a two's complement checksum is given in Section 5.15.

Table 17.7. *Details of Status bytes.*

Byte	Bit	Meaning
Byte 1	bit-0	High O_2 alarm
	bit-1	Low O_2 alarm
	bit-2	Apnoea alarm
	bit-3	Low patient MV alarm
	bit-4	High pressure alarm
	bit-5	Low pressure alarm
	bit-6	1
	bit-7	Not used—set to 0
Byte 2	bit-0	Sustained pressure alarm
	bit-1	Sub-atmospheric pressure alarm
	bit-2	AC failure (primary supply voltage low)
	bit-3	Low battery alarm
	bit-4	O_2 limit set error
	bit-5	Ventilator setting range error
	bit-6	1
	bit-7	Not used—set to 0
Byte 3	bit-0	O_2 sensor failure alarm
	bit-1	Volume failure alarm
	bit-2	Maximum pressure >60 cm H_2O
	bit-3	Reverse flow
	bit-4	Low gas supply pressure alarm
	bit-5	Apnoea alarm off
	bit-6	1
	bit-7	Not used—set to 0

17.7 Example interactive program

The following interactive QuickBASIC 4.5 utility program indicates how to send command messages interactively from the keyboard, collect the reply, save data and messages to a log file, and extract specific parameter values from a data-string.

The program starts by making the ventilator enter the Auto-output mode using Printer format. While in Auto-output mode, the data format can be switched by pressing either <Q> (Compressed format) or <P> (Printer format). When using the Printer format, a subset of the data is extracted from the data-string and printed in full (e.g. TV = 526).

Table 17.7 cont. Details of Status bytes.

Byte	Bit	Meaning
Byte 4	bit-0	A/D conversion failure
	bit-1	CPU failure
	bit-2	ROM checksum failure
	bit-3	RAM read/write failure
	bit-4	Gas supply <30 psi gauge
	bit-5	Power loss
	bit-6	1
	bit-7	Not used—set to 0
Byte 5	bit-0	Flow output incorrect or continuously on
	bit-1	Exh. valve not on/off in insp/exp
	bit-2	Gas supply control solenoid not on
	bit-3	D/A write/read failure
	bit-4	Pressure transducer board failure
	bit-5	7.5 volt supply out of range
	bit-6	1
	bit-7	Not used—set to 0
Byte 6	bit-0	Flow table values 0,FF or non-increasing
	bit-1	Inspiratory pause on
	bit-2	Volume monitor standby
	bit-3	Ventilation switch on
	bit-4	Volume sensor cartridge coasting (end of breath not detected)
	bit-5	Alarms are silenced
	bit-6	1
	bit-7	Not used—set to 0

Slave mode is entered by pressing <S>, whereupon the program prompts the operator for a command-code. After entering a command-code, the program transmits the command and then displays both the full command and the reply. Sending the command-code X (or entering A†) will return the ventilator to Auto-output mode.

---

† Note that the option to use A to switch to Auto-output mode actually results in sending the command-code X—see the example program.

Program points

- Since only three lines are used for communications, there is no hardware handshaking, and so the CS and DS parameters need to be used in the OPEN COM statement.
- In the subroutine SEND there is no ⟨CR⟩ in the string to be sent to the ventilator (s$ = CHR$(27) + "VT" + UCASE$(s$) + CHR$(32)) since the PRINT# statement is not followed by a semicolon (see Section 5.3.1).
- All Ohmeda 7800 command-codes are in uppercase.
- dataformat$ is a shared variable since its value (either 'printer' or 'compressed') determines whether specific parameter values are extracted and printed while in Auto-output mode (see the subroutine AUTOOUTPUT).
- Since the letter Q is a command-code (change to Compressed format) the program requires the user to press <T> to terminate (quit) the program.

Example program

```
REM [ohm7800.bas]
REM interactive program for Ohmeda 7800 ventilator
DECLARE SUB emptybuffer ()
DECLARE SUB getreply ()
DECLARE SUB send (s$)
DECLARE SUB slavemode ()
DECLARE SUB autooutputmode ()
COMMON SHARED dataformat$
CLS
OPEN "COM1:1200,0,7,1,CS,DS" FOR RANDOM ACCESS READ WRITE
                                                       AS #1
OPEN "7800log.dat" FOR OUTPUT AS #2
PRINT "communications open OK"
REM   send data in Printer format (P-code)
PRINT "switching to Printer format"
PRINT #2, "switching to printer format"
PRINT #1, CHR$(27) + "VTP" + CHR$(32)
CALL getreply
dataformat$ = "printer"
```

```
CALL autooutputmode
END



SUB autooutputmode
    CLS
    REM switch to auto-output mode
    PRINT "entering AUTO-OUTPUT mode", , , "press <T> to quit"
    PRINT #2, "entering auto-output mode"
    PRINT #1, CHR$(27) + "VTX" + CHR$(32)
    CALL getreply
    DO
        DO
            a$ = a$ + INPUT$(LOC(1), #1)
            L% = INSTR(1, a$, CHR$(13))
            key$ = INKEY$
            SELECT CASE UCASE$(key$)
                CASE "T"
                    CLOSE #1, #2
                    END
                CASE "S"
                    PRINT #1, CHR$(27) + "VTS" + CHR$(32)
                    PRINT "entering slave mode"
                    PRINT #2, "entering slave mode"
                    CALL getreply
                    CALL slavemode
                CASE "Q"
                    dataformat$ = "compressed"
                    PRINT #1, CHR$(27) + "VTQ" + CHR$(32)
                    PRINT "switching to compressed format"
                    PRINT #2, "switching to compressed format"
                    CALL getreply
                CASE "P"
                    dataformat$ = "printer"
                    PRINT #1, CHR$(27) + "VTP" + CHR$(32)
                    PRINT "switching to Printer format"
                    PRINT #2, "switching to printer format"
                    CALL getreply
```

```
            END SELECT
        LOOP UNTIL L% > 0
        data$ = MID$(a$, 1, L% - 1):
        PRINT data$
        PRINT #2, data$
        a$ = RIGHT$(a$, LEN(a$) - L%)
        IF dataformat$ = "printer" THEN
            REM printing data
            TV$ = MID$(data$, 6, 4)
            MV$ = MID$(data$, 11, 5)
            RR$ = MID$(data$, 17, 3)
            FIO2$ = MID$(data$, 21, 3)
            PMAX$ = MID$(data$, 25, 3)
            PMIN$ = MID$(data$, 33, 3)
            PRINT "Time     = "; TIME$, , , "press <T> to quit"
            PRINT "TV       = "; TV$
            PRINT "Min Vol  =    "; MV$
            PRINT "Resp Rate = "; RR$
            PRINT "FIO2     = "; FIO2$
            PRINT "Pressure = "; PMAX$; "/"; PMIN$
            PRINT : PRINT : PRINT
        END IF
    LOOP
END SUB



SUB emptybuffer
    REM empties the receive buffer
    DO WHILE NOT EOF(1)
        buff$ = INPUT$(LOC(1), #1)
    LOOP
    PRINT "buffer emptied OK"
END SUB



SUB getreply
    REM wait 1 sec
    REM because of the second compressed data-string
    SLEEP 1
```

```
        a$ = ""
        timezero = TIMER
        DO
            DO
                a$ = a$ + INPUT$(LOC(1), #1)
                IF TIMER > timezero + 5 THEN
                    PRINT "time-out - no reply: press key to
continue"
                    SLEEP: z$ = INKEY$
                    END
                END IF
                L% = INSTR(1, a$, CHR$(13))
            LOOP UNTIL L% > 0
            reply$ = MID$(a$, 1, L% - 1)
            PRINT "reply = "; reply$
            PRINT #2, "reply$ = "; reply$
            a$ = RIGHT$(a$, LEN(a$) - L%)
        LOOP UNTIL LEN(a$) = 0
END SUB


SUB send (s$)
    REM sends the command string
    CALL emptybuffer
    thiscommand$ = CHR$(27) + "VT" + s$ + CHR$(32)
    PRINT #1, thiscommand$
    PRINT #2, thiscommand$
    PRINT "sending command ", thiscommand$
END SUB


SUB slavemode
    CLS
    PRINT "SLAVE mode"
    PRINT #2, "SLAVE mode"
    DO
        PRINT
        INPUT "enter command-code"; commandcode$
        SELECT CASE commandcode$
            CASE "T", "t"
```

```
                CLOSE #1, #2
                END
            CASE "A", "X"
                PRINT "entering auto-output mode"
                PRINT #2, "entering auto-output mode"
                PRINT #1, CHR$(27) + "VTX" + CHR$(32)
                CALL getreply
                CALL autooutputmode
            CASE "P"
                dataformat$ = "printer"
                PRINT "switching to Printer format"
                PRINT #2, "switching to Printer format"
            CASE "Q"
                dataformat$ = "compressed"
                PRINT "switching to Compressed  format"
                PRINT #2, "switching to Compressed format"
        END SELECT
        CALL send(commandcode$)
        CALL getreply
        PRINT
        PRINT "press a key to continue (T to quit)"
        SLEEP: a$ = INKEY$
    LOOP
END SUB
```

18

The Dräger Evita intensive care ventilator

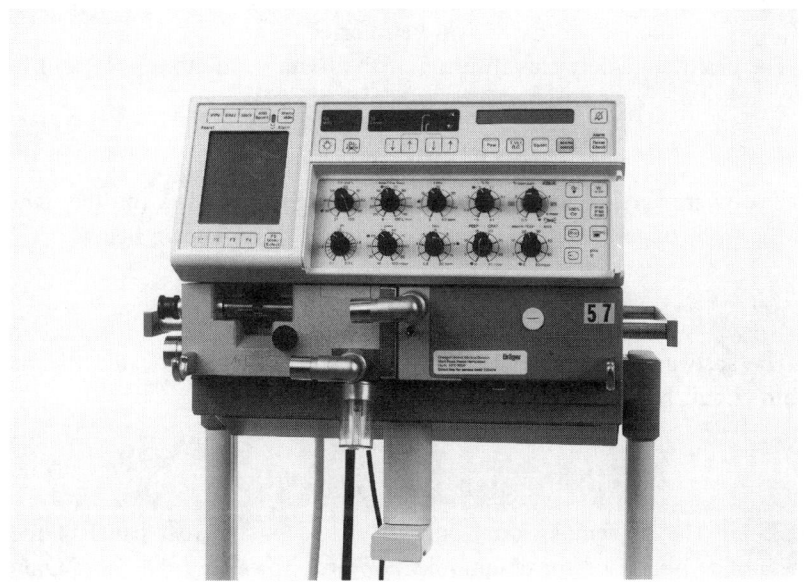

18.1 Introduction

The Evita† is a time-cycled intensive care ventilator for both adults and infants. Waveform, current parameter values and alarm settings are displayed on two LCD screens.

Comprehensive information regarding a wide range of measured parameters and alarm settings is available via the serial port. In addition, the Evita has a Drägerbus analogue interface which allows two Evitas to be linked together to deliver synchronised bilateral ventilation.

There are currently two Evita ventilators. The earlier model is known simply as the 'Evita'; the subsequent model is called the Evita 2. Where it

---

† Drägerwerk Aktiengesellschaft, Moislinger Allee 53–55, D-23542 Lübeck 1, Germany. Tel: +49–(0)451–8820. Fax: +49–(0)451–8822080.

Table 18.1. *Evita serial port (25-pin)*.

Pin No.	Name	Comments
1	Shield	Connected to Evita housing
2	TxD	Transmits data
3	RxD	Receives data
7	GND	Signal ground

is necessary in this Chapter to distinguish unambiguously between these two models, the earlier 'Evita' will be referred to as the Evita 1.

The electrical safety classification of the Evita ventilators is Type B.†

18.1.1 Software version

The software version is displayed in the small LCD window (on the right of the front panel) when the Evita is switched on, as shown below.

> Evita version 11.01

The software version is also printed on the EPROM located on the main circuit board.

18.2 Serial port

A 25-pin D-type female serial port is located on the rear-panel of the Evita. The pins used for communication are shown in Table 18.1. Only four pins are used for communications. The serial interface satisfies both the RS-232-C and the CCITT V.24 standards. A small booklet on the serial interface is available from Dräger Limited.‡

18.2.1 Protocol options

The protocol and available bit rates are shown in Table 18.2. The bit rate is set at the factory to 1200 bps since the Evita can only process incoming commands at the rate of one character per 8.5 ms.

Other bit rates can be used if necessary, but in order to do this the four DIP switches on the serial interface board which control the bit rate (switches 9–12) will have to be reset according to Table 18.3.

† See Chapter 7 for further details.
‡ *RS-232 Interface for Dräger Medical Equipment* (1992).

Table 18.2. *Evita protocol.*

Bit rate	50, 75, 150, 300, 600, 1200 (standard factory setting,) 1800, 2400, 3600, 4800, 7200, 9600, 19200
Data bits	7
Parity	Even
Stop bits	2

Table 18.3. *Evita bit rate DIP switch settings.*

	Switch No.			
Bit rate	9	10	11	12
Not used	0	0	0	0
50	1	0	0	0
75	0	1	0	0
150	1	0	1	0
300	0	1	1	0
600	1	1	1	0
1200	0	0	0	1
1800	1	0	0	1
2400	0	1	0	1
3600	1	1	0	1
4800	0	0	1	1
7200	1	0	1	1
9600	0	1	1	1
19200	1	1	1	1

18.2.2 Cable connections

Figure 18.1 indicates the wiring configuration for interfacing to a PC.

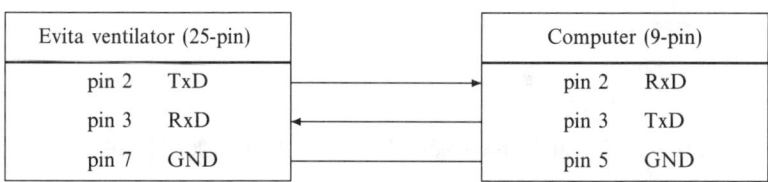

Fig. 18.1. Evita wiring configuration.

Table 18.4. *Evita command-codes.*

Code	ASCII (dec)	Meaning
⟨ACK⟩	6	Get Identification data telegram
⟨ENQ⟩	5	Get Measured data telegram
⟨NAK⟩	21	Get Status data telegram
⟨DC1⟩	17	Data enable (XON)
⟨DC3⟩	19	Data disable (XOFF)
⟨DC2⟩	18	Alarm enable
⟨DC4⟩	20	Alarm disable

18.3 Command format

The Evita responds to a number of command-codes which control the alarm status and initiate the output of data telegrams (see Table 18.4). Note that all the command-codes recognised by the Evita are ASCII control characters.† The Evita responds to command errors by returning the control code ⟨DLE⟩.

The three command-codes used for accessing data are the ASCII control codes ⟨ACK⟩, ⟨ENQ⟩, and ⟨NAK⟩, which request the Identification data, Measured data, and Status data respectively, as shown in Table 18.4.

The Evita does not have a special command format; all that is necessary is to send the appropriate command-code, the command string transmitted by the PC being as follows. Note that the Evita disregards extra ⟨CR⟩ or ⟨LF⟩ characters.

⟨command-code⟩

For example, if the command-code ⟨ENQ⟩ is to be sent, this can be sent using QuickBASIC as follows, where the serial port is designated as #1.

```
ENQ$ = CHR$(5)
PRINT #1, ENQ$
```

The serial port must be opened FOR RANDOM ACCESS READ WRITE since data is being transmitted and received via the same serial port.

† See Appendix 1 for details of ASCII control characters.

Table 18.5. *Evita telegram formatting codes.*

Telegram	Heading	Data separators	End
Identification data	⟨STX⟩	⟨ESC⟩, ⟨RS⟩	⟨EOT⟩
Measured data	⟨SOH⟩	⟨ESC⟩, ⟨GS⟩, ⟨FS⟩	⟨EOT⟩
Status data	⟨SOH⟩	⟨FS⟩, ⟨GS⟩	⟨EOT⟩
Alarm data	⟨BEL⟩	⟨ESC⟩	⟨EOT⟩

18.4 Reply format

The Dräger RS-232 interface manual refers to each group of data output in response to a command-code as a **telegram**. There are four telegrams as follows.

- Identification data telegram
- Measured data telegram
- Status data telegram
- Alarm data telegram

The ASCII control characters used in formatting the data within each telegram are shown in Table 18.5. All telegrams have a **header code** (the first character) which is either ⟨STX⟩, ⟨SOH⟩ or ⟨BEL⟩, and all end with the 'end of transmission' control character ⟨EOT⟩.

The second field of a telegram is the three-character **equipment identification number**, which varies according to the particular ventilator and the software version as shown in Table 18.6. The first character is currently set to zero (0), and is designed to be used in future expansions. The third field is a single-character **channel number**, which is currently always set to zero (0).

All telegrams are made up of a number of data blocks (e.g. time, compliance etc.) separated by the ⟨ESC⟩ control character. The separate items of data within each data block are separated by other control characters which are specific to the particular telegram; i.e. different data separators are used for different telegrams—see Table 18.5.

Table 18.6. *Evita equipment identification numbers.*

Model	Software version	Equipment ident. no.
Evita-1	7.00–14.01	015
Evita-1	13.02–14.02	016
Evita-2	—	040
Evita-2 + CO_2 monitoring	—	041

Table 18.7. *Identification data telegram.*

Element	Characters	Meaning
⟨BEL⟩		
Equip. ident. no.	nnn	Evita-1 (015, 016) Evita-2 (040, 041) see Table 18.6
Channel no.	n	unallocated (= 0)
⟨ESC⟩		
⟨equipment name⟩	max. 15 characters	Evita-1, Evita-2
⟨ESC⟩		
Measured data code	nn	00–14
⟨RS⟩		
Long name	max. 22 characters	
⟨RS⟩		
Short name	max. 4 characters	
⟨RS⟩		
Units	max. 10 characters	
⟨RS⟩		
Least possible value	max. 5 characters	
⟨RS⟩		
Greatest possible value	max. 5 characters	
⟨EOT⟩		

18.4.1 Identification data telegram

This telegram is transmitted in response to the command-code ⟨ACK⟩ (see Table 18.4), and gives details of all the measured parameters,† namely the parameter code (0–14), full parameter name, abbreviated name, units, and the range of possible values. The various fields of the Identification telegram are separated using the control characters ⟨ESC⟩ and ⟨RS⟩. Details

† Note that the measured values of these parameters are returned in the Measured data telegram.

of the fields are given in Table 18.7 The format of this telegram is as follows.

⟨STX⟩⟨equip. ident. no.⟩⟨channel no.⟩⟨ESC⟩⟨equipment name⟩⟨ESC⟩ ⟨Measured data code⟩⟨RS⟩⟨long name⟩⟨RS⟩⟨short name⟩ ⟨RS⟩⟨units⟩⟨RS⟩⟨least possible value⟩⟨RS⟩⟨greatest possible value⟩ ⟨ESC⟩...⟨EOT⟩

The format of a typical Identification data telegram is shown below, where the space character is represented by the symbol ␣.

⟨STX⟩0150
⟨ESC⟩Evita
⟨ESC⟩00⟨RS⟩Time⟨RS⟩t⟨RS⟩h:min⟨RS⟩␣0,00⟨RS⟩23,59
⟨ESC⟩01⟨RS⟩Exp.␣tidal␣volume⟨RS⟩VTe⟨RS⟩L⟨RS⟩0,00⟨RS⟩2,00
⟨ESC⟩02⟨RS⟩Breathing␣frequency⟨RS⟩f⟨RS⟩1/min⟨RS⟩␣0⟨RS⟩60
⟨ESC⟩03⟨RS⟩MV⟨RS⟩MV⟨RS⟩L/min⟨RS⟩␣0,0⟨RS⟩41,0
⟨ESC⟩04⟨RS⟩Peak-pressure⟨RS⟩Peak⟨RS⟩mbar⟨RS⟩␣0⟨RS⟩99
⟨ESC⟩05⟨RS⟩Plateau-pressure⟨RS⟩Plat⟨RS⟩mbar⟨RS⟩␣0⟨RS⟩99
⟨ESC⟩06⟨RS⟩PEEP-pressure⟨RS⟩PEEP⟨RS⟩mbar⟨RS⟩␣0⟨RS⟩99
⟨ESC⟩07⟨RS⟩Minimum-pressure⟨RS⟩Pmin⟨RS⟩mbar⟨RS⟩−20⟨RS⟩99
⟨ESC⟩08⟨RS⟩Mean-pressure⟨RS⟩Mean⟨RS⟩mbar⟨RS⟩␣0⟨RS⟩99
⟨ESC⟩09⟨RS⟩Insp.␣O2-concentration⟨RS⟩FIO2⟨RS⟩%⟨RS⟩15⟨RS⟩99
⟨ESC⟩10⟨RS⟩Compliance⟨RS⟩C⟨RS⟩mL/mbar⟨RS⟩␣␣0⟨RS⟩255
⟨ESC⟩11⟨RS⟩Resistance⟨RS⟩R⟨RS⟩mbar/(L/s)⟨RS⟩␣0⟨RS⟩99
⟨ESC⟩12⟨RS⟩Spont.␣minute␣volume⟨RS⟩MVs⟨RS⟩L/min⟨RS⟩␣0,0⟨RS⟩41,0
⟨ESC⟩13⟨RS⟩Spont.␣frequency⟨RS⟩f␣s⟨RS⟩1/min⟨RS⟩␣0⟨RS⟩60
⟨ESC⟩14⟨RS⟩Airway␣temperature⟨RS⟩Temp⟨RS⟩deg␣C⟨RS⟩18⟨RS⟩45
⟨EOT⟩

18.4.2 Measured data telegram

This telegram is transmitted in response to the command-code ⟨ENQ⟩ (see Table 18.4), and gives the values of all the Measured parameters (prefixed by the ⟨ESC⟩ character), as well as details of any changes in the status of the set parameters (i.e. Status data) made since the last Measured data telegram was transmitted (prefixed by the ⟨GS⟩ character).

The various parameters (either Measured data or Status data) are identified using both the relevant parameter code, and the parameter's abbreviated name.†

† Note that the parameter codes for the 14 Measured parameters are returned in the Identification data telegram. The parameter codes for the Status data are returned in the Status data telegram.

The general format is as follows.

⟨SOH⟩⟨equip. ident. no.⟩⟨channel no.⟩⟨ESC⟩⟨00⟩nn,nn⟨ESC⟩⟨01⟩n,nn
⟨ESC⟩⟨02⟩nn⟨ESC⟩⟨03⟩nn,n⟨ESC⟩⟨04⟩nn⟨ESC⟩⟨05⟩nn⟨ESC⟩⟨06⟩nn
⟨ESC⟩⟨07⟩nn⟨ESC⟩⟨08⟩nn⟨ESC⟩⟨09⟩nn⟨ESC⟩⟨10⟩nnn⟨ESC⟩⟨11⟩nn
⟨ESC⟩⟨12⟩nn,n⟨ESC⟩⟨13⟩nn⟨ESC⟩⟨14⟩nn⟨GS⟩⟨status message⟩
⟨GS⟩...⟨EOT⟩

The format of a typical Measured data telegram is shown below. Note that the values of the Measured parameters are transmitted first, followed by any Status changes. Where a parameter is not measured, each digit in the parameter field is replaced by a bar (–).

⟨SOH⟩0150
⟨ESC⟩0016,47
⟨ESC⟩010,80
⟨ESC⟩0211
⟨ESC⟩03␣8,6
⟨ESC⟩0446
⟨ESC⟩0541
⟨ESC⟩06␣0
⟨ESC⟩07– – –
⟨ESC⟩0811
⟨ESC⟩0951
⟨ESC⟩10␣19
⟨ESC⟩11␣16
⟨ESC⟩12– –, –
⟨ESC⟩13– –
⟨ESC⟩14– –
⟨GS⟩20MV␣low␣limit␣=␣⟨FS⟩␣9,0⟨FS⟩␣L/min
⟨GS⟩21MV␣high␣limit␣=␣⟨FS⟩15,0⟨FS⟩␣L/min
⟨EOT⟩

18.4.3 Status data telegram

This telegram is transmitted in response to the command-code ⟨NAK⟩ (see Table 18.4). A full list of the possible Status messages is shown in Table 18.8. The general format is as follows.

⟨SOH⟩⟨equip. ident. no.⟩⟨channel no.⟩
⟨GS⟩⟨status parameter code⟩⟨status message⟩
⟨GS⟩...⟨EOT⟩

The Dräger Evita intensive care ventilator 321

The format of a typical Status data telegram is shown below. Note that each Status category is prefixed by ⟨GS⟩ followed by the Status parameter code.

⟨SOH⟩0150
⟨GS⟩00date␣:␣⟨FS⟩22⟨FS⟩-⟨FS⟩␣4⟨FS⟩-⟨FS⟩93⟨FS⟩
⟨GS⟩01O2␣setting-value␣=␣⟨FS⟩␣49⟨FS⟩␣%
⟨GS⟩02Max.␣inspiratory␣flow␣=␣⟨FS⟩␣54⟨FS⟩␣L/min
⟨GS⟩03Insp.␣tidal␣volume␣=␣⟨FS⟩0,81⟨FS⟩␣L
⟨GS⟩04Frequency␣IPPV␣=␣⟨FS⟩10⟨FS⟩␣1/min
⟨GS⟩06I␣:␣E␣=␣⟨FS⟩1,0⟨FS⟩␣:␣⟨FS⟩2,0⟨FS⟩
⟨GS⟩07Max.␣breathing␣pressure␣=␣⟨FS⟩␣50⟨FS⟩␣mbar
⟨GS⟩08Frequency␣IMV␣=␣⟨FS⟩␣7,5⟨FS⟩␣1/min
⟨GS⟩09PEEP␣/␣CPAP␣=␣⟨FS⟩␣0⟨FS⟩␣mbar
⟨GS⟩10ASB␣=␣⟨FS⟩␣0⟨FS⟩␣mbar
⟨GS⟩11Interm.␣PEEP␣=␣⟨FS⟩␣0⟨FS⟩␣mbar
⟨GS⟩12BIPAP_P_level_1␣=␣⟨FS⟩␣0⟨FS⟩␣mbar
⟨GS⟩13BIPAP_P_level_2␣=␣⟨FS⟩10⟨FS⟩␣mbar
⟨GS⟩14BIPAP_leveltime_1␣=␣⟨FS⟩␣1,8⟨FS⟩␣s
⟨GS⟩15BIPAP_leveltime_2␣=␣⟨FS⟩␣3,0⟨FS⟩␣s
⟨GS⟩16Apnoea␣time␣=␣⟨FS⟩15⟨FS⟩␣s
⟨GS⟩20MV␣low␣limit␣=␣⟨FS⟩␣9,0⟨FS⟩␣L/min
⟨GS⟩21MV␣high␣limit␣=␣⟨FS⟩15,0⟨FS⟩␣L/min
⟨GS⟩22Triggerlevel␣off
⟨GS⟩54O2␣monitoring␣on␣
⟨GS⟩23Tachypnoea␣warning␣off
⟨GS⟩30Mode␣IPPV
⟨GS⟩50Audio␣alarm␣inactive␣off
⟨GS⟩51Nebulizer␣off
⟨GS⟩52Screen␣frozen␣off
⟨GS⟩53O2␣calibration␣off
⟨GS⟩55Suction␣off
⟨EOT⟩

18.4.4 Alarm telegrams

All Alarm telegrams are prefixed by ⟨BEL⟩, followed by the equipment identification number (015 for the Evita), and terminated with ⟨EOT⟩. Details of the fields are given in Table 18.9. The format of Alarm data telegrams is as follows.

Table 18.8. *Evita Status messages. Integers are indicated by n, d, m, y.*

Status code	Status message
00	date␣␣␣⟨FS⟩dd⟨FS⟩mm⟨FS⟩-⟨FS⟩yy⟨FS⟩
01	On␣setting-value␣=␣⟨FS⟩nnn⟨FS⟩␣%
02	Max␣inspiratory␣flow␣=␣⟨FS⟩nnn⟨FS⟩␣L/min
03	Insp.␣tidal␣volume␣=␣⟨FS⟩n,nn⟨FS⟩␣L
04	Frequency␣IPPV␣=␣⟨FS⟩nn⟨FS⟩nn/min
05	Triggerlevel␣=␣⟨FS⟩n,n⟨FS⟩mbar
06	I␣:␣E␣=␣⟨FS⟩n,n⟨FS⟩␣:␣␣⟨FS⟩n,n⟨FS⟩
07	Max␣breathing␣pressure␣=␣⟨FS⟩nnn⟨FS⟩␣mbar
08	Frequency␣IMV␣=␣⟨FS⟩nn,n⟨FS⟩␣L/min
09	PEEP␣/␣CPAP␣=␣⟨FS⟩nn⟨FS⟩␣mbar
10	ASB␣=␣⟨FS⟩nn⟨FS⟩␣mbar
11	Interm.␣PEEP␣=␣⟨FS⟩nn⟨FS⟩␣mbar
12	BIPAP␣P␣level␣1␣=␣⟨FS⟩nn⟨FS⟩␣mbar
13	BIPAP␣P␣level␣2␣=␣⟨FS⟩nn⟨FS⟩␣mbar
14	BIPAP␣leveltime␣1␣=␣⟨FS⟩nn,n⟨FS⟩␣s
15	BIPAP␣leveltime␣2␣=␣⟨FS⟩nn,n⟨FS⟩␣s
16	Apnoea␣time␣=␣⟨FS⟩nn⟨FS⟩␣s
17	Tachypnoea␣warning␣=␣⟨FS⟩nn⟨FS⟩␣bpm⟨FS⟩␣s
20	MV␣low␣limit␣off
21	MV␣high␣limit␣off
22	Triggerlevel␣off
23	Tachypnoea␣warning␣off
30	Mode␣IPPV
31	Mode␣IPPV/Assist
32	Mode␣CPPV
33	Mode␣CPPV/Assist
34	Mode␣SIMV
35	Mode␣SIMV/ASB

Table 18.8 cont.

Status code	Status message
36	Mode␣SB
37	Mode␣ASB
38	Mode␣CPAP
39	Mode␣CPAP/ASB
40	Mode␣MMV
41	Mode␣MMV/ASB
42	Mode␣BIPAP
43	Mode␣Sync.␣Master
44	Mode␣Sync.␣Slave
45	Mode␣Apnoea ventilation
50	Audio␣alarm␣inactive␣off/on
51	Nebulizer␣off/on
52	Screen␣frozen␣off/on
53	O2␣calibration␣off/on
54	O2␣monitoring␣off/on
55	Suction␣off/on
60	Sigh␣active
61	Breathing␣system␣vented
62	O2␣supply␣down
63	O2␣measurement␣inop
64	FIO2␣high
65	FIO2␣low
66	Flow␣measurement␣inop
67	Mixer␣inop
68	Time␣limited
69	Pressure␣limited
70	Malfunction␣fan

Table 18.9. *Evita alarm data telegram.*

Element	Characters	Meaning
⟨BEL⟩ Equip. ident. no.	nnn	Evita-1 (015, 016) Evita-2 (040, 041) see Table 18.6
Channel no.	n	unallocated (= 0)
⟨ESC⟩ Alarm/warning	n	1 = alarm; 0 = warning
Alarm status	n	1 = alarm activated 0 = alarm cancelled
Alarm code	nn	see Table 18.10
Alarm message ⟨EOT⟩	max. 50 characters	see Table 18.10

⟨BEL⟩⟨equip. ident. no.⟩⟨channel no.⟩⟨ESC⟩⟨alarm/warning⟩⟨status⟩ ⟨alarm code⟩⟨alarm message⟩⟨EOT⟩

Alarm data telegrams are not transmitted in response to a command-code, but are normally output automatically as and when alarms are triggered, since the alarm data outflow facility is automatically enabled when the Evita is powered on.

A full list of possible Alarm messages is shown in Table 18.10. Note that the automatic outflow of alarm data can be disabled if necessary by sending the command-code ⟨DC4⟩. The outflow of alarm data can subsequently be enabled using the command-code ⟨DC2⟩.

When an alarm limit is violated, the relevant Alarm data telegram has the 'alarm/warning' bit set to 1 (= alarm message) and the status bit set to 1 (= alarm activated), as shown in the following example.

⟨BEL⟩0150⟨ESC⟩1128Airway␣pressure␣high⟨EOT⟩

When the parameter falls within the alarm limits again, another Alarm data telegram is transmitted with the status bit set to 0 (= alarm discontinued), as follows.

⟨BEL⟩0150⟨ESC⟩1028Airway␣pressure␣high⟨EOT⟩

Table 18.10. *Evita Alarm messages.*

Alarm code	Alarm message
01	Device failure
02	Air supply down
03	O2 supply down
04	Pressure meas. inop
05	O2 measurement inop
06	Flow measurement inop
07	Mixer inop
08	Exp. valve inop
09	Fan defect
10	Temperature meas. inop
11	Temperature sensor ?
12	Temperature high
22	Apnoea
23	FIO2 high
24	FIO2 low
25	MV low
26	MV high
27	Airway pressure low
28	Airway pressure high
29	Fail to cycle
30	High frequency
31	Synchronization inop

18.5 Interactive program for accessing telegrams

The following example QuickBASIC 4.5 program indicates how to send command messages interactively from the keyboard, and collect the reply telegram from the Evita. The program prompts the operator to press a key as follows.

---
press <I> for Identification data telegram
press <D> for Measured data telegram
press <S> for Status data telegram
press <Q> to quit

The program then displays the telegram, and also saves all data to a file (evita.dat) in the same directory. This file can be viewed by pressing <V>. When alarms are triggered the Evita automatically transmits an Alarm telegram, which is then displayed on the screen.

The Dräger Evita intensive care ventilator 325

Telegrams are printed to the screen with all control characters converted into an appropriate text code for convenience (e.g. File Separator is printed as <FS>)† since some control characters will otherwise be actioned (e.g. backspace) and make reading the telegram difficult.

When a telegram is viewed from the file (e.g. using a text editor) all control characters are displayed using either IBM graphics characters (e.g. ☺) or the MS-DOS system (e.g. ^A). For example when IBM graphics control characters are being used, a typical Measured data telegram will be viewed from the file as follows, where the symbols ☺, ←, ↔, ᒪ, ♦ represent the control characters ⟨SOH⟩, ⟨ESC⟩, ⟨GS⟩, ⟨FS⟩, ⟨EOT⟩ respectively (see Appendix 1).

```
☺0150←0016,47←010,80←0211←03 8,6←0446←0541←06 0←0
7- - -←0811←0951←10 19←11 16←12- -, -←13- -←14-
-↔20MV low limit = ᒪ 9,0ᒪ L/min↔21MV high limit =
ᒪ15,0ᒪ L/min♦
```

Where the MS-DOS system is used, the above Measured data telegram will appear as follows.

```
^A0150^[0016,47^[010,80^[0211^[03 8,6^[0446^[0541^[
06 0^[07- - -^[0811^[0951^[10 19^[11 16^[12- -, -^[13-
-^[14- -^]20MV low limit = ^\ 9,0^\ L/min^]21MV
high limit = ^\ 15,0^\ L/min^D
```

The process of extracting specific data values from the telegrams involves extensive string manipulation, and an example of how this may be done is given in a later Section which describes a program to analyse the Measured data telegram.

Program points

- Since no hardware handshaking lines are used for communications, the CS and DS options need to be used in the OPEN COM statement.
- Since the same serial port is being used for transmitting and receiving data it must be opened FOR RANDOM ACCESS READ WRITE in the OPEN COM statement.

† See Appendix 1 for details of the short codes for control characters.

- When a telegram is printed to the screen all control characters are represented by the standard short codes (see Appendix 1) in anglebrackets, e.g. <FS>.
- Pressing <V> will view the data file evita.dat using the file viewer VIEW.EXE.† In practice any appropriate file viewer can be used to view the datafile—see Chapter 5 for further details.

  In view of the QuickBASIC SHELL 'bug' (data is lost from the buffer when using the SHELL command), the example program gets all outstanding buffer data written to the file by first closing the file (CLOSE #2), then using the SHELL command, and then reopening the file FOR APPEND as follows.

```
CLOSE #2
SHELL "view evita.dat"
OPEN "evita.dat" FOR APPEND ACCESS READ WRITE AS #2
```

- The buffer is emptied at the beginning of the SEND subroutine.
- A loop generating a time-out of 5 seconds is placed at the beginning of the GETREPLY subroutine.

Example program

```
REM [evita-I.bas]
REM interactive program for Evita ventilator
DECLARE SUB emptybuffer ()
DECLARE SUB getreply ()
DECLARE SUB send (s$)
COMMON SHARED reply$
CLS
OPEN "COM1: 1200,E,7,2,CS,DS" FOR RANDOM ACCESS
                                        READ WRITE AS #1
OPEN "evita.dat" FOR OUTPUT AS #2
PRINT #2, "DATA FROM EVITA VENTILATOR", DATE$, TIME$
LOCATE 5, 1
PRINT "program to access data from EVITA"
PRINT "data saved in file EVITA.DAT"
PRINT "serial port open OK"
PRINT
EOT$ = CHR$(4): REM end of transmission
```

† See Section 5.10.

```
ACK$ = CHR$(6)
ENQ$ = CHR$(5)
NAK$ = CHR$(21)
PRINT "press <I> for Identification Data Telegram"
PRINT "press <D> for Measured Data Telegram"
PRINT "press <S> for Status Data Telegram"
PRINT "press <Q> to quit"
PRINT
DO
    key$ = INKEY$
    IF UCASE$(key$) = "I" THEN CALL send(ACK$)
    IF UCASE$(key$) = "D" THEN
        CALL send(ENQ$)
    END IF
    IF UCASE$(key$) = "S" THEN CALL send(NAK$)
    IF UCASE$(key$) = "V" THEN
        CLOSE #2
        SHELL "view evita.dat"
        OPEN "evita.dat" FOR APPEND ACCESS READ WRITE AS #2
    END IF
    IF UCASE$(key$) = "Q" THEN
        CLOSE #1, #2
        END
    END IF
    REM collect ALARM Telegrams
    IF LOC(1) > 2 THEN CALL getreply
LOOP
END


SUB emptybuffer
    DO WHILE NOT EOF(1)
        buff$ = INPUT$(LOC(1), #1)
        PRINT buff$
    LOOP
    REM PRINT "Buffer emptied OK"
END SUB
```

```
SUB getreply
    timezero = TIMER
    REM implement a 5 sec time-out (increase if necessary)
    DO WHILE LOC(1) = 0
        IF TIMER > timezero + 5 THEN
            PRINT "No reply after 5 secs"
            CLOSE
            END
        END IF
    LOOP
    PRINT "data being transmitted by EVITA"
    DO
        DO
            char$ = INPUT$(1, #1)
            SELECT CASE char$
                CASE CHR$(1)
                    char$ = "<SOH>"
                CASE CHR$(2)
                    char$ = "<STX>"
                CASE CHR$(4)
                    char$ = "<EOT>"
                CASE CHR$(7)
                    char$ = CHR$(10) + "ALARM TELEGRAM:"
+ CHR$(10) + "<BEL>"
                CASE CHR$(27)
                    char$ = "<ESC>"
                CASE CHR$(28)
                    char$ = "<FS>"
                CASE CHR$(29)
                    char$ = "<GS>"
                CASE CHR$(30)
                    char$ = "<RS>"
            END SELECT
            a$ = a$ + char$
            REM look for end of transmission marker <EOT>
            L% = INSTR(1, a$, "<EOT>")
        LOOP UNTIL L% > 0
        REM include the final <EOT> character in the data
        reply$ = MID$(a$, 1, L% + 4)
        PRINT reply$
```

```
        PRINT #2, reply$
        PRINT
        REM set the string a$ to zero length
        a$ = ""
        REM loop until only 1 char left (<EOF>)
    LOOP UNTIL LOC(1) <= 1
    CALL emptybuffer
    PRINT
    PRINT "press <I> for Identification Data Telegram"
    PRINT "press <D> for Measured Data Telegram"
    PRINT "press <S> for Status Data Telegram"
    PRINT "press <V> to view data using VIEW.EXE"
    PRINT "press <Q> to quit"
END SUB


SUB send (s$)
    CALL emptybuffer
    IF s$ = CHR$(6) THEN message$ = "Identification
Data Telegram"
    IF s$ = CHR$(5) THEN message$ = "Measured Data
Telegram"
    IF s$ = CHR$(21) THEN message$ = "Status Data
Telegram"
    PRINT
    PRINT "requesting" + " " + message$
    PRINT #1, s$
    PRINT #2,
    PRINT #2, TIME$
    PRINT #2, message$
    CALL getreply
END SUB
```

18.6 Program to access the Measured data telegram

The following example QuickBASIC 4.5 program shows how to extract and display the data values embedded within the Measured Data telegram, using a variety of string manipulation techniques. The values are placed in a variable, and then printed to screen and file as shown in

```
MEASURED DATA / equipment = EVITA
00  Time               = 16.49   h:m
01  Exp Tidal vol      = 0.39    L
02  Resp freq          = 41      /min
03  Min vol            = 19.6    L/min
04  Peak-pressure      = 16      mbar
05  Plateau-pressure   = --      mbar
06  PEEP-pressure      = 2       mbar
07  Min-pressure       = 0       mbar
08  Mean-pressure      = 5       mbar
09  Insp O2 conc       = 49      %
10  Compliance         = ---     mL/mbar
11  Resistance         = ---     mbar/L/s
12  Spont. Min Vol     = 19.6    L/min
13  Spont. freq        = 42      /min
14  Airway temp        = --      deg C
STATUS DATA
10  ASB = 16   mbar
11  Interm PEEP =  16  mbar
```

Fig. 18.2. Example screen view using the program **evita-md.bas** to analyse the Measured data telegram. The numbers on the left-hand side are the parameter codes.

Figure 18.2. The values can then be easily used for other purposes if necessary.

Note that the following example program processes only the Measured Data telegram; the other telegrams can be processed in a largely similar way.

The program uses two subroutines; one to clear the buffer (EMPTYBUFFER), and the other to print each of the telegram's component data-strings READDATASTRING).

The general structure and order of the program is as follows.

(1) Start.
(2) Open the serial port.
(3) Send the command-code ENQ to access the Measured data telegram.
(4) Collect the telegram from the buffer one character at a time, changing commas to decimal points, and changing ⟨FS⟩ control characters to spaces.
(5) Save the telegram (a$) to a temporary file.
(6) Save the telegram (a$) to the main data file.
(7) Analyse the data stored in the temporary file by breaking it down

The Dräger Evita intensive care ventilator 331

into the component strings between the ASCII control characters, and calling the READDATASTRING subroutine to print the strings to the screen, and to the main data file.

(8) Prompt the operator to get another telegram, view all the data in the main data file, or quit the program.

(9) End.

Program points

- Since no hardware handshaking lines are used for communications, the CS and DS options need to be used in the OPEN COM statement.
- Since the same serial port is being used for transmitting and receiving data it must be opened FOR RANDOM ACCESS READ WRITE in the OPEN COM statement.
- The telegram is analysed by breaking it up into the strings which lie between the control characters ⟨ESC⟩, ⟨FS⟩, and ⟨GS⟩. The number of characters up to and including a particular character is determined using the INSTR function.
- The program determines whether or not to print the heading STATUS DATA by looking for a ⟨GS⟩ control character, and using a string variable (status$) and a counter (counter).
- The saved data can be viewed by pressing <V>, which invokes the file viewer VIEW.EXE (see Section 5.10 for details of commercial file-viewing utilities.)

Example program

```
REM [evita-md.bas]
REM collects Measured data telegram from Evita
DECLARE SUB readdatastring ()
DECLARE SUB emptybuffer ()
COMMON SHARED data$, status$
CLS
OPEN "COM1: 1200,E,7,2,CS,DS" FOR RANDOM ACCESS
                                        READ WRITE AS #1
OPEN "alldata.dat" FOR OUTPUT AS #3
PRINT "serial port open OK"
EOT$ = CHR$(4)
ENQ$ = CHR$(5)
SOH$ = CHR$(1)
```

```
GS$ = CHR$(29)
FS$ = CHR$(28)
ESC$ = CHR$(27)
LOCATE 7
PRINT "press <ENTER> for Measured Data Telegram"
PRINT "press    <Q>    to quit"
CALL emptybuffer
REM send command-code ENQ
DO
    key$ = INKEY$
    IF UCASE$(key$) = CHR$(13) THEN
        PRINT #1, CHR$(5): REM ENQ
        EXIT DO
    END IF
    IF UCASE$(key$) = "Q" THEN
        CLOSE
        END
    END IF
LOOP
repeatline:
REM collect Telegram from buffer
CLS
a$ = ""
timezero = TIMER
DO
    REM 10 sec time-out
    DO WHILE LOC(1) = 0
        IF TIMER > timezero + 10 THEN
            PRINT "No reply for 10 secs"
            CLOSE
            END
        END IF
    LOOP
    REM input 1 character at a time
    char$ = INPUT$(1, #1)
    REM change <,> to <.>
    IF char$ = CHR$(44) THEN char$ = CHR$(46)
    REM change <FS> to <SPACE> for convenience
    IF char$ = FS$ THEN char$ = CHR$(32)
    a$ = a$ + char$
```

```
LOOP UNTIL char$ = EOT$
REM save the data to a temporary file TEMPFILE.dat (#2)
OPEN "tempfile.dat" FOR OUTPUT AS #2
PRINT #2, a$
CLOSE #2
REM save all data to a file ALLDATA.dat (#3)
PRINT #3,
PRINT #3, "DATE "; DATE$ + "/" + "TIME "; TIME$
PRINT #3, a$
REM analyse data saved in TEMPFILE.dat
OPEN "tempfile.dat" FOR INPUT AS #2
k = 0
n = LEN(a$)
counter = 0
status$ = "measured data"
DO
    REM determine no. of chars (E%) up to <ESC> char
    E% = INSTR(a$, ESC$)
    REM determine no. of chars (G%) up to <GS> char
    G% = INSTR(a$, GS$)
    REM determine no. of chars (EOT%) up to <EOT> char
    EOT% = INSTR(a$, EOT$)
    lengthofstring% = E%
    REM if no <ESC> then string is up to <GS>
    IF E% = 0 THEN lengthofstring% = G%
    REM if no <ESC> and no <GS> then string up to <EOT>
    IF E% = 0 AND G% = 0 THEN lengthofstring% = EOT%
    datastring$ = INPUT$(lengthofstring%, #2)
    REM look at the first character
    firstchar$ = LEFT$(datastring$, 1)
    IF firstchar$ = SOH$ THEN
        equip.id.no$ = MID$(datastring$, 3, 2)
        SELECT CASE equip.id.no$
            CASE "15", "16"
                name$ = "EVITA-1"
            CASE "40", "41"
                name$ = "EVITA-2"
        END SELECT
        PRINT "MEASURED DATA" + SPACE$(30) + "equipment
= "; name$
```

```
            PRINT #3, "MEASURED DATA / equipment = "; name$
        END IF
        data$ = MID$(datastring$, 1, lengthofstring% - 1)
        lastchar$ = RIGHT$(datastring$, 1)
        CALL readdatastring
        REM if there is a <GS> char then print STATUS DATA
        IF lastchar$ = GS$ AND counter = 0 THEN
            status$ = "status"
            PRINT "STATUS DATA"
            PRINT #3, "STATUS DATA"
            counter = 1
        END IF
        k = k + lengthofstring%
        IF lastchar$ = EOT$ THEN
            EXIT DO
            ELSE a$ = RIGHT$(a$, n - k)
        END IF
LOOP UNTIL EOF(2)
PRINT
PRINT "   enter <R> to repeat; <V> to view Measured Data
                                    Telegram; <Q> to quit"
DO
    key$ = INKEY$
    IF UCASE$(key$) = "R" THEN
        REM send for a new telegram
        CLOSE #2
        CALL emptybuffer
        PRINT #1, ENQ$
        GOTO repeatline
    END IF
    IF UCASE$(key$) = "V" THEN
        REM view the data using the VIEW.EXE file viewer
        CLOSE #3
        SHELL "view alldata.dat"
        OPEN "alldata.dat" FOR APPEND ACCESS READ WRITE
AS #3
    END IF
    IF UCASE$(key$) = "Q" THEN
        CLOSE
        END
```

```
      END IF
LOOP
END


SUB emptybuffer
DO WHILE NOT EOF(1)
   buff$ = INPUT$(LOC(1), #1)
   PRINT buff$
LOOP
END SUB


SUB readdatastring
    id$ = LEFT$(data$, 2)
    d$ = RIGHT$(data$, LEN(data$) - 2)
    IF status$ = "measured data" THEN
        SELECT CASE id$
        CASE "ØØ"
            PRINT id$ + SPACE$(2) + "Time" + SPACE$(13) + "="
+ SPACE$(1) + d$ + SPACE$(1) + "h:m"
            PRINT #3, id$ + SPACE$(2) + "Time" + SPACE$(13) +
"=" + SPACE$(1) + d$ + SPACE$(1) + "h:m"
        CASE "Ø1"
            PRINT id$ + SPACE$(2) + "Exp Tidal vol" + SPACE$(4)
+ "=" + SPACE$(2) + d$ + SPACE$(1) + "L"
            PRINT #3, id$ + SPACE$(2) + "Exp Tidal vol"
+ SPACE$(4) + "=" + SPACE$(2) + d$ + SPACE$(1) + "L"
        CASE "Ø2"
            PRINT id$ + SPACE$(2) + "Resp freq" + SPACE$(8)
+ "=" + SPACE$(2) + d$ + SPACE$(3) + "/min"
            PRINT #3, id$ + SPACE$(2) + "Resp freq" + SPACE$(8)
+ "=" + SPACE$(2) + d$ + SPACE$(3) + "/min"
        CASE "Ø3"
            PRINT id$ + SPACE$(2) + "Min vol" + SPACE$(1Ø) +
"=" + SPACE$(2) + d$ + SPACE$(1) + "L/min"
            PRINT #3, id$ + SPACE$(2) + "Min vol" + SPACE$(1Ø)
+ "=" + SPACE$(2) + d$ + SPACE$(1) + "L/min"
        CASE "Ø4"
            PRINT id$ + SPACE$(2) + "Peak-pressure" + SPACE$(4)
```

```
              + "=" + SPACE$(2) + d$ + SPACE$(3) + "mbar"
                PRINT #3, id$ + SPACE$(2) + "Peak-pressure"
         + SPACE$(4) + "=" + SPACE$(2) + d$ + SPACE$(3) + "mbar"
                CASE "05"
                PRINT id$ + SPACE$(2) + "Plateau-pressure"
         + SPACE$(1) + "=" + SPACE$(2) + d$ + SPACE$(3) + "mbar"
                PRINT #3, id$ + SPACE$(2) + "Plateau-pressure"
         + SPACE$(1) + "=" + SPACE$(2) + d$ + SPACE$(3) + "mbar"
                CASE "06"
                PRINT id$ + SPACE$(2) + "PEEP-pressure"
         + SPACE$(4) + "=" + SPACE$(2) + d$ + SPACE$(3) + "mbar"
                PRINT #3, id$ + SPACE$(2) + "PEEP-pressure"
         + SPACE$(4) + "=" + SPACE$(2) + d$ + SPACE$(3) + "mbar"
                CASE "07"
                PRINT id$ + SPACE$(2) + "Min-pressure"
         + SPACE$(5) + "=" + SPACE$(1) + d$ + SPACE$(3) + "mbar"
                PRINT #3, id$ + SPACE$(2) + "Min-pressure"
         + SPACE$(5) + "=" + SPACE$(1) + d$ + SPACE$(3) + "mbar"
                CASE "08"
                PRINT id$ + SPACE$(2) + "Mean-pressure"
         + SPACE$(4) + "=" + SPACE$(2) + d$ + SPACE$(3) + "mbar"
                PRINT #3, id$ + SPACE$(2) + "Mean-pressure"
         + SPACE$(4) + "=" + SPACE$(2) + d$ + SPACE$(3) + "mbar"
                CASE "09"
                PRINT id$ + SPACE$(2) + "Insp O2 conc"
         + SPACE$(5) + "=" + SPACE$(2) + d$ + SPACE$(3) + "%"
                PRINT #3, id$ + SPACE$(2) + "Insp O2 conc"
         + SPACE$(5) + "=" + SPACE$(2) + d$ + SPACE$(3) + "%"
                CASE "10"
                PRINT id$ + SPACE$(2) + "Compliance" + SPACE$(7)
         + "=" + SPACE$(1) + d$ + SPACE$(3) + "mL/mbar"
                PRINT #3, id$ + SPACE$(2) + "Compliance"
         + SPACE$(7) + "=" + SPACE$(1) + d$ + SPACE$(3) + "mL/mbar"
                CASE "11"
                PRINT id$ + SPACE$(2) + "Resistance" + SPACE$(7)
         + "=" + SPACE$(1) + d$ + SPACE$(3) + "mbar/L/s"
                PRINT #3, id$ + SPACE$(2) + "Resistance"
         + SPACE$(7) + "=" + SPACE$(1) + d$ + SPACE$(3) + "mbar/L/s"
                CASE "12"
                PRINT id$ + SPACE$(2) + "Spont. Min Vol"
```

```
             + SPACE$(3) + "=" + SPACE$(2) + d$ + SPACE$(1) + "L/min"
             PRINT #3, id$ + SPACE$(2) + "Spont. Min Vol"
             + SPACE$(3) + "=" + SPACE$(2) + d$ + SPACE$(1) + "L/min"
          CASE "13"
             PRINT id$ + SPACE$(2) + "Spont freq" + SPACE$(7)
             + "=" + SPACE$(2) + d$ + SPACE$(3) + "L/min"
             PRINT #3, id$ + SPACE$(2) + "Spont freq"
             + SPACE$(7) + "=" + SPACE$(2) + d$ + SPACE$(3) + "L/min"
          CASE "14"
             PRINT id$ + SPACE$(2) + "Airway temp" + SPACE$(6)
             + "=" + SPACE$(2) + d$ + SPACE$(3) + "Deg C"
             PRINT #3, id$ + SPACE$(2) + "Airway temp"
             + SPACE$(6) + "=" + SPACE$(2) + d$ + SPACE$(3) + "Deg C"
          END SELECT
       END IF
       IF status$ = "status" THEN
          PRINT id$ + SPACE$(2) + d$
          PRINT #3, id$ + SPACE$(2) + d$
       END IF
END SUB
```

PART IV
APPENDICES

(1) ASCII control and graphic characters

(2) Serial port connector pin-outs

(3) Key codes

(4) The null modem

(5) Program for a device simulator

(6) QuickBASIC 4.5 OPEN and OPEN COM statements

(7) Plotting data using GNUPLOT

(8) Binary and hexadecimal notation

(9) Glossary of terms and abbreviations

Appendix 1
ASCII control and graphic characters

Table A1.1. *ASCII control characters.*

Dec	Code	Hex	Name	Character[a]	DOS
0	NUL	00h	Null	—	^@
1	SOH	01h	Start of heading	☺	^A
2	STX	02h	Start of text	☻	^B
3	ETX	03h	End of text	♥	^C
4	EOT	04h	End of transmission	♦	^D
5	ENQ	05h	Enquiry	♣	^E
6	ACK	06h	Acknowledge	♠	^F
7	BEL	07h	Bell	•	^G
8	BS	08h	Back space	◘	^H
9	HT	09h	Horizontal tab	○	^I
10	LF	0Ah	Line feed	◙	^J
11	VT	0Bh	Vertical tab	♂	^K
12	FF	0Ch	Form feed	♀	^L
13	CR	0Dh	Carriage return	♪	^M
14	SO	0Eh	Shift out	♫	^N
15	SI	0Fh	Shift in	☼	^O
16	DLE	10h	Data link escape	►	^P
17	DC1	11h	Device control 1 (XON)	◄	^Q
18	DC2	12h	Device control 2	↕	^R
19	DC3	13h	Device control 3 (XOFF)	‼	^S
20	DC4	14h	Device control 4	¶	^T
21	NAK	15h	Negative acknowledge	§	^U
22	SYN	16h	Synchronous idle	▬	^V
23	ETB	17h	End transmission block	↨	^W
24	CAN	18h	Cancel	↑	^X
25	EM	19h	End of medium	↓	^Y
26	SUB	1Ah	Substitute (EOF)	→	^Z
27	ESC	1Bh	Escape	←	^[
28	FS	1Ch	File separator	∟	^\
29	GS	1Dh	Group separator	↔	^]
30	RS	1Eh	Record separator	▲	^^
31	US	1Fh	Unit separator	▼	^_

[a] The characters in this table were printed using the TeX ASCII font in conjunction with the style-option ASCII.STY (Ramasubramanian, Nickalls & Reed; 1993, 1994).

Table A1.2. *ASCII graphic characters*

Dec	Character	Hex	Dec	Character	Hex
32	SPACE [a]	20h	80	P	50h
33	!	21h	81	Q	51h
34	"	22h	82	R	52h
35	#	23h	83	S	53h
36	$	24h	84	T	54h
37	%	25h	85	U	55h
38	&	26h	86	V	56h
39	'	27h	87	W	57h
40	(	28h	88	X	58h
41	)	29h	89	Y	59h
42	*	2Ah	90	Z	5Ah
43	+	2Bh	91	[	5Bh
44	,	2Ch	92	\	5Ch
45	-	2Dh	93	]	5Dh
46	.	2Eh	94	^	5Eh
47	/	2Fh	95	_	5Fh
48	0	30h	96	`	60h
49	1	31h	97	a	61h
50	2	32h	98	b	62h
51	3	33h	99	c	63h
52	4	34h	100	d	64h
53	5	35h	101	e	65h
54	6	36h	102	f	66h
55	7	37h	103	g	67h
56	8	38h	104	h	68h
57	9	39h	105	i	69h
58	:	3Ah	106	j	6Ah
59	;	3Bh	107	k	6Bh
60	<	3Ch	108	l	6Ch
61	=	3Dh	109	m	6Dh
62	>	3Eh	110	n	6Eh
63	?	3Fh	111	o	6Fh
64	@	40h	112	p	70h
65	A	41h	113	q	71h
66	B	42h	114	r	72h
67	C	43h	115	s	73h
68	D	44h	116	t	74h
69	E	45h	117	u	75h
70	F	46h	118	v	76h
71	G	47h	119	w	77h
72	H	48h	120	x	78h
73	I	49h	121	y	79h
74	J	4Ah	122	z	7Ah
75	K	4Bh	123	{	7Bh
76	L	4Ch	124	|	7Ch
77	M	4Dh	125	}	7Dh
78	N	4Eh	126	~	7Eh
79	O	4Fh	127	␣ (DEL)	7Fh

[a] Throughout this book the symbol ␣ is used to indicate the SPACE character.

ASCII control and graphic characters

Classification of ASCII control characters

The control characters of the 7-bit coded character set are classified into six categories as follows.†

Transmission control characters (SOH, STX, ETX, EOT, ENQ, ACK, DLE, NAK, SYN, ETB)

Transmission control characters are intended to control or facilitate transmission of information over telecommunication networks. Procedures for the use of the transmission control characters on telecommunication networks are the subjects of other standards and correspond to Open Systems Interconnection (OSI) levels 1 through 4 (see ANSI X3.28-1976 and Appendix E of ANSI X3.4-1986). Transmission control characters may also be referred to as *communication* control characters.

Format effectors (BS, HT, LF, VT, FF, CR)

Format effectors are mainly intended to control the layout and positioning of information on character-imaging devices, such as printing and display devices.

Code extension control characters (SO, SI, ESC)

Code extension control characters are used to extend the character set of the code. They may alter the meaning of one or more bit combinations that follow them in the data stream. Procedures for the use of the code extension control characters are specified in ANSI X3.41-1974.

Device control characters (DC1, DC2, DC3, DC4)

Device control characters are intended to control local or remote devices or ancillary devices connected to a data processing or data communication system. These control characters are not intended to control data communication systems; this should be achieved by the use of transmission control characters.

† This material is reproduced with permission from American National Standard ANSI X3.4-1986 (Coded character sets—7-bit American National Standard Code for Information Interchange; 7-bit ASCII), copyright 1986 by the American National Standards Institute. Copies of this standard may be purchased from the American National Standards Institute at 11 West 42nd Street, New York, N.Y. 10036, USA.

Information separators (FS, GS, RS, US)

Information separators are used to separate and qualify data logically. There are four such characters. They may be used in either hierarchical or non-hierarchical order; in the latter case, their specific meanings depend on the application.

Other control characters (NUL, BEL, CAN, EM, SUB, DEL)

These are the control characters that fall outside the preceding categories.

Description of the control characters

The control characters are described in the order they appear in the ASCII table. It should be noted that the control characters of ASCII are identical to those of ISO 646-1983.†

- **0: NUL (null)** A control character used to accomplish media-fill or time-fill. NUL characters may be inserted into or removed from a stream of data without affecting the information content of that stream, but such action may affect the information layout and/or the control of equipment.
- **1: SOH (start of heading)** A transmission control character used as the first character of a heading of an information message.
- **2: STX (start of text)** A transmission control character that precedes a text and that is used to terminate a heading.
- **3: ETX (end of text)** A transmission control character that terminates a text.
- **4: EOT (end of transmission)** A transmission control character used to indicate the conclusion of the transmission of one or more texts.
- **5: ENQ (enquiry)** A transmission control character used as a request for a response from a remote station—the response may include station identification and/or station status. When a 'who are you?' function is required on a switched transmission network, the first use of ENQ after the connection is established shall have the meaning 'who are you?' (station identification). Subsequent use of ENQ may or may not include the function 'who are you?,' as determined by agreement.

† This material is reproduced with permission from American National Standard ANSI X3.4-1986 (Coded character sets—7-bit American National Standard Code for Information Interchange; 7-bit ASCII), copyright 1986 by the American National Standards Institute. Copies of this standard may be purchased from the American National Standards Institute at 11 West 42nd Street, New York, N.Y. 10036, USA.

- **6: ACK (acknowledge)** A transmission control character transmitted by a receiver as an affirmative response to the sender.
- **7: BEL (bell)** A control character that is used when there is a need to call for attention; it may control alarm or attention devices.
- **8: BS (backspace)** A format effector that causes the active position to move one character position backwards.
- **9: HT (horizontal tabulation)** A format effector that causes the active position to advance to the next predetermined character position.
- **10: LF (line feed)** A format effector that causes the active position to advance to the corresponding character position of the next line.
- **11: VT (vertical tabulation)** A format effector that causes the active position to advance to the corresponding character position on the next predetermined line.
- **12: FF (form feed)** A format effector that causes the active position to advance to the corresponding character position on a predetermined line of the next form or page.
- **13: CR (carriage return)** A format effector that causes the active position to move to the first character position on the same line.
- **14: SO (shift-out)** A control character that is used in conjunction with SI and ESC to extend the graphic character set of the code. It may alter the meaning of the bit combinations that follow it until an SI character is reached. The effect of this character is described in ANSI X3.41-1974.
- **15: SI (shift-in)** A control character that is used in conjunction with SI and ESC to extend the graphic character set of the code. It may reinstate the standard meanings of the bit combinations that follow it. The effect of this character is described in ANSI X3.41-1974.
- **16: DLE (data link escape)** A transmission control character that changes the meaning of a limited number of contiguously following bit combinations. It is used exclusively to provide supplementary transmission control functions. Only graphic characters and transmission control characters may be used in DLE sequences. Appropriate sequences are defined in ANSI X3.28-1976.
- **17: DC1 (device control one)** A device control character that is primarily intended for turning on or starting an ancillary device. If it is not required for this purpose, it may be used to restore a device to the basic mode of operation (see also DC2 and DC3), or for any other device control function not provided by any other DCs.
- **18: DC2 (device control two)** A device control character that is primarily intended for turning on or starting an ancillary device. If it

is not required for this purpose, it may be used to set a device to a special mode of operation (in which case DC1 is used to restore the device to the basic mode), or for any other device control function not provided by any other DCs.
- **19: DC3 (device control three)** A device control character that is primarily intended for turning off or stopping an ancillary device. This function may be a secondary level stop, for example, wait, pause, standby, or halt (in which case DC1 is used to restore normal operation). If it is not required for this purpose, it may be used for any other ancillary device control function not provided by other DCs.
- **20: DC4 (device control four)** A device control character that is primarily intended for turning off, stopping, or interrupting an ancillary device. If it is not required for this purpose, it may be used for any other device control function not provided by other DCs.
- **21: NAK (negative acknowledge)** A transmission control character transmitted by a receiver as a negative response to the sender.
- **22: SYN (synchronous idle)** A transmission control character used by a synchronous transmission system in the absence of any other character (idle condition) to provide a signal from which synchronism may be achieved or retained between data terminal equipment.
- **23: ETB (end of transmission block)** A transmission control character used to indicate the end of a transmission block of data where data is divided into such blocks for transmission purpose.
- **24: CAN (cancel)** A character, or the first character of a sequence, indicating that the data preceding it is in error. As a result, this data is to be ignored. The specific meaning of this character shall be defined for each application and/or defined between sender and recipient.
- **25: EM (end of medium)** A control character that may be used to identify the physical end of a medium, the end of a used portion of a medium, or the end of the wanted portion of data recorded on a medium. The position of this character does not necessarily correspond to the physical end of the medium.
- **26: SUB (substitute character)** A control character used in the place of a character that has been found to be invalid or in error. SUB is intended to be introduced by automatic means, as for example, when a transmission error is detected.
- **27: ESC (escape)** A control character that is used to provide additional characters (code extension). It alters the meaning of a limited number of contiguously following bit combinations. The use of this character is specified in ANSI X3.41-1974.

ASCII control and graphic characters

- **28: FS (file separator)** A control character used to separate and qualify data logically; its specific meaning has to be defined for each application. If this character is used in hierarchical order, as specified in the general definition of the information separators (see above), it delimits a data item called a 'file'.
- **29: GS (group separator)** A control character used to separate and qualify data logically; its specific meaning has to be defined for each application. If this character is used in hierarchical order, as specified in the general definition of the information separators (see above), it delimits a data item called a 'group'.
- **30: RS (record separator)** A control character used to separate and qualify data logically; its specific meaning has to be defined for each application. If this character is used in hierarchical order, as specified in the general definition of the information separators (see above), it delimits a data item called a 'record'.
- **31: US (unit separator)** A control character used to separate and qualify data logically; its specific meaning has to be defined for each application. If this character is used in hierarchical order, as specified in the general definition of the information separators (see above), it delimits a data item called a 'unit'.
- **127: DEL (delete)** A character used primarily to erase or obliterate an erroneous or untoward character in punched tape. DEL characters may also serve to accomplish media-fill or time-fill. They may be inserted into or removed from a stream of data without affecting the information content of that stream, but such action may affect the information layout and/or the control of equipment. If media-fill or time-fill is required, it is preferable that the NULL character be used.

Appendix 2
Serial port connector pin-outs

Table A2.1. *EIA/TIA-232-E pin assignments for 25/26-pin connectors.*

Pin No.	Code	Descriptive name
1		Shield
2	TxD	Transmits data
3	RxD	Receives data
4	RTS	Request to send/ready for receiving
5	CTS	Clear to send
6	DSR	Data set ready (DCE ready)
7	GND	Signal ground
8	DCD	Data carrier detect (received line signal detector)
9		RESERVED FOR TESTING
10		RESERVED FOR TESTING
11		UNASSIGNED
12		Secondary received line signal detector
13		Secondary clear to send
14		Secondary transmitted data
15		Transmitter signal element timing—DCE source
16		Secondary received data
17		Receiver signal element timing
18		Local loopback
19		Secondary request to send
20	DTR	Data terminal ready (DTE ready)
21		Remote loopback/signal quality detector
22	RI	Ring indicator
23		Data signal rate selector
24		Transmitter signal element timing—DTE source
25		Test mode
26		Alt A connector only—not connected

Table A2.2. *Pin assignments for 9-pin serial port connectors.*

Pin No.	Code	Descriptive name
1	DCD	Data carrier detect
2	RxD	Receives data
3	TxD	Transmits data
4	DTR	Data terminal ready
5	GND	Signal ground
6	DSR	Data set ready
7	RTS	Request to send
8	CTS	Clear to send
9	RI	Ring indicator

Appendix 3
Key codes

When a key is pressed a 1-byte **scan code** is generated which allows the computer to identify the key. The ROM BIOS then interprets the scan code and places a two-byte code in the keyboard buffer. The nature of the first byte depends on the key pressed; if it is a *character* key, then the first byte is the ASCII code; if it is an *extended* key, then the first byte is zero. The second byte is the scan code itself (Aitken, 1992).

QuickBASIC identifies key strokes using the INKEY$ function which returns a string consisting of either one or two bytes depending on the key pressed. When a character key is pressed then INKEY$ returns a one-byte string corresponding to the ASCII code of the character associated with the key. However, when an extended key is pressed (e.g. a FUNCTION-key) then INKEY$ returns the two-byte string ⟨0⟩⟨scan code⟩.

In order to determine which key has been pressed when using QuickBASIC it is therefore necessary to first determine the length of the string returned by INKEY$, and then test whether the byte (when only one byte is returned), or the second byte (if two bytes are returned) represents the relevant key (i.e. the key to be 'trapped'). If the value of the first byte returned is zero, then the key pressed must have been an extended key. See Section 5.14 for details on using key codes for trapping keys.

Since keyboards vary (e.g. PC, PC/AT, enhanced, laptops etc.), some of the values given in Table A3.1 below may not be valid for all computers. It is therefore important to check the keyboard directly for the correct key code, and the following short QuickBASIC program can be used to do this.

The example program waits for a key to be pressed, and then prints to the screen the decimal equivalent of the byte (or bytes) returned by the INKEY$ function (firstcode%, secondcode%). Pressing <Q> will quit the program.

Example program

```
REM [keycode.bas]
REM QuickBASIC test program for keyboard scan codes
CLS
LOCATE 5, 5
PRINT "press a key or key combination (<Q> to quit)"
PRINT
DO
    DO: key$ = INKEY$: LOOP WHILE key$ = ""
    L% = LEN(key$)
    firstcode% = ASC(LEFT$(key$, 1))
    IF UCASE$(key$) = "Q" THEN END
    SELECT CASE L%
        CASE 1
            PRINT "Length ="; LEN(key$); "  key = ";
key$; "   key code = "; firstcode%
        CASE 2
            secondcode% = ASC(RIGHT$(key$, 1))
            PRINT "Length = 2  (extended key)   key code
= "; firstcode%; " ; "; secondcode%
    END SELECT
    PRINT
LOOP
END
```

For example, pressing the keys j and F2 gives the following output.

```
Length = 1   key = j   key code = 106
Length = 2   (extended key)   key code = 0 ; 60
```

Some keys are handled differently by different PCs. For example, when the 'R anglebracket' key (. >) is pressed, QuickBASIC returns the two bytes ⟨0⟩⟨83⟩ on a Toshiba 2000sx, but returns the single byte ⟨62⟩ on a Dell 325sx.

In Table A3.1 brackets () are used to indicate that the enclosed codes may not apply to some keyboards, particularly laptop and notebook PCs. An asterisk * indicates that the code is generated on *release* of the Alt key. Where two different codes are given (e.g. 62/0;83), this indicates that some variation exists with respect to the key.

Table A3.1. *Key codes.*

Key		Code	Shift	Ctrl	Alt
Escape		27	27	27	—
F1		0 ; 59	0 ; 84	0 ; 94	0 ; 104
F2		0 ; 60	0 ; 85	0 ; 95	0 ; 105
F3		0 ; 61	0 ; 86	0 ; 96	0 ; 106
F4		0 ; 62	0 ; 87	0 ; 97	0 ; 107
F5		0 ; 63	0 ; 88	0 ; 98	0 ; 108
F6		0 ; 64	0 ; 89	0 ; 99	0 ; 109
F7		0 ; 65	0 ; 90	0 ; 100	0 ; 110
F8		0 ; 66	0 ; 91	0 ; 101	0 ; 111
F9		0 ; 67	0 ; 92	0 ; 102	0 ; 112
F10		0 ; 68	0 ; 93	0 ; 103	0 ; 113
F11		0 ; 133	0 ; 135	0 ; 137	0 ; 139
F12		0 ; 134	0 ; 136	0 ; 138	0 ; 140
7 Home	(white)	0 ; 71	55	0 ; 119	7*
8 Up Arrow	(white)	0 ; 72	56	(0 ; 141)	8*
9 Page Up	(white)	0 ; 73	57	0 ; 132	9*
4 Left Arrow	(white)	0 ; 75	52	0 ; 115	4*
6 Right Arrow	(white)	0 ; 77	54	0 ; 116	6*
1 End	(white)	0 ; 79	49	0 ; 117	1*
2 Down Arrow	(white)	0 ; 80	50	(0 ; 145)	2*
3 Page Down	(white)	0 ; 81	51	0 ; 118	3*
0 Insert	(white)	0 ; 82	48	(0 ; 146)	—
. Delete	(white)	0 ; 83	46	(0 ; 147)	—
Home	(grey)	0 ; 71	0 ; 71	0 ; 119	(0 ; 151)
Up Arrow	(grey)	0 ; 72	0 ; 72	(0 ; 141)	(0 ; 152)
Page Up	(grey)	0 ; 73	0 ; 73	0 ; 132	(0 ; 153)
Left Arrow	(grey)	0 ; 75	0 ; 75	0 ; 115	(0 ; 155)
Right Arrow	(grey)	0 ; 77	0 ; 77	0 ; 116	(0 ; 157)
End	(grey)	0 ; 79	0 ; 79	0 ; 117	(0 ; 159)
Down Arrow	(grey)	0 ; 80	0 ; 80	(0 ; 145)	(0 ; 154)
Page Down	(grey)	0 ; 81	0 ; 81	0 ; 118	(0 ; 161)
Insert	(grey)	0 ; 82	0 ; 82	(0 ; 146)	(0 ; 162)
Delete	(grey)	0 ; 83	0 ; 83	(0 ; 147)	(0 ; 163)
Print Screen		—	—	0 ; 114	—
Pause/Break		—	—	0 ; 0	—
Backspace		8	8	127	(0)
Enter		13	13	10	(0 ; 28)
Tab		9	0 ; 15	(0 ; 148)	(0 ; 165)
(Null)		0 ; 3	—	—	—
Enter	(keypad)	13	13	10	(0 ; 166)
/	(keypad)	47	47	(0 ; 142)	(0 ; 74)
*	(keypad)	42	42	(0 ; 78)	—
−	(keypad)	45	45	—	—
+	(keypad)	43	43	(0 ; 150)	(0 ; 55)
5	(keypad)	(53)	53	(0 ; 143)	—

Table A3.1 *cont.*

Key	Code	Shift	Ctrl	Alt
A a	97	65	1	0 ; 30
B b	98	66	2	0 ; 48
C c	99	67	3	0 ; 46
D d	100	68	4	0 ; 32
E e	101	69	5	0 ; 18
F f	102	70	6	0 ; 33
G g	103	71	7	0 ; 34
H h	104	72	8	0 ; 35
I i	105	73	9	0 ; 23
J j	106	74	10	0 ; 36
K k	107	75	11	0 ; 37
L l	108	76	12	0 ; 38
M m	109	77	13	0 ; 50
N n	110	78	14	0 ; 49
O o	111	79	15	0 ; 24
P p	112	80	16	0 ; 25
Q q	113	81	17	0 ; 16
R r	114	82	18	0 ; 19
S r	115	83	19	0 ; 31
T t	116	84	20	0 ; 20
U u	117	85	21	0 ; 22
V v	118	86	22	0 ; 47
W w	119	87	23	0 ; 17
X x	120	88	24	0 ; 45
Y y	121	89	25	0 ; 21
Z z	122	90	26	0 ; 44
1 !	49	33	—	0 ; 120
2 "	50	34	0 ; 3	0 ; 121
3 £	51	156	—	0 ; 122
4 $	52	36	—	0 ; 123
5 %	53	37	—	0 ; 124
6 ^	54	94	30	0 ; 125
7 &	55	38	(0, 119)	0 ; 126
8 *	56	42	—	0 ; 127
9 (	57	40	(9, 132)	0 ; 128
0)	48	41	—	0 ; 129
− _	45	95	31	0 ; 130
= +	61	43	—	0 ; 131
[{	91	123	27	(0 ; 26)
] }	93	125	29	(0 ; 27)
# ~	35	126	—	—
\ ¦	92	124	(28)	(0 ; 43)
; :	59	(58/43)	—	(0 ; 39)
' @	39	64	—	(0 ; 40)
, <	44	60	—	(0 ; 51)
. >	46	(62/0;83)	—	(0 ; 52)
/ ?	47	(63/47)	—	(0 ; 53)
` ¬	96	170	28	(0 ; 41)

Appendix 4
The null modem

It is often convenient to connect two PCs together via their serial ports (see Appendix 5). However, the wiring depends on a number of factors such as the particular handshaking lines required, and whether a full or half-duplex system is used. There is, therefore, no 'perfect' null modem configuration which works in all cases. Thus Goodwin (1992), Perry (1993), Gofton (1986), and Van Gilluwe (1994) all give slightly different configurations for a null modem. An excellent discussion on this topic is that by Perry (1993).

However, if both PCs are using QuickBASIC then the simple three-wire configuration shown in Figure A4.1 will suffice for transferring files between computers, since using the CS, DS options in the OPEN COM statement eliminates the need for all the other connections. If hardware handshaking has to be used for control then the appropriate lines can be added as required.

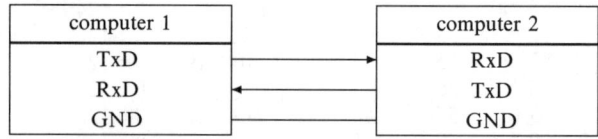

Fig. A4.1. A three-wire connection for use with QuickBASIC.

Example programs to transmit and receive files

The following example QuickBASIC 4.5 programs illustrate a method of transmitting ASCII files from one computer to another via the serial port, using the wiring configuration shown in Figure A4.1.

The transmitting program prompts the operator to press a key when ready to send the datafile. Pressing <Q> will quit the program.

Program points

- Insert the name of the file to be transmitted into the OPEN...FOR INPUT statement of the transmitting program.
- Insert the new name of the received file into the OPEN...FOR OUTPUT statement of the receiving program.
- Start the receiving program (**nulmod-r.bas**) before transmitting the datafile.
- Make sure both programs are using the same Protocol. Most PCs nowadays are able to use 19200 bps.
- The programs assume that the wiring configuration shown in Figure A4.1 is being used.
- Since hardware handshaking is not used, the CS and DS options need to be used in the OPEN COM statement.
- The receive and transmit buffers have been increased to 20000 bytes using the TB20000 and RB20000 options in the OPEN COM statement.
- The 'end of transmission' character (EOT, ♦, ASCII 4) is sent following the end of the transmitted datafile using the PRINT# statement as follows.

```
PRINT #1, CHR$(4)
```

When the ⟨EOT⟩ character is detected, the receive program exits the data-collecting loop using the following line.

```
IF data$ = CHR$(4) THEN EXIT DO
```

- Both the transmitting and receiving programs give the file size on completion of the transfer as a check that the complete file has been transferred. The time taken is also given.

Example programs

```
REM [nulmod-t.bas]
REM this is the transmitting program
CLEAR
CLS
```

```
LOCATE 5
PRINT "press any key when ready to send the datafile"
PRINT "press <Q> to quit"
SLEEP: z$ = INKEY$
OPEN "COM1:19200,N,8,1,CS,DS,ASC,TB20000" FOR OUTPUT AS #1
OPEN "c:file_to_transmit" FOR INPUT AS #2
time1 = TIMER
DO
   key$ = INKEY$
   IF UCASE$(key$) = "Q" THEN
       PRINT #1,
       PRINT #1, STRING$(30, "*") + "TRANSMISSION ERROR"
+ STRING$(30, "*")
       REM send EOT character
       PRINT #1, CHR$(4)
       CLOSE
       END
   END IF
   LINE INPUT #2, line$
   PRINT line$
   PRINT #1, line$
LOOP UNTIL EOF(2)
PRINT #1, CHR$(4): REM end of transmission character
PRINT STRING$(50, "*")
PRINT "transmission complete"
PRINT "size of file ="; LOF(2)
PRINT "time taken = "; TIMER - time1; " secs"
CLOSE
END
```

```
REM [nulmod-r.bas]
REM program to receive the datafile
CLEAR
CLS
LOCATE 5
OPEN "COM1:19200,N,8,1,CS,DS,RB20000" FOR INPUT AS #1
OPEN "c:received_filename" FOR OUTPUT AS #2
PRINT "computer ready: waiting for data to arrive"
PRINT "(press <Q> to quit)"
```

```
DO
    DO
        key$ = INKEY$
        IF UCASE$(key$) = "Q" THEN
            CLOSE
            END
        END IF
        a$ = a$ + INPUT$(LOC(1), #1)
        L% = INSTR(1, a$, CHR$(13))
    LOOP UNTIL L% > 0
    data$ = MID$(a$, 1, L% - 1)
    IF data$ = CHR$(4) THEN EXIT DO
    PRINT data$
    PRINT #2, data$
    a$ = RIGHT$(a$, LEN(a$) - L%)
LOOP UNTIL L% = 0
PRINT STRING$(30, "*")
PRINT "END OF TRANSMISSION"
PRINT "size of received file = "; LOF(2)
CLOSE
END
```

Appendix 5
Program for a device simulator

If a second PC is available, it is often convenient to use it to simulate a peripheral device (e.g. the Evita ventilator), and so allow work on a serial interface program even when the peripheral device itself is not available. Once a number of sample data outputs from the peripheral device have been downloaded and stored in files, the second PC can be used to transmit the data in these files in response to the appropriate command-codes, and so appear to behave just as if it were the peripheral device.

When the following example QuickBASIC 4.5 program is run on a second PC, it waits until it receives a command-code via the serial port. When the command-code is received (e.g. code$ in this example), the remote program transmits the contents of a data file (datafile.dat) back to the first PC, as well as printing it to its own screen to indicate that the data is being transmitted. See Appendix 4 for details of a null modem wiring configuration.

Note that the following example program assumes that the received command-code (code$) is followed by the ⟨CR⟩ control character, i.e. it was sent using PRINT #1, code$. Pressing <Q> will quit the program.

Example program

```
REM [a-sim.bas]
REM program run by second PC simulating remote device
CLS
OPEN "COM1:1200,E,7,2,CS,DS" FOR RANDOM ACCESS
                                        READ WRITE AS #1
LOCATE 10, 25
```

```
PRINT "REMOTE DEVICE SIMULATOR"
CR$ = CHR$(13) : REM carriage return character
REM collect data as it arrives at the serial port
DO
    DO
        a$ = a$ + INPUT$(LOC(1), #1)
        L% = INSTR(1, a$, CR$)
        key$ = INKEY$
        IF UCASE$(key$) = "Q" THEN END
    LOOP UNTIL L% > 0
    REM send contents of file in response to command-code
    IF a$ = code$ + CR$ THEN
        OPEN "datafile.dat" FOR INPUT AS #2
        DO
            LINE INPUT #2, line$
            PRINT line$       :REM print to screen
            PRINT #1, line$   :REM print to serial port
        LOOP UNTIL EOF(2)
        CLOSE #2
    END IF
    a$ = RIGHT$(a$, LEN(a$) - L%)
LOOP
CLOSE
END
```

If it is only necessary for the second PC to reply with a short string (say, datastring$), then the conditional loop could be replaced by the following statements. Note the use of the semicolon on the end of the PRINT# statement to prevent an additional ⟨CR⟩ character being sent.

```
IF a$ = code$ + CR$ THEN
    PRINT datastring$
    PRINT #1, datastring$;
END IF
```

Appendix 6
QuickBASIC 4.5 OPEN and OPEN COM statements

The following Sections from the QuickBASIC 4.5 *BASIC language reference* (Microsoft, 1988) are reproduced with permission from Microsoft Corporation.

OPEN Statement

ACTION
Enables I/O to a file or device.

SYNTAX 1
OPEN *file* [FOR *mode1*] [ACCESS *access*][*lock*] AS[#]*filenum* [LEN=*reclen*]

SYNTAX 2
OPEN *mode2*,[#]*filenum,file*[,*reclen*]

The *file* is a string expression that specifies an optional device, followed by a file name or path name conforming to the DOS file-naming conventions.

You must open a file before any I/O operation can be performed on it. OPEN allocates a buffer for I/O to the file or device and determines the mode of access used with the buffer.

Syntax 1

In the first syntax, *mode1* is one of the following:

Mode	Description
OUTPUT	Specifies sequential output mode.
INPUT	Specifies sequential input mode.

QuickBASIC 4.5 OPEN and OPEN COM statements

APPEND
: Specifies sequential output mode and sets the file pointer to the end of the file and the record number to the last record of the file. A PRINT# or WRITE# statement then extends (appends to) the file.

RANDOM
: Specifies random-access file mode, the default mode. In RANDOM mode, if no ACCESS clause is present, three attempts are made to open the file when the OPEN statement is executed. Access is attempted in the following order:
  1. Read/write
  2. Write-only
  3. Read-only

BINARY
: Specifies binary file mode. In binary mode, you may read or write information to any byte position in the file using GET and PUT.

   In binary mode, if no ACCESS clause is present, three attempts are made to open the file. The attempts follow the same order as those for RANDOM files.

If *mode1* is omitted, the default random-access mode is assumed.

The *access* expression specifies the operation performed on the opened file. If the file is already opened by another process and the specified type of access is not allowed, the OPEN fails and an error message is generated that reads PERMISSION DENIED. The ACCESS clause works in an OPEN statement only if you are using a version of DOS that supports networking (DOS versions 3.0 or later). In addition, you must run the SHARE.EXE program (or the network startup program must run it) to perform any locking operation. If ACCESS is used with OPEN, earlier versions of DOS return an error message that reads ADVANCED FEATURE UNAVAILABLE.

The *access* argument can be one of the following:

Access Type	Description
READ	Opens the file for reading only.
WRITE	Opens the file for writing only.

READ WRITE   Opens the file for both reading and writing. This mode is valid only for RANDOM and BINARY files and files opened for APPEND.

The *lock* clause works in a multiprocessing environment to restrict access by other processes to an open file. The lock types are as follows:

Lock Type	**Description**
Default	If *lock* type is not specified, the file may be opened for reading and writing any number of times by this process, but other processes are denied access to the file while it is opened.
SHARED	Any process on any machine may read from or write to this file. Do not confuse the SHARED lock type with the SHARED statement or the SHARED attribute appearing in other statements.
LOCK READ	No other process is granted read access to this file. This access is granted only if no other process has a previous READ access to the file.
LOCK WRITE	No other process is granted write access to this file. This lock is granted only if no other process has a previous WRITE access to the file.
LOCK READ WRITE	No other process is granted either read or write access to this file. This access is granted only if READ or WRITE access has not already been granted to another process, or if a LOCK READ or LOCK WRITE is not already in place.

When the OPEN is restricted by a previous process, it generates error 70, PERMISSION DENIED, under DOS.

The *filenum* (file number) argument is an integer expression whose value is between 1 and 255. When an OPEN is executed, the file number is associated with the file as long as it is open. Other I/O statements may use the number to refer to the file.

The *reclen* (record length) argument is an integer expression that, if included, sets the record length (number of characters in one record) for random-access files. For sequential files, the default length for records is

512 bytes; for random-access files, the default is 128 bytes. The value of *reclen* cannot exceed 32,767 bytes. If the file mode is binary, then the LEN clause is ignored.

For sequential files, *reclen* need not correspond to an individual record size, since a sequential file may have records of different sizes. When used to open a sequential file, *reclen* specifies the number of characters to be loaded into the buffer before the buffer is written to, or read from, the disk. A larger buffer means more room taken from BASIC, but faster file I/O. A smaller buffer means more room in memory for BASIC, but slower I/O. The default buffer size is 512 bytes.

Syntax 2

In the second form of the OPEN syntax, *mode2* is a string expression, the first character of which must be one of the following:

Mode	Description
O	Specifies sequential output mode.
I	Specifies sequential input mode.
R	Specifies random-access file input/output mode.
B	Specifies binary file mode.
A	Specifies sequential output mode and sets the file pointer to the end of the file and the record number to the last record of the file. A PRINT# or WRITE# statement extends (appends to) the file.

NOTE: The second form of the OPEN syntax does not support any of the access and file-sharing options found in the first syntax and is supported for compatibility with programs written in earlier versions of BASIC.

The following devices are supported by BASIC and can be named and opened with the *file* argument: KYBD:, SCRN:, COM*n*:, CONS:.

The BASIC file I/O system allows you to take advantage of user-installed devices (see your DOS manual for information on character devices).

Character devices are opened and used in the same manner as disk files. However, characters are not buffered by BASIC as they are for disk files. The record length for the device files is set to one.

BASIC only sends a carriage return at the end of a line. If the device requires a line feed, the driver must provide it. When writing device drivers, keep in mind that other BASIC users will want to read and write control information. The writing and reading of device control data is handled by the IOCTL statement and IOCTL$ function.

None of the BASIC devices directly supports binary mode. However, the line printer devices (LPT1:, LPT2:) can be opened in binary mode by adding the BIN keyword.

```
OPEN "LPT1:BIN" FOR OUTPUT AS #1
```

Opening a printer in BIN mode eliminates printing a carriage return at the end of a line.

NOTE: In INPUT, RANDOM, and BINARY modes you can open a file under a different file number without first closing the file. In OUTPUT or APPEND mode you must close a file before opening it with a different file number.

OPEN COM statement

ACTION

Opens and initializes a communications channel for I/O.

SYNTAX

OPEN "COM*n: optlist1 optlist2*" [FOR *mode*] AS[#]*filenum* [LEN=*reclen*]

COM*n*: is the name of the device to be opened. The *n* argument is the number of a legal communications device, such as COM1: or COM2:. The first list of options, *oplist1*, has the following form:

[*speed*][,[*parity*][,[*data*][,[*stop*]]]]

The following list describes the possible options:

Option	Description
speed	The 'baud' rate (baud means 'bits per second') of the device to be opened. Valid speeds are 75, 110, 150, 300, 600, 1200, 1800, 2400, 4800, 9600, 19200. The default is 300 bps.

QuickBASIC 4.5 OPEN and OPEN COM statements

parity The parity of the device to be opened. Valid entries for parity are: N (none), E (even), O (odd), S (space), or M (mark).

data The number of data bits per byte. Valid entries are 5, 6, 7, or 8.

stop The number of stop bits. Valid entries are 1, or 2. The 1.5 stop bit option is not supported (Microsoft, 1990f).

Options from this list must be entered in the order shown; moreover, if any options from *optlist2* are chosen, comma placeholders must still be used even if none of the options from *optlist1* are chosen. For example:

OPEN "COM1: ,,,,CD1500" FOR INPUT AS #1

If you set the data bits per byte to eight, you must specify no parity (N). Because QuickBASIC uses complete bytes (eight bits) for numbers, you must specify eight data bits when transmitting or receiving numeric data.

The choices for *optlist2* are described in the following list. The argument *m* is given in milliseconds; the default value for *m* is 1000.

Option	**Description**
ASC	Opens the device in ASCII mode. In ASCII mode, tabs are expanded to spaces, carriage returns are forced at end-of-line, and CTRL+Z is treated as end-of-file. When the channel is closed, CTRL+Z is sent over the RS-232 line.
BIN	Opens the device in binary mode. This option supersedes the LF option. BIN is selected by default unless ASC is specified. In the BIN mode, tabs are not expanded to spaces, a carriage return is not forced at the end-of-line, and CTRL+Z is not treated as end-of-file. When the channel is closed, CTRL+Z will not be sent over the RS-232 line.

CD[*m*]   Controls the timeout on the Data Carrier Detect line (DCD). If DCD is LOW for more than *m* milliseconds, a device timeout occurs.

CS[*m*]   Controls the timeout on the Clear To Send line (CTS). If CTS is LOW (there is no signal) for more than *m* milliseconds, a device timeout occurs.

DS[*m*]   Controls the timeout on the Data Set Ready line (DSR). If DSR is LOW for more than *m* milliseconds, a device timeout occurs.

LF   Allows communication files to be printed on a serial line printer. When LF is specified, a line feed character (0Ah) is automatically sent after each carriage return character (0Dh). This includes the carriage return sent as a result of the width setting. Note that INPUT and LINE INPUT, when used to read from a COM file that was opened with the LF option, stop when they see a carriage return, ignoring the line feed.

OP[*m*]   Controls how long the statement waits for the open to be successful. The parameter *m* is a value in the range 0 to 65,535 representing the number of milliseconds to wait for the communication lines to become active. If OP is specified without a value, the statement waits indefinitely. If OP is omitted, OPEN COM waits for ten times the maximum value of the CD or DS timeout values.

PE   The PE option enables parity checking during communications. If the PE option is used, and the communications system is using different parity options, then a DEVICE I/O ERROR occurs (Microsoft, 1990i).

RB[*m*]   Sets the size of the receive buffer to *n* bytes. If *n* is omitted, or the option is omitted, the current value is used. The current value can be set by the /C option on the QuickBASIC or BC command line. The default is 512 bytes. The maximum size is 32,767 bytes.

RS   Suppresses detection of Request To Send (RTS).

TB[*m*]   Sets the size of the transmit buffer to *n* bytes. If *n* is omitted, or the option is omitted, the current value is used. The default is 512 bytes.

The options from the list above can be entered in any order, but they must be separated from one another by commas. For CS[*m*], DS[*m*], and CD[*m*], if there is no signal within *m* milliseconds, a timeout occurs. The value of *m* may range from 0 to 65,535, with 1000 as the default value (the CD default is 0). If *m* is equal to 0 for any of these options the option is ignored. The CTS line is checked whenever there is data in the transmit buffer if the CS option is specified. The DSR and DCD lines are continuously checked for timeouts if the corresponding options (DS, CD) are specified.

The *mode* argument is one of the following string expressions:

Mode	Description
OUTPUT	Specifies sequential output mode.
INPUT	Specifies sequential input mode.
RANDOM	Specifies random-access mode.

If the *mode* expression is omitted, it is assumed to be random-access input/output. The *filenum* is the number used to open the file. The OPEN COM statement must be executed before a device can be used for communication using an RS-232 interface.

If the device is opened in RANDOM mode, the LEN option specifies the length of an associated random-access buffer. The default value for length is 128. You can use any of the random-access I/O statements, such as GET and PUT, to treat the device as if it were a random-access file. The OPEN COM statement performs the following steps in opening a communications device.

(1) The communications buffers are allocated and interrupts are enabled.
(2) The Data Terminal Ready line (DTR) is set HIGH.
(3) If either the OP or DS options is nonzero, the statement waits up to the indicated time for the Data Set Ready line (DSR) to be HIGH. If a timeout occurs, the process goes to step 6.

(4) The Request To Send line (RTS) is set HIGH if the RS option is not specified.

(5) If either of the OP or CD options is nonzero, OPEN COM waits up to the indicated time for the Data Carrier Detect line (DCD) to be HIGH. If a timeout occurs, the process goes to step 6. Otherwise, OPEN COM has succeeded.

(6) The open has failed due to a timeout. The process deallocates the buffers, disables interrupts, and clears all of the control lines.

NOTE: Use a relatively large value for the OP option compared to the CS, DS, or CD options. If two programs are attempting to establish a communications link, they both need to attempt an OPEN during at least half of the time they are executing.

Any syntax errors in the OPEN COM statement produce an error message that reads BAD FILE NAME.

Appendix 7
Plotting data using GNUPLOT

Introduction

This Appendix illustrates the use of the remarkable 'freeware' package GNUPLOT.† It is a command-driven interactive function plotting package which is freely available for downloading by 'anonymous ftp' from **dartmouth.edu**.‡

GNUPLOT covers the full range of mathematical functions (e.g. complex numbers, Bessel functions, 3-dimensional surfaces), and supports an extensive range of graphics devices and modes (e.g. MS Windows, PostScript, HP LaserJet series, TeX and LaTeX picture environments).§ Numerous extensions to GNUPLOT are available (via ftp) in the files **gpcontrib.tar.z**. An extensive user manual is also available.

The current version at the time of writing is 3.5, which is a 'bug-fix' release over version 3.4.

Formatting the data

GNUPLOT accepts input data formatted in columns, so it is best to arrange that the data collecting program outputs the data in a file in columns with at least one space separating the columns, as shown in Table A7.1. This data-file can then be the input-file for the GNUPLOT program, which will then plot the graph and either output it to the screen or a printer, or save it in a format required by a typesetting system (e.g. TeX or LaTeX).

---

† Copyright © 1986–1993 Thomas Williams & Colin Kelley.
‡ Search for the file **/pub/gnuplot/gnuplot.3.5.tar.z**. General information regarding GNUPLOT is available via the Usenet newsgroup **comp.graphics.gnuplot**.
§ The GNUPLOT 3.4 quick reference manual lists 74 supported devices and modes.

Table A7.1. *Time, blood pressure, heart rate, and saturation data, arranged in columns in the file* anaes.dat.

T(mins)	BP(s)	BP(d)	HR	SaO$_2$
2	127	72	73	96
4	131	72	68	97
6	141	81	70	96
8	138	78	71	95
10	136	77	79	95
12	142	82	79	98
14	137	79	80	98
16	140	77	77	98
18	138	79	80	97
20	136	77	82	95
22	144	80	78	96
24	139	79	78	93
26	135	77	58	90
28	137	75	61	89
30	142	79	60	89
32	145	83	62	91
34	148	86	63	97
36	144	85	62	98
38	143	83	61	97

Plotting the graph

GNUPLOT is easy to use, and excellent graphs can be generated with very little effort. All the labels are defined using a range of set commands, and the graph(s) are drawn using the plot command. Comments can be added to the program by prefixing the line with the # symbol.

Once the data-file is formatted in columns GNUPLOT will plot one column against any other column. If several curves are to be displayed on the same graph, then the instructions for each curve are grouped within the same plot command.

As an example, the following GNUPLOT program draws on the data shown in Table A7.1 (held in the file anaes.dat), and generates the graph shown in Figure A7.1 exactly as it appears in this book. Since this book was typeset using LaTeX, the example GNUPLOT program outputs the graph in a format compatible with the LaTeX Picture environment (set terminal emtex). Similarly, the caption and labels for the x-axis and y-axis are written in LaTeX format.

The graph was saved in a file (hr-sa02.pic) on drive C (set output "c:\emtex\texinput\hr-sao2.pic"). The other set commands are self explanatory. Note that in Table A7.1 the time data is in column 1, HR data in column 4, and SaO_2 data in column 5. Thus the instruction using 1:5 results in the data in columns 1 and 5 being plotted against each other, i.e. the SaO_2 vs. Time plot.

Automating the process

Since GNUPLOT is available as a text based program, it can therefore be written by a general computer program, e.g. QuickBASIC. In practice this means that the whole process of data collection, analysis, and display, can be controlled by a single computer program. This can be useful since it allows such a program to tailor graphics and text to the data.

There are, therefore, advantages of using packages which are completely text based (e.g. GNUPLOT, TeX, LaTeX). For example, a single computer program could save data to a file, write appropriate GNUPLOT and LaTeX programs to plot the data and write text, save these programs to files, and then invoke these programs itself later.

Example GNUPLOT program

```
# gnuplot file for plotting saturation vs time.
set terminal emtex
set output "c:\emtex\texinput\hr-sao2.pic"
set nokey
set ylabel "Sa0$_2$ $\diamond$\\ {\ }\\HR $\bullet$"-1
set xlabel "Time (mins)"
set title "{\large Saturation (Sa0$_2$)\& heart rate (HR)}"
set size 0.787, 0.787
set xtics 0,10,40
set ytics 40,10,100
xmin=0; xmax=40
ymin=40;ymax=100
plot [xmin:xmax]  [ymin:ymax]\
    90 with lines 1,\
    "anaes.dat" using 1:5 with linespoints 1 1,\
    "anaes.dat" using 1:4 with linespoints 1 12
```

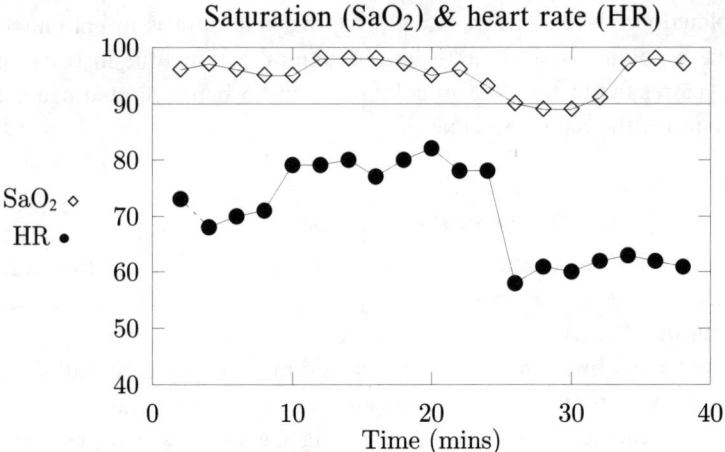

Fig. A7.1. Graph of SaO$_2$ and heart rate data drawn using GNUPLOT 3.4.

Appendix 8
Binary and hexadecimal notation

Binary notation

An ordered group of 8 bits is known as a byte. It is usual to number the 8 bits from 0–7, and such a group is always written with the least significant bit (bit-0) on the right. This notation is useful since the value of any particular bit is then given by raising 2 to the power of the bit-position. Thus the value of a 1 in the bit-4 position is given by $2^4 = 16$, as shown in Figure A8.1.

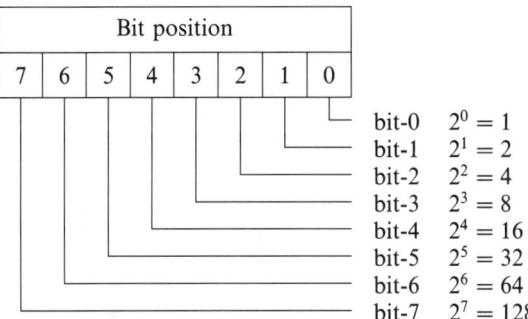

Fig. A8.1.

Thus the value of 10100110b is calculated as follows.

$$10100110 = 2^7 + 2^5 + 2^2 + 2^1$$
$$= 128 + 32 + 4 + 2$$
$$= 166$$

Hexadecimal notation

Hexadecimal notation uses 0–9 and A–F to represent the values 0–15 as shown in Table A8.1. Note that each hexadecimal value 0–F represents 4 bits. In view of this, binary numbers are commonly split into groups of 4 bits with each group then being represented by its hexadecimal equivalent. Thus a byte is often represented as two hexadecimal values. Similarly, a 2-byte word (16-bit number) is commonly represented in terms of four hexadecimal values.

For example, the byte 10100110b can be written as two groups of four bits as 1010 0110, which can then be regarded as being equivalent to the hexadecimal pair A6h.

Table A8.1. *Decimal, hex and binary equivalents.*

Dec	Hex	Binary
0	0h	0000b
1	1h	0001b
2	2h	0010b
3	3h	0011b
4	4h	0100b
5	5h	0101b
6	6h	0110b
7	7h	0111b
8	8h	1000b
9	9h	1001b
10	Ah	1010b
11	Bh	1011b
12	Ch	1100b
13	Dh	1101b
14	Eh	1110b
15	Fh	1111b

Appendix 9
Glossary of terms and abbreviations

- **ACK** A control character (ASCII 6) meaning 'acknowledge'. Used for error-checking purposes. See also NAK.
- **address** A numeric value representing a memory location.
- **analog signal** A continuously varying signal, such that its magnitude is proportional to the magnitude of the parameter being measured.
- **AND** A logical operation which gives logic 1 when *all* inputs are logic 1.
- **ANSI** American National Standards Institute. This is an organisation concerned with the development of standards for computing and electronic communications.
- **ARQ** Automatic Repeat Request. A common system for error-checking used in data transmission. ARQ systems request the retransmission of a data block if an error is detected.
- **ASCII** American Standard Code for Information Interchange. This was formerly known as USASCII. It is a seven-bit code which represents each of 128 upper and lower-case letters, numbers and symbols as a number from 0 to 127. An 'extended' ASCII code provides for a further 128 commonly used symbols, making a total of 256 codes.
- **ASCII file** Otherwise known as a 'text' file—a file made up entirely of symbols and characters from the ASCII character set.
- **asynchronous communication** A variety of serial communication for which data transmission is independent of a common timing mechanism.
- **AT** A term applied to a PC which handles 16-bit data.
- **BASIC** Beginner's All-purpose Symbolic Instruction Code. A high-level programming language established at Dartmouth College, USA. Several versions have evolved, with QuickBASIC 4.5 being one of the more recent structured and compilable versions.

- **baud rate** The rate of signal elements transmitted per second. It is commonly, but incorrectly, used to mean the bit rate. The term Baud is named after Jean Maurice Emile Baudot (1845–1903).
- **BCD** Binary Coded Decimal. This is a system whereby each digit of a decimal number is coded separately in binary. For example, although the decimal number 31 is equivalent to 11111 in binary, it is represented as 0011 0001 in BCD notation.
- **bell** A control character (ASCII 7), which causes the computer to sound a buzzer, or beep.
- **binary** A coding system which uses only two states; e.g. on and off, positive and negative voltages. These states are represented by the digits 1 and 0. Binary numbers are usually written in groups of four, followed by the letter b or B to avoid confusion with decimal numbers. For example, the binary equivalent of the decimal number 4 is 0100b. See also BCD.
- **BIOS** Basic Input-Output System. Refers to a system of computer programs which are used by the PC to control the basic functions of the associated elements of the computer, for example the keyboard or screen.
- **BIPAP** Biphasic Intermittent Positive Airway Pressure.
- **bit** A contraction of Binary Digit. A bit represents a unit of information (1 or 0) which can be processed by the computer. An ordered group of 4 bits is known as a nibble. An ordered group of 8 bits is known as a byte.
- **bit time** The duration of 1 bit. The bit time therefore varies with the clock speed.
- **bits per second** Usually contracted to bps. The number of bits transmitted per second.
- **block** A group of transmitted data having a certain general structure which includes checksums, identification codes etc. Data transmitted in this way facilitates error-checking.
- **block length** The length of a data block, usually expressed in bytes.
- **BP** Blood pressure.
- **BPS** Bits per second.
- **BRDH** Baud Rate Divisor High byte. One of the UART registers.
- **BRDL** Baud Rate Divisor Low byte. One of the UART registers.
- **break** A signal sent to the remote device to indicate that it should stop the current operation. The hardware break signal is defined as setting a positive voltage (logic 0) on the RS-232 data line for longer

than the time taken to transmit a single character. Ctrl-C (^C) is the usual internal break signal for PCs.
- **BS** British Standards Institution, London, UK.
- **buffer** A memory area which is used to temporarily store data or information.
- **bug** A defect or error in either software (software bug) or hardware (hardware bug).
- **byte** An ordered group of 8 bits. A byte can therefore be represented by two hexadecimal characters.
- **carriage return** ⟨CR⟩ A control character (ASCII 13), which causes the receiving terminal to move the cursor to the beginning of the line (column 1). The carriage return character is commonly associated with the linefeed character ⟨LF⟩.
- **CCITT** Comité Consultatif International Télégraphique et Téléphonique. A standards organisation based in Geneva.
- **CENELEC** Comité Européen de Normalisation Electrotechnique (European Committee for Electro-technical Standardisation).
- **checksum** An error-checking device used in data communications.
- **chip** An integrated circuit.
- **CMOS** Complementary Metal-Oxide Semiconductor. CMOS chips have a low power consumption and a wide operating supply voltage range (+3V to +18V). CMOS chips are therefore ideal for battery-powered devices.
- **CO_2** Carbon dioxide.
- **COM port** The term used to refer to a serial communications port. Thus COM1 refers to the first serial communications port.
- **compiler** A program which converts a high-level language program (the source code) into the machine code used by the computer.
- **control character** Name for certain ASCII characters (ASCII 0–31) which have control functions. For example, carriage return ⟨CR⟩ and linefeed ⟨LF⟩ are control characters.
- **CPAP** Continuous Positive Airway Pressure.
- **CRC** Cyclic Redundancy Check. A form of error checking used in data communications.
- **CTS** Clear To Send. One of the communication channels of the serial port.
- **data bits** The bits which code for an ASCII character.
- **DC1, DC2, DC3, DC4** Device control characters (ASCII 17–20). See Appendix 1 for details.

- **DCD** Data Carrier Detect. One of the communication channels of the serial port.
- **DCE** Data Communications Equipment. A Standards term for devices like modems and monitors which process data at the end of a communications channel.
- **digital signal** A signal which can take one of only two states, either on or off, 1 or 0.
- **DIP** Dual In-line Pins. DIP switches are small switches mounted on a device having two rows of pins designed to fit into a circuit board.
- **DMA** Direct Memory Access. Relates to access to memory areas without involving the microprocessor.
- **DOS** Disk Operating System.
- **DSR** Data Set Ready. One of the communication channels of the serial port.
- **DTE** Data Terminal Equipment. A Standards term for devices like a computer which can output digital data.
- **DTR** Data Terminal Ready. One of the communication channels of the serial port.
- **EBCDIC** Extended Binary Coded Decimal Interchange Code. An 8-bit code used mainly by large computers.
- **ECG** Electrocardiogram.
- **EIA** Electronic Industries Association.
- **EISA** Extended Industry Standard Architecture. The term EISA indicates compatibility with 32-bit data handling.
- **EOF** The End-Of-File marker
- **EOR** The logical operation Exclusive OR. The equivalent command in QuickBASIC is XOR.
- **EPROM** Erasable Programmable Read-Only Memory. Non-volatile memory chips which are programmed after manufacture.
- **escape** A control character (ASCII 27) used to indicate that the letters or codes following it have a special meaning.
- **EtAA** End-tidal concentration of an anaesthetic agent.
- **EtCO$_2$** End-tidal carbon dioxide concentration.
- **EtN$_2$O** End-tidal nitrous oxide concentration.
- **EtO$_2$** End-tidal oxygen concentration.
- **FCR** FIFO Control Register. One of the UART registers.
- **FiAA** Fractional inspired concentration of an anaesthetic agent.
- **FiCO$_2$** Fractional inspired carbon dioxide concentration.
- **FIFO** First In First Out. FIFO buffers hold data in a queue such that the data enters and leaves the buffer in the same order.

- **file** A body of data having a specific format, usually stored on a disk. For example, ASCII file or binary file.
- **FiN$_2$O** Fractional inspired nitrous oxide concentration.
- **FiO$_2$** Fractional inspired oxygen concentration.
- **framing bits** These are the bits (start, stop, parity) which enclose the data bits, and together with the data bits constitute the data frame, or character frame.
- **freeware** Often applied to programs or utilities which can be used without payment *and* where the author retains the copyright.
- **ftp** File Transfer Protocol. A system of transferring files from one computer to another.
- **full-duplex** A system which allows communication in both directions at the same time.
- **FVC** Forced Vital Capacity. The maximum volume of air which can be breathed out in a single breath when executed as fast as possible.
- **half-duplex** A system which allows communication in both directions, but only in one direction at a time.
- **handshaking** The system by which computers and peripheral devices communicate with one another. There are both software and hardware methods of handshaking.
- **hex** Hexadecimal. This is a base-16 code used by computers. The characters 0–9, A–F are used to represent the numbers 0–15. For example, the decimal number 12 is represented in hexadecimal notation as the letter C.
- **high byte** The most significant 8 bits of a 2-byte group, i.e. bits 8–15.
- **HR** Heart Rate.
- **IC** Integrated Circuit.
- **IEC** International Electrotechnical Commission (3, rue de Varembe, Geneva, Switzerland).
- **IEEE** Institute of Electrical and Electronics Engineers.
- **IER** Interrupt Enable Register. One of the UART registers.
- **IIR** Interrupt Identification Register. One of the UART registers.
- **I/O** Input / Output.
- **IPPV** Intermittent Positive Pressure Ventilation.
- **ISO** International Organisation for Standardisation.
- **Kermit** A popular and very reliable, albeit slow, file transfer protocol, which allows data to be transferred between computers.
- **kilobyte** A unit of memory size, equivalent to 1024 bytes (= 2^{10}). Kilobyte is often abbreviated to KB or Kb.
- **LCR** Line Control Register. One of the UART registers.

- **LED** Light Emitting Diode. Small low current lights which are commonly used to indicate that a circuit is active. Often used to indicate which RS-232 circuits are active.
- **line feed** ⟨LF⟩ A control character (ASCII 10) which makes the computer or printer move the cursor to the next line. This control character is commonly associated with the carriage return character ⟨CR⟩.
- **log** A record of what has happened. A log-file is a file in which the computer writes details of its actions during the running of a program.
- **low byte** The least significant 8 bits of a 2-byte group, i.e. bits 0–7.
- **LPT** Line Printer. Thus LPT1, LPT2 are the names used by MS-DOS for the first and second parallel printer ports.
- **LSB** Least Significant Bit. The rightmost bit of a binary number.
- **LSR** Line Status Register. One of the UART registers.
- **mask** A binary number used in combination with logical operators (AND, OR, XOR) to alter individual bits of another binary number.
- **MB** Megabyte. 1048576 bytes ($= 2^{20}$).
- **MCR** Modem Control Register. One of the UART registers.
- **MMV** Mandatory Minute Volume.
- **modem** Contraction of MOdulator/DEModulator. A communications device which allows computer output to be relayed down telephone lines.
- **modulo** An operation which determines the remainder of a division. Thus, 10 (*modulo* 3) = 1 since 10 divided by 3 leaves the remainder 1. Modulo is often shortened to 'mod', for example, 300(*mod* 128)= 44.
- **ms** Millisecond.
- **MSB** Most Significant Bit. The leftmost bit of a binary number.
- **MS-DOS** Microsoft Disk Operating System.
- **MSR** Modem Status Register. One of the UART registers.
- **MV** Minute Volume. The volume of a gas mixture breathed per minute.
- **N_2O** Nitrous oxide.
- **NAK** A control character (ASCII 21) which is transmitted to indicate that data was received incorrectly. NAK stands for Negative AcKnowledge.
- **nibble** An ordered group of 4 bits. A nibble can therefore be represented by a single hexadecimal character.
- **NIBP** Non-Invasive Blood Pressure measurement.
- **NOT** A logical operation making the output have the reverse logical state to the input. Thus 1 = NOT 0.

- **null modem** A cable connecting two computers, which is wired in such a way as to allow the two computers to communicate with one another *without* the need for a modem.
- **O_2** Oxygen.
- **OR** A logical operation making the output have logic 1 if *any* of the inputs has logic 1.
- **OS/2** A protected-mode multitasking operating-system.
- **parity** A simple error-checking technique, whereby an additional parity bit is added to the data bits in order to make the total number of 1 bits conform to a common system, for example adding up to either an odd number (Odd parity), or an even number (Even parity). Other common parity systems are Mark and Space parity, where the parity bit is always set to either 0 (Space parity) or 1 (Mark parity). The parity bit is often not used at all (parity None).
- **PEEP** Positive End-Expiratory Pressure.
- **PEF** Peak Expiratory Flow rate.
- **PIA** Peripheral Interface Adapter. A chip incorporating all the circuitry to interface a port to the microprocessor.
- **port** The interface between the computer and the peripheral device. The serial and parallel ports are examples of digital ports.
- **protocol** The conditions to be adhered to in order for communications to proceed. For example, the serial protocol specifies a certain bit rate, parity system, number of stop-bits and start-bits.
- **public domain** Often applied to programs or utilities which can be used without payment *and* where the author does not retain the copyright.
- **RAM** Random Access Memory.
- **raw data** Unprocessed data—exactly as it was collected by the computer.
- **RDR** Received Data Register. One of the UART registers.
- **register** An area of memory holding a relatively small number of bytes. Individual bytes in a register are usually referred to by their offset from the first byte in the register.
- **ROM** Read Only Memory.
- **RR** Respiratory Rate.
- **RS-232** Recommended Standard No. 232. A standard for serial interfaces established in 1960. The latest revision (July 1991) is termed EIA/TIA-232-E.
- **RTS** Ready To Send. One of the communication channels of the serial port.

- **RxD** Receive data line. One of the communication channels of the serial port.
- **SaO$_2$** Oxygen saturation of arterial blood.
- **serial communication** A system of communication between computers and devices, in which information is transferred one bit at a time.
- **serial port** A communications port which transfers information one bit at a time.
- **start-bit** The first bit of a character-frame. It is used to indicate the start of a character in asynchronous serial communications.
- **stop-bit** The last bit of a character-frame. It is used to indicate the end of a character in asynchronous serial communications. Sometimes two stop-bits are used.
- **THR** Transmitter Holding Register. One of the UART registers.
- **TIA** Telecommunications Industry Association.
- **time-stamp** A note of the current time (and sometimes date) saved with data.
- **Trend data** Sequential data stored over a period of time. Usually refers to data measured by a device over 8–24 hours and temporarily stored in its memory. The data is downloaded to a PC at a later time.
- **TTL** Transistor-Transistor Logic. TTL chips operate within the voltage range 0–5 volts, and have a relatively high power consumption, when compared to CMOS chips.
- **TV** Tidal Volume. The volume of a gas mixture breathed in a single breath.
- **TxD** Transmit data line. One of the communication channels of the serial port.
- **UART** Universal Asynchronous Receiver/Transmitter. The term UART has become a generic term for any chip which controls the interface between the microprocessor and the serial port. There is a wide variety of UARTs, all with slightly different capabilities.
- **V(1.0)** Volume of air breathed out during the first second of expiration.
- **VC** Vital Capacity. The maximum volume of air which can be breathed in or out in a single breath.
- **word** A group of bits used for storing data. For example, different computer systems may use an 8-bit word (a byte), or 16-bit word (two bytes).
- **Xmodem** An early file-transfer protocol invented by Ward Christensen.
- **XON/XOFF** A software handshaking system.

- **XOR** The logical operation Exclusive OR. QuickBASIC uses the code XOR for Exclusive OR.
- **XT** A term applied to a PC which handles 8-bit data.
- **Ymodem** An improved version of Xmodem, incorporating CRC error checking.
- **Zmodem** A fast and popular file-transfer protocol for PCs, which is very reliable owing to the advanced error checking technique that it employs.

References

Aitken, P. G. (1992). *Essential guide to MS-DOS 5 programming.* (Microsoft Press, Richmond, Washington, USA). [See chapters on 'Serial and parallel ports', pp. 311–335; 'The keyboard', pp. 41–81.]

Alford, R. C. (1992). How interrupts work. *Byte*, February, 249–256.

Al-Shaikh, B. (1991). Effect of inspired oxygen concentration on the incidence of desaturation in patients undergoing total hip replacement. *British Journal of Anaesthesia*, **66**, 580–582.

American Thoracic Society (1987). Standardization of spirometry—1987 update. *American Review of Respiratory Disease*, **136**, 1285–1298.

ANSI X3.32. (1973). *American national standard graphic representation of the control characters of American National Standard Code for Information Interchange.* (American National Standards Institute, New York, USA).

ANSI X3.41. (1974). *Code extension techniques for use with the 7-bit coded character set of American National Standard Code for Information Interchange.* (American National Standards Institute, New York, USA).

ANSI X3.28. (1976). *Procedures for the use of the communication control characters of American National Standard Code for Information Interchange in specified data communication links.* (American National Standards Institute, New York, USA).

ANSI X3.4. (1986). *Coded character sets: 7-bit American National Standard Code for Information Interchange (7-bit ASCII).* (American National Standards Institute, New York, USA).

Appleby, D. (1992). Classic languages, part 6: BASIC. *Byte*, March, 155–158.

Appleman, D. (1993). *Visual Basic programmer's guide to the Windows API.* (Ziff-Davis Press, Emeryville, California, USA).

Avent, R. K. & Charlton, J. D. (1990). A critical review of trend-detection methodologies for biomedical monitoring systems. *Critical reviews in Biomedical Engineering*, **17**, 621–659.

Banks, M. A. (1990). *The modem reference.* (Simon & Schuster, New York, USA).

Baran, N. (1991). Data acquisition: PCs on the bench. *Byte*, May, 145–149.

Beard, N. (1992). Visualisation. *Personal Computer World*, Part I, Inner vision, November, 380–384; Part II, Tunnel vision, December, 374–382; Part III, Filling a tool bag, January 1993, 350–374; Part IV, Art for art's sake, February 1993, 350–354. [Articles on visualising data]

Beard, N. (1993). Software for scientists. *Personal Computer World*, Part I, The

art and craft of good science, June, 350–354; Part II, Soft options, July, 280–292. [Articles on mathematical and statistical software]
Bedford, M. (1991). Breakfast serial. *Computer Shopper*, Part I, June, 229–233; Part II, July, 273–278. [Articles on serial interfacing]
Bedford, M. (1992a). Under control. *Computer Shopper*, Part I, December 1992, 364–372; Part II, January 1993, 368–376. [Articles on interfacing]
Bedford, M. (1992b). Scientific computing. *Computer Shopper*, Part I, June, 323–331 [scientific text processors]; Part II, July, 358–364 [maths packages].
Bedford, M. (1993a). Only make believe. *Computer Shopper*, August, 378–386; September, 362–372; October, 406–415. [Articles on computer modelling and simulation]
Bedford, M. (1993b). Winning formulae. *Computer Shopper*, May, 372–381. [Article on mathematical text processors]
Beydon, L., Hassapopoulos, J., Quera, M. A., Rauss, A., Becquemin, J. P., Bonnet, F., Harf, A. & Goldenberg, F. (1992). Risk factors for oxygen desaturation during sleep, after abdominal surgery. *British Journal of Anaesthesia*, **69**, 137-142.
Beynon, R. J. (1984). Communicating with microcomputers. In *Microcomputers in biology: a practical approach*, eds. C. R. Ireland and S. P. Long, pp. 17–42. (IRL Press, Oxford, UK).
Brown, R. & Kyle, J. (1991). *PC Interrupts—a programmer's reference to BIOS, DOS, and third-party calls.* (Addison-Wesley Publishing Company Inc., New York, USA).
Campbell, J. (1989a). *The RS-232 solution: how to use your serial port*, 2nd edn. (Sybex Inc., Alameda, California, USA).
Campbell, J. (1989b). *C programmer's guide to serial communications.* (Howard W. Sams & Company, Carmel, Indiana, USA).
Carr, J. J. (1991). *Microcomputer interfacing: a practical guide for technicians, engineers and scientists.* (Prentice-Hall Inc., London, UK).
Chaput de Saintonge, D. M. & Carter, D. W. (1974). Why don't doctors use CUSUMs ? *Lancet*, **i**, 120-121.
Chatfield, C. (1975). *Time series.* (Chapman and Hall Ltd., London, UK).
Church, J. A., Stanton, P. D., Kenny, G. N. C. & Anderson, J. R. (1991). Propofol for sedation during endoscopy: assessment of a computer-controlled infusion system. *Gastrointestinal Endoscopy*, **37**, 175–179.
Collin, S. (1992). Activating the 16550A UART for quicker comms. *PC Magazine*, **1**, June, 250–251.
Crawford, M., Pollock, J., Anderson, K., Glavin, R. J., Macintyre, D. & Vernon, D. (1993). Comparison of midazolam with propofol for sedation in outpatient bronchoscopy. *British Journal of Anaesthesia*, **70**, 419–422.
Cripps, M. (1989). *Computer interfacing: connection to the real world.* (Edward Arnold, London, UK).
Cullimore, I. (1987). *Communicating with microcomputers.* (Sigma Press, Wilmslow, UK).
D'Hulster, D., Dardenne, G., Evrards, A. M., Fritschke, J. M., Henin, J. C., Lavergne, L., Lippens, R., Mourisse, P., Naud, J. L., Nihoul, J. Parys, T. & Wellemans, W. M. (1991). Induction of anaesthesia with an infusion of propofol using the Ohmeda 9000 syringe driver. In *Focus on infusion: intravenous anaesthesia*, ed. C. Prys-Roberts, pp. 97–100. (Current Medical Literature Ltd., London, UK).

References

Da Cruz, F. (1987). *Kermit: a file transfer protocol.* (Digital Press, Bedford, MA, USA).

Dettmann, T. R. (1989). *DOS programmer's reference*, 2nd edn. (Que Corporation, Carmel, Indiana, USA).

Dottrens, M., Rifat, K. & Morel, D. R. (1992). Comparison of extradural administration of sufentanil, morphine and sufentanil-morphine combination after caesarean section. *British Journal of Anaesthesia*, **69**, 9–12.

Dougherty, D. (1990). *Sed and awk.* (O'Reilly and Associates Inc., Sebastopol, California, USA).

Duncan, R. (1988). *The MS-DOS encyclopedia.* (Microsoft Press, Richmond, Washington, USA).

Duncan, R. (1989). *Advanced OS/2 programming.* (Microsoft Press, Richmond, Washington, USA).

Dvorak, J. C. & Anis, N. (1992). *Dvorak's guide to PC telecommunications*, 2nd edn. (McGraw-Hill Publishing Company, New York, USA).

Eggebrecht, L. C., (1990). *Interfacing to the IBM personal computer*, 2nd edn. (Sams publishing, Carmel, Indiana, USA).

Endresen, J. & Hill, D. W. (1977). The present state of trend detection and prediction in patient monitoring. *Intensive Care Medicine*, **3**, 15–26.

Entwistle, M. D., Roe, P. G., Sapsford, D. J., Berrisford, R. G. & Jones, J. G. (1991). Patterns of oxygenation after thoracotomy. *British Journal of Anaesthesia*, **67**, 704–711.

Evans, R. J., Wilhoit, S. C. & Suratt, P. M. (1984). A microcomputer system for monitoring and analysing oxyhaemoglobin saturation during sleep. *Computer Methods and Programs in Biomedicine*, **18**, 227–234.

Freedman, A. M., Buneman, O. P., Peckham, G. & Trattner, A. (1979). Automatic recognition of significant events in the vital signs of neonatal infants. *Computers and Biomedical Research*, **12**, 141–148.

Friend, G. E., Fike, J. L., Baker, H. C. & Bellamy, J. C., (1988). *Understanding data communications*, 2nd edn. (Howard W. Sams & Co., Indianapolis, USA).

Genois, M. (1992). CHK_UART.COM *version 1.0. A utility to check the UART used by the serial port.* CompuServe, IBMCOM forum, library 7 (search for UART.ZIP).

Gershon, N. & Dozier, J. (1993). The difficulty with data. *Byte*, April, 143-146.

Gianone, C. M. (1992). *Using MS-DOS Kermit*, 2nd edn. (Digital Press, Bedford, MA, USA).

Gianone, C., da Cruz, F. & Doupnik, J. R. (1988). *MS-DOS Kermit user guide for the IBM PC family, compatibles and other MS-DOS systems; version 2.32.* (Trustees of Columbia University, New York, USA).

Gill, N. P., Wright, B. & Reilly, C. S. (1992). Relationship between hypoxaemia and cardiac ischaemic events in the perioperative period. *British Journal of Anaesthesia*, **68**, 471–473.

Godfrey, K. (1985). Simple linear regression in medical research. *New England Journal of Medicine*, **313**, 1629–1636.

Gofton, P. W. (1986). *Mastering serial communications.* (Sybex Inc., Alameda, California, USA).

Goodwin, M. (1992). *Serial communications in C and C++.* (MIS Press, New York, USA).

Halsal, F. (1992). *Data communications, computer networks, and open systems.* (Addison-Wesley Publishing Company Inc., New York, USA).

Harrison, P. J. & Stevens, C. F. (1976). Bayesian forecasting. *Journal of the Royal Statistical Society*, Series B, **38**, 205–247.

Harvey, G. & Nelson, K. Y. (1990). *Encyclopaedia WordPerfect 5.1.* (Sybex Inc., Alameda, California, USA).

Haynes, S. R., Allsop, J. R. & Gillies, G. W. A. (1992). Arterial oxygen saturation during induction of anaesthesia and laryngeal mask insertion: prospective evaluation of four techniques. *British Journal of Anaesthesia*, **68**, 519–522.

Hogan, T. (1991). *The programmer's PC source book: reference tables for IBM PCs and compatibles, PS/2 systems, EISA-based systems, MS-DOS operating system through version 5, Microsoft Windows through version 3*, 2nd edn. (Microsoft Press, Richmond, Washington, USA).

Honig, D. A. & Hoover, K. A. (1990). *Desktop communications: IBM PC, PS/2, and compatibles.* (John Wiley & Sons, Inc., New York, USA).

Hoskins, J. (1990). *IBM PS/2: A business perspective.* (John Wiley & Sons Inc., New York, USA).

Hughes, L. E. (1989). *A practical guide to RS-232 interfacing.* E390 (e390RS232.boo), National Public Domain Software Library, Lancaster University, England, UK.

Jackson, P. (1992). File transfer protocols: how to achieve speed and data integrity. *PC Magazine*, **1**, June, 286–287.

Jones, J. G., Bembridge, J. L., Sapsford, D. J. & Turney, J. H. (1992). Continuous measurements of oxygen saturation during haemodialysis. *Nephrology, Dialysis, Transplantation*, **7**, 110–116.

Kenny, G. N. C. (1991). Computer controlled infusion of propofol. In *Focus on infusion: intravenous anaesthesia*, ed. C. Prys-Roberts, pp. 91–93. (Current Medical Literature Ltd., London, UK).

Kenny, G. N. C. & White, M. (1990). A portable computerized infusion system for Propofol. *Anaesthesia*, **45**, 692–693.

Kenny, G. N. C. & White, M. (1992). A portable target controlled propofol infusion system. *International Journal of Clinical Monitoring and Computing*, **9**, 179–182.

Knapp, M. S., Gordon, K. & Smith, A. F. M. (1986). The Kalman filter for monitoring clinical problems. (Abstract). *International Journal of Clinical Monitoring and Computing*, **3**, 47.

Lanigan, C. J. (1992). Oxygen desaturation after dental anaesthesia. *British Journal of Anaesthesia*, **68**, 142–145.

Livingstone, B. & Livingstone, M. (1993). *Windows gizmos.* (IDG Books, Worldwide Inc., USA). [See section on the RS-232 serial monitor.]

Madej, T. H., Wheatley, R. G., Jackson, I. J. B. & Hunter, D. (1992). Hypoxaemia and pain relief after lower abdominal surgery: comparison of extradural and patient-controlled analgesia. *British Journal of Anaesthesia*, **69**, 554–557.

Maine, A. C. (1986). *International standards for computers.* (IEEIE, London, UK).

Margolis, A. (1989). The thinking programmer's guide to UARTs. *.EXE Magazine*, December, 18–24.

Margolis, A. (1990). If I may interrupt? *.EXE Magazine*, March, 24–30. [Article on interrupt-driven serial communications]

Marjot, R. & Valentine, S. J. (1990). Arterial oxygen saturation following premedication for cardiac surgery. *British Journal of Anaesthesia*, **64**, 737–740.

Marsh, B. J., Morton, N. S., White, M. & Kenny, G. N. C. (1990). A computer controlled infusion of Propofol for induction and maintenance of anaesthesia in children. *Canadian Journal of Anaesthesia*, **37**, S97.

McCarthy, J. P. & Potter, R. (1985). Connecting Computers to Medical Equipment. *The HPA Bulletin*, June, 34.

Microsoft, (1988). *Microsoft QuickBASIC language reference (version 4.5) for IBM personal computers and compatibles.* (Microsoft Corporation, USA).

Microsoft, (1989a). *Communications 'Device timeout': increase CS and DS time limit.* Document No. Q31432, (Microsoft Corporation, USA).

Microsoft, (1989b). *'Device unavailable'; PS/2 SETUP doesn't recognise COM2 port.* Document No. Q43895, (Microsoft Corporation, USA).

Microsoft, (1989c). *QuickBASIC program to send a BREAK through COM1 port.* Document No. Q43746, (Microsoft Corporation, USA).

Microsoft, (1989d). *How to pipe input into a QuickBASIC program.* Document No. Q46376, (Microsoft Corporation, USA).

Microsoft, (1989e). *Must use A$=INKEY$ after SLEEP to clear keyboard buffer.* Document No. Q36397, (Microsoft Corporation, USA).

Microsoft, (1989f). *List of run-time error numbers and messages for QuickBASIC.* Document No. Q47753, (Microsoft Corporation, USA).

Microsoft, (1989g). *Numerical calculations and loops are faster with integers.* Document No. Q36901, (Microsoft Corporation, USA).

Microsoft, (1989h). *How to calculate absolute address; DEF SEG and PEEK examples.* Document No. Q41531, (Microsoft Corporation, USA).

Microsoft, (1990a). *How to solve common QuickBASIC communication port problems.* Document No. Q39342, (Microsoft Corporation, USA).

Microsoft, (1990b). *Description of serial port transmission and break signals.* Document No. Q63597, (Microsoft Corporation, USA).

Microsoft, (1990c). *Toggling DTR handshaking line (pin 20) with OUT statement.* Document No. Q37093, (Microsoft Corporation, USA).

Microsoft, (1990d). *Explanation of why BASIC programs can open devices as files.* Document No. Q65935, (Microsoft Corporation, USA).

Microsoft, (1990e). *How to use CALL INTERRUPT to diagnose COM device I/O error.* Document No. Q67315, (Microsoft Corporation, USA).

Microsoft, (1990f). *Error message explanations when using COM1 and COM2.* Document No. Q39386, (Microsoft Corporation, USA).

Microsoft, (1990g). *SHELL statement loses current data in serial port input buffer.* Document No. Q37417, (Microsoft Corporation, USA).

Microsoft, (1990h). *ON KEY key trap with INKEY$: loop requires additional key presses.* Document No. Q64785, (Microsoft Corporation, USA).

Microsoft, (1990i). *PE option in OPEN COM statement enables parity checking.* Document No. Q51076, (Microsoft Corporation, USA).

Microsoft, (1991a). *XON/XOFF communication protocol not supported in QuickBASIC.* Document No. Q22019, (Microsoft Corporation, USA).

Microsoft, (1991b). *MSJ TSRCOMM: a replacement for Interrupt 14.* Document No. Q42119, (Microsoft Corporation, USA).

Microsoft, (1991c). *How to calculate a segmented executable checksum value.* Document No. Q71971, (Microsoft Corporation, USA).

Microsoft, (1991d). *COM1 - COM4 may be accessed from BASIC through DOS service.* Document No. Q76742, (Microsoft Corporation, USA).
Microsoft, (1991e). *Answers to common questions about QuickBASIC 4.5.* Document No. Q58531, (Microsoft Corporation, USA).
Microsoft, (1991f). *No EOF (CTRL Z) marker written at end of sequential file.* Document No. Q25996, (Microsoft Corporation, USA).
Microsoft, (1992a). *Finding the COM1 serial port on PC/XT/AT and PS/2 machines.* Document No. Q44126, (Microsoft Corporation, USA).
Microsoft, (1992b). *Toggling RTS handshaking line (pin 4) with OUT statement.* Document No. Q79957, (Microsoft Corporation, USA).
Microsoft, (1992c). *Why BASIC doesn't support COM3 or COM4 serial port.* Document No. Q21789, (Microsoft Corporation, USA).
Microsoft, (1992d). *'Input past End of File' with INPUT#; use LINE INPUT#.* Document No. Q82001, (Microsoft Corporation, USA).
Mitchell, P. (1988). *Control applications of microcomputers.* (Edward Arnold, London, UK).
Moller, J. T., Johannessen, N. W., Berg, H., Espersen, K. & Larsen, L. E. (1991). Hypoxaemia during anaesthesia – an observer study. *British Journal of Anaesthesia,* **66**, 437–444.
Moller, J. T., Jensen, P. F., Johannessen, N. W. & Espersen, K. (1992). Hypoxaemia is reduced by pulse oximetry monitoring in the operating theatre and in the recovery room. *British Journal of Anaesthesia,* **68**, 146–150.
Monk, T. S. (1992). *Windows programmer's guide to serial communications.* (Sams publishing, Carmel, Indiana, USA).
Nameroff, S. (1989). *QuickBASIC: the complete reference.* (Osborne McGraw-Hill, USA).
Nance, B. (1992). Opening the lines of communications: a functional INT 14h replacement to fill the communications gap in PC BIOS services. *Byte,* July, 301.
Nelson, S.B., Reed, M., Gardner, R.M., Crapo, R.O. & Jensen, R.L. (1990). Performance evaluation of contemporary spirometers. *Chest,* **97**, 288–297.
Novisoff, M. (1991). QUIRKS.TXT. CompuServe Microsoft Systems forum (MSSYS).
O'Brien, D. (1992). Serial Killer. *Personal Computer World,* March, 318–322. [Article on the serial port and UARTS]
Oliver, V. (1993). Upgrading your serial port. *PC Direct,* July, 442–444. [Includes a program for detecting 16550 UARTs]
Pasterkamp, H. & Daien, D. (1988). The use of a personal computer for trend analysis with Ohmeda 3700 pulse oximeter. *Journal of Clinical Monitoring,* **4**, 215–222.
Peacock, J. E. (1991). Manual infusion schemes for the spontaneously breathing patient. In *Focus on infusion: intravenous anaesthesia,* ed. C. Prys-Roberts, pp. 82–84. (Current Medical Literature Ltd., London, UK).
Penfold, R. A. (1992). *Interfacing PCs and compatibles.* (Bernard Babini Publications Ltd., London, UK).
Perry, R. (1993). Straight talking. *Computer Shopper,* October, 319–322. [Article on the Null Modem]
Pettitt, A. N. (1979). A non-parametric approach to the change point problem. *Applied Statistics,* **28**, 126–135.
Phoenix (1991). *System Bios for IBM PC's, compatibles, and EISA computers:*

the complete guide to ROM-based System software, 2nd edn, Phoenix Technologies Ltd. (Addison-Wesley Publishing Company Inc., New York, USA).
Pollock, J. S. S. & Kenny G. N. C. (1993). Effects of lorazepam on oxygen saturation before cardiac surgery. *British Journal of Anaesthesia*, **70**, 219–220.
Prosise, J. (1989). PC Lab notes: RS-232 monitoring. *PC Magazine*, April, 128–134. [Describes the LITES utility program for monitoring the serial port]
Ramasubramanian, R., Nickalls, R. W. D. & Reed, M. (1993). ASCII.STY version 1. [computer program] MS-DOS version. Comprehensive TEX Archive Network, Aston University, UK. [Search the CTAN archive (ftp.tex.ac.uk) for the directory /pub/archive/fonts/ascii]
Ramasubramanian, R., Nickalls, R. W. D. & Reed, M. (1994). A new style-option and encoded font with IBM graphics control characters for use with TEX & LATEX. *TUGboat*, **15** (2), June, 98–103.
Reeder, M. K., Muir, A. D., Foex, P., Goldman, M. D., Loh, L. & Smart, D. (1991). Postoperative myocardial ischaemia: temporal association with nocturnal hypoxaemia. *British Journal of Anaesthesia*, **67**, 626–631.
Reeder M. K., Goldman, M. D., Loh, L., Muir, A. D., Foex, P., Casey, K. R. & McKenzie, P. J. (1992). Postoperative hypoxaemia after major abdominal vascular surgery. *British Journal of Anaesthesia*, **68**, 23–26.
Ribarsky, W. (1993). Navigating the data flood. *Byte*, April, 129–135.
Roberts, F. L., Dixon, J., Lewis, G. T. R., Tackley, R. M. & Prys-Roberts, C. (1988). Induction and maintenance of propofol anaesthesia; a manual infusion scheme. *Anaesthesia*, **43**, Supplement, 14–17.
Roget, J. A. & Shield, C. M. (1986). Evaluation of the Vitalograph Compact spirometer. Annual Scientific Meeting, Australasian Society of Respiratory Technology.
Ronald, A. L., Ramayya, G. P. & Chambers, W. A. (1992). Continuous collection of pulse oximetry data: a new, inexpensive, portable computerised method. *British Journal of Anaesthesia*, **69**, 105–107.
Rosenberg, J., Rasmussen, V., von Jessen, F., Ullstad, T. & Kehlet, H. (1990). Late postoperative episodic and constant hypoxaemia and associated ECG abnormalities. *British Journal of Anaesthesia*, **65**, 684–691.
Rosenberg, J., Pedersen, M. H., Gebuhr, P. & Kehlet, H. (1992). Effect of oxygen therapy on late postoperative episodic and constant hypoxaemia. *British Journal of Anaesthesia*, **68**, 18–22.
Sainsbury, D. (1992). *Communicating with the Datex Cardiocap^{TM} II CG-series monitors*. Available from: D. Sainsbury, Department of Anaesthesia, Adelaide Children's Hospital, North Adelaide, South Australia 5006, Australia.
Sainsbury, D. (1993). *Communicating with the Ohmeda 9000 syringe pump.* Available from: D. Sainsbury, Department of Anaesthesia, Adelaide Children's Hospital, North Adelaide, South Australia 5006, Australia.
Schildt, H. (1989). *Born to code in C*. (Osborne McGraw-Hill, USA).
Schwaderer, W. D. (1986). *Modems and communication on IBM PCs*. (John Wiley & Sons Inc., New York, USA).
Schofield, S. (1993). *The PC Plus modem and communications guidebook*. (Future Publishing Ltd., Bath, UK).
Seyer, M. D. (1991). *RS-232 made easy: connecting computers, printers, terminals,*

and modems, 2nd edn. (Prentice-Hall International (UK) Ltd., London, UK).

Shanley, T. (1991). *The IBM PS/2 from the inside out*. (Addison-Wesley Publishing Company Inc., New York, USA).

Sinclair, I. (1990). *PC troubleshooter*. (Sigma Press, Wilmslow, Cheshire, UK).

Skipsey, I. G., Colvin, J. R., Mackenzie, N. & Kenny, G. N. C. (1993). Sedation with propofol during surgery under local blockade: assessment of a target controlled infusion system. *Anaesthesia*, **48**, 210–213.

Slater, E. J. (1985). Electrical Safety. *Intensive Care World*, June, 38–40.

Slutsky, A. S. & Strohl, K. P. (1980). Quantification of oxygen saturation during episodic hypoxemia. *American Review of Respiratory Disease*, **121**, 893–895.

Smith, B. (1993). Data from the depths. *Byte*, July, 69–78.

Starfield, A. M., Smith, K. A. & Bleloch, A. L. (1990). *How to model it: problem solving for the computer age*. (McGraw-Hill Publishing Company, New York, USA).

Stephenson, A. P. (1983). *Computing for the hobbyist and small business*. (Granada Publishing, London, UK).

Stokes, D. N., Peacock, J. E., Lewis, R. & Hutton, P. (1990). The Ohmeda 9000 syringe pump: the first of a new generation of syringe pumps. *Anaesthesia*, **45**, 1062–1066.

Stoodley, K. D. C. & Mirnia, M. (1979). The automatic detection of transients, step changes and slope changes in the monitoring of medical time series. *The Statistician*, **28**, 163–170.

Suresh, D., Purdy, G., Wainwright, A. P. & Flynn, P. J. (1991). Use of continuous positive airway pressure in paediatric dental extraction under general anaesthesia. *British Journal of Anaesthesia*, **66**, 200–204.

Taylor, R. J. (1991). The retrieval, storage, numerical and graphical trending of data from an Ohmeda 3700e pulse oximeter by personal computer. *Clinical Physics and Physiological Measurement*, **12**, 185–189.

Taylor, I., White, M. & Kenny, G. N. C. (1993). Assessment of the value and pattern of use of a target controlled propofol infusion system. *International Journal of Clinical Monitoring and Computing*, **10**, 175–180.

Thompson, B. G. & Kuckles, A. F. (1989). *IBM-PC in the laboratory*. (Cambridge University Press, Cambridge, UK). [See chapter on interrupts, pp. 108–120.]

Tischer, M. (1991). *PC systems programming: an in depth reference for the DOS programmer*. (Abacus, Grand Rapids, MI, USA).

Tooley, M. (1989). *Data communications pocket book*. (Heinemann Newnes, London, UK).

Townsend, J. J. (1992). *Introduction to databases*. (Que Corporation, Carmel, Indiana, USA).

Trimble, I. M., West, M., Knapp, M. S., Pownall, R. & Smith, A. F. M. (1983). Detection of renal allograft rejection by computer. *British Medical Journal*, **286**, 1695–1699.

Tufte, E. R. (1983). *The visual display of quantitative information*. (Graphics Press, Connecticut, USA).

Tukey, J. (1977). *Exploratory Data Analysis*. (Addison-Wesley Publishing Company Inc., New York, USA).

Van Gilluwe, F. (1994). *The undocumented PC: a programmer's guide to I/O, CPUs, and fixed memory areas*. (Addison-Wesley Publishing Company Inc.,

References

New York, USA). [see the excellent chapter entitled 'Serial ports', p. 563–615]

Vears, R. (1990). *Microprocessor interfacing.* (Heinemann Newnes, London, UK).

Waite, M., Arnson, R., Gemmell, C. & Henderson, H. (1990). *The Waite Group's Microsoft QuickBASIC bible.* (Microsoft Press, Richmond, Washington, USA).

Wayner, P. (1993). Image building. *Byte*, April, 137–141.

Weber, J. (1993). Visualisation: seeing is believing. *Byte*, April, 121–128.

Wheatley, R. G., Somerville, I. D., Sapsford, D. J. & Jones, J. G. (1990). Postoperative hypoxaemia: comparison of extradural, i.m. and patient-controlled opioid analgesia. *British Journal of Anaesthesia*, **64**, 267–275.

Wheatley, R. G., Shepherd, D., Jackson, I. J. B., Madej, T. H. & Hunter, D. (1992). Hypoxaemia and pain relief after upper abdominal surgery: comparison of i.m and patient-controlled analgesia. *British Journal of Anaesthesia*, **69**, 558–561.

Wideman, G. (1986). *Computer connection mysteries solved.* (Howard W. Sams & Co., Indianapolis, USA).

Wohl, H. (1977). The CUSUM plot: its utility in the analysis of clinical data. *New England Journal of Medicine*, **296**, 1044–1045.

Wyatt, A. L. (1990). *Using assembly language*, 2nd edn. (Que Corporation, Carmel, Indiana, USA).

Index

8250, 25
16450, 25
16C1450, 33
16550, 25
  FIFO buffers, 26
16C1550, 33
82510, 26

ACIA, 25
ACK control character, 19, 20, 345
analysis of pulse oximetry data, 102
AND, 73, 75, 76, 78, 79
  logic table, 76
& prefix, 73
&H prefix, 73
ANSI Standards, 3
applied parts, 89
ARQ protocol, 19, 20
ASC option, 48, 365
ASCII, 12
  ASC option, 48, 365
  classification of control characters, 343
  description of control characters, 344
  table of control characters, 341
  table of graphic characters, 342
asynchronous transmission, 13
autocorrelation, 99

baud, 14
baud rate divisor, 28, 31, 34
  diagram of low & high registers, 40
  high byte, 28, 31, 34
  low byte, 28, 31, 34
  table of, 28
Baudot code, 12
Baudot, Jean Maurice Emile, 14
BEL control character, 345
BIN option, 365
binary notation, 373
bit, 12

bit-encoded registers, 31
bit-mapped registers, 31
bit-mask, 74–76, 78, 79
bit-rate, 14
  and ON COM statement, 46
break, 34, 42
  and line control register, 34
  and line status register, 36
  break interrupt, 36
BS control character, 345
buffer
  buffer overflow error, 69
  emptying the receive buffer, 64
  FIFO, 26
  RB option, 48, 366
  TB option, 48, 367
byte, 12

cable length for RS-232, 11
CAN control character, 346
capacitance of RS-232 cable, 11
Capnomac Ultima series, 176
Cardiocap series, 176
category AP equipment, 94
category APG equipment, 94
CD option, 47, 366
character interface, 3
character-frame, 13
  diagram of, 14
chassis ground, 7
checksum, 21
  7-bit, 22, 72
  8-bit, 22, 71
  CHECKSUMHEX$ function, 71
  cyclic redundancy check, 18, 21, 24
  HEX$, 71
  hexadecimal, 71
  *modulo*128, 22, 72
  *modulo*256, 22, 71
  Σ-checksum, 22, 71

396   *Index*

Graseby 3400 pump, 220
Nellcor N-200E, 138
QuickBASIC programs for, 71
TC-checksum, 22, 23, 72
Ohmeda 7800 ventilator, 304
Ohmeda 9000 pump, 249
two's complement, 22, 23, 72, 249, 304
TWOSCHECKSUM$ function, 72
CHECKSUMHEX$ function, 71
circuits
  control, 7, 8
  data, 7, 8
  diagram of RS-232 circuits, 8
  ground, 7, 8
  input, 8
  output, 8
class I electrical equipment, 91
class II electrical equipment, 91
clear to send, *see* CTS
clock
  master clock, 28
  receive clock, 16
  reference clock, 28
  resident clock, 17
  table of baud rate divisors, 28
code extension control characters, 343
COLLECT.EXE, 177
COM port, 25
COMMANDER program, 112
Compact II spirometer, 272
compressed spectral array plot, 102, 105
connectors, 9
  pin-outs for 9-pin connectors, 6, 349
  pin-outs for 25/26-pin connectors, 6, 348
control characters
  code extension characters, 343
  device control characters, 343
  format effectors, 343
  information separators, 344
  transmission control characters, 343
control circuits, 7, 8
  monitoring input control lines, 78
  setting output control lines, 72
  testing for line status, 80
CR control character, 345
CRC, *see* cyclic redundancy check
CS option, 47, 50, 366
CTS, 8, 9
  and data output, 50
  and device time-out error, 69
  and modem status register, 35
  CS option, 47, 50, 366
  monitoring CTS status, 78
  set HIGH to enable data output, 41
  time-out parameter, 42
cumulative distribution plot, 102, 104
cumulative sum test (CUSUM), 99

cyclic redundancy check (CRC), 18, 21, 24

DART, 25
data analysis, 98
data bits, 13–15, 34
  and line control register, 34
  and ON COM statement, 46
data carrier detect, *see* DCD
data circuits, 7, 8
data file
  opening a data file, 56
  SHOW.COM, 65
  VIEW.EXE, 65
  viewing a data file, 65
data frame, 13
  diagram of, 14
data packet, 21
data set request, *see* DSR
data transmission, 12
  asynchronous, 13
  enchronous, 13
  isochronous, 13
  synchronous, 13
data transmit ready, *see* DTR
data visualisation, 99
database packages, 100
DATE$, 57
Datex anaesthesia monitors, 176
  COLLECT.EXE, 177
DC1 control character, 20, 345
DC2 control character, 345
DC3 control character, 20, 346
DC4 control character, 346
DCD, 8, 9
  and device time-out error, 69
  and modem status register, 35
  CD option, 47, 366
  monitoring DCD status, 78
DEL control character, 347
descriptive procedures, 98
device control characters, 343
DLAB, 27, 31, 34
  and line control register, 34
DLE control character, 345
double insulation, 91, 92
Dräger Evita ventilator, 313
DS option, 47, 366
DSR, 8, 9
  and device time-out error, 69
  and modem status register, 35
  DS option, 47, 366
  monitoring DSR status, 78
  set HIGH to enable data input, 42
  time-out parameter, 42
DTR, 8, 77
  and modem control register, 33, 72
  control line subroutine SETDTR, 77

Index

programming the DTR status, 72
serial port on/off status, 41
SETDTR subroutine, 77

earthing, 91
EBCDIC code, 12
edge sensitive
 Capnomac Ultima CTS, 181
 modem status register bit-2 (RI), 35
EIA, *see* Electronic Industries Association
EIA Standards, 3
ELAPSEDTIME$ function, 66
electrical safety, 88
 and the PC, 88
 applied parts
  table of, 94
  types, 93
 category AP equipment, 94
 category APG equipment, 94
 caution with type B equipment, 96
 class I equipment, 91
 class II equipment, 91
 definitions
  applied parts, 89
  medical electrical equipment, 89
  patient circuit, 90
  patient connection, 89
  patient environment, 90
 double insulation, 91, 92
 F-type isolation, 92
 general aspects, 90
 general precautions, 95
 guidelines for safe use of PCs, 97
 isolating transformer, 88, 96
 isolation circuits, 92
 leakage current, 92, 95
 single fault condition, 90
 Standards, 88
 table of applied part types, 94
 type B equipment, 93, 96
 type BF equipment, 93
 type CF equipment, 93
Electronic Industries Association, 3
EM control character, 346
EMPTYBUFFER subroutine, 65
ENQ control character, 344
EOR 77, *see also* XOR
EOT control character, 344
ERDEV, 68
ERDEV$, 68
ERR, 68
errors
 and line status register, 36
 buffer overflow error, 69
 error messages, 69
 error trapping, 68
 framing error, 36, 69

overrun error, 36, 69
parity error, 36, 69
time-out error, 36, 42
ESC control character, 346
escape sequence, 19
ETB control character, 346
ETX control character, 19–21, 344
Evans *et al.* oximetry program, 103
Evita ventilator, 313
exclusive OR, *see* XOR
exit routine, 70
exploratory data analysis, 98
extended keys, 70

F-type isolation, 92
FCR, *see* FIFO control register
FF control character, 345
FIFO buffer, 26
FIFO control register, 27, 39
file viewing utilities, 65
flow control, 18
format effectors, 343
frame, 13
 diagram of, 14
framing error, 17, 36
 and device I/O error, 69
 and line status register, 36
frequency distribution plot, 102, 104
FS control character, 347
FULLCODE subroutine, 52, 57, 58, 280

GETREPLY subroutine, 63, 64
glossary, 375
GND, 7, 8
GNUPLOT, 369
graphics packages, 101
Graseby 3400 syringe pump, 211
 Σ-checksum, 220
ground
 chassis ground, 7
 circuits, 7
 errors with differences in potential, 11
 shield, 7
 signal ground, 7, 8
GS control character, 21, 347
guidelines for safe use of PCs, 97

H prefix, 73
handshaking, 18
 hardware, 18
 software, 19
hardware break, *see* break
hardware handshaking, 18
HEX$, 71
hexadecimal notation, 374
HT control character, 345

Index

I/O control by PC, 41
  break signal, 42
  role of DSR, 42
  role of DTR, 41
  role of RTS/CTS, 41
IBMCOM forum, 29
IER, *see* interrupt enable register
IIR, *see* interrupt identification register
inferential procedures, 98, 99
information separators, 344
INKEY$, 70
INP, 30, 73
INPUT#, 56
INPUT$, 52
INSTR, 55
interrupt enable register, 38
interrupt identification register, 37
isolating transformer, 88, 96
isolation circuits, 92

Kalman filter, 99
Kermit, 83
  capture, 84
  control codes, 86
  initialisation file, 85
  log session, 84
  problems, 87
  protocol, 84
  terminal emulation, 85
key
  INKEY$, 70
  trapping extended keys, 70
  trapping keys, 70
key codes, 350
  table of, 352

LCR, *see* line control register
leakage current, 92, 95
least significant bit, 14
LF option, 48, 366
LF control character, 345
line control register, 34
line status register, 36
LOC, 65
LOF, 50
long integer (&) notation, 73
loopback, 33
  and modem control register, 33
LSB, *see* least significant bit
LSR, *see* line status register
LTRIM$, 66

mark/marking, 9
master clock, 28
  table of baud rate divisors, 28
mathematical packages, 102
MCR, *see* modem control register

memory address, 30
MID$, 71
Minolta Pulsox-7 pulse oximeter, 160
MOD, 66, 71
modem control register, 8, 33, 72
modem status register, 9, 35, 78
modulo arithmetic, *see* checksum
most significant bit, 14
moving average, 99
MSB, *see* most significant bit
MSR, *see* modem status register
Murray code, 12

NAK control character, 20, 346
Nellcor N-200E pulse oximeter, 129
  Σ-checksum, 138
NOT, 24, 73, 75
  logic table, 76
  one's complement, 24
  two's complement, 24
Novametrix
  500 pulse oximeter, 155
  505 pulse oximeter, 155
  515A pulse oximeter, 154
  520A pulse oximeter, 155
NUL control character, 344

O2SAT.COM program, 113
offset, 30
Ohmeda
  3700 pulse oximeter, 111
  3740 pulse oximeter, 111
  7800 ventilator, 295
  9000 syringe pump, 241
ON COM(n) GOSUB, 60
ON ERROR GOTO, 68
one's complement, 24
OP option, 47, 48, 366
OPEN, 56, 360
OPEN COM, 45, 364
  bad file-name error, 69
  execution of, 49
opening a data file, 56
opening the serial port, 45
OR, 73
  logic table, 74
  OR, 74, 75
OR, 74, 75
OS/2 and the serial port, 25
OUT, 30, 73
overrun error, 36
  and device I/O error, 69
  and line status register, 36
oximetry data, *see* pulse oximetry data

parity, 14, 15, 34
  and line control register, 34

Index

and ON COM statement, 46
errors and line status register, 36
parity error, 36, 69
PE option, 48, 366
table of parity options, 15
Pasterkamp & Daien program, 103, 112
patient circuit, 90
patient connection, 89
patient environment, 90
PC
  and electrical safety, 88
  and electrical Standards, 88, 95
  guidelines for safe use of PCs, 97
PE option, 48, 366
PEEK, 30
Pettitt's non-parametric test, 99
piecewise linear regression, 99
pin-outs
  table for 9-pin connectors, 6, 349
  table for 25/26-pin connectors, 6, 348
plotting the data, 369
  see also data analysis
POKE, 30
predictive procedures, 98, 99
PRINT, 50
PRINT#, 50
problems with RS-232, 10
programming, 29
protocol, 16
  ARQ protocol, 19, 20
  parameters, 46
  table of protocol options, 16
protocol options, 29
pulse oximeter
  Minolta Pulsox-7, 160
  Nellcor N-200E, 129
  Novametrix 500, 155
  Novametrix 505, 155
  Novametrix 515A, 154
  Novametrix 520A, 155
  Ohmeda 3700, 111
  Ohmeda 3740, 111
pulse oximetry data
  analysis, 102
  COLLECT.EXE, 177
  COMMANDER program, 112
  compressed spectral array plot, 102, 105
  cumulative distribution plot, 102, 104
  desaturation index, 103
  Evans *et al.* program, 103
  frequency distribution plot, 102, 104
  index of severity, 102
  inferential procedures, 105
  O2SAT.COM program, 113
  Pasterkamp & Daien program, 103, 112
  Taylor program, 103
  time plot, 102, 103
Pulsox-7 pulse oximeter, 160

QBserial 2.0 program, 20
QuickBASIC
  adding date & time, 57
  advantage over QBASIC, 44
  AND, 75, 76
    logic table, 76
  &H prefix, 73
  ASC option, 48, 365
  BIN option, 365
  CD option, 47, 366
  checksum, 71
  CHECKSUMHEX$ function, 71
  collecting reply codes, 63
  controlling output control lines, 72
  CS option, 47, 366
  data-bits, 46
  DATE$, 57
  DS option, 47, 366
  ELAPSEDTIME$ function, 66
  EMPTYBUFFER subroutine, 65
  EOR, *see* XOR
  ERDEV, 68
  ERDEV$, 68
  ERR, 68
  error messages, 69
  error trapping, 68
  exclusive OR, *see* XOR
  exit routine, 70
  FULLCODE subroutine, 57
  GETREPLY subroutine, 63, 64
  GNUPLOT, 371
  hexadecimal numbers, 73
  INKEY$, 70
  INP, 73
  input control line status, 80
  INPUT#, 56
  INPUT$, 52
  inputting data from the serial port, 51
  LaTeX, 371
  LF option, 48, 366
  LOC, 65
  LOF, 50
  LTRIM$, 66
  MID$, 71
  MOD, 71
  monitoring input control lines, 78
  NOT, 75
    logic table, 76
  ON COM(n) GOSUB, 60
  ON ERROR GOTO, 68
  OP option, 47, 366
  OPEN, 56, 360
  OPEN COM, 45, 364
  opening a data file, 56
  opening the serial port, 45

400 Index

optional OPEN COM parameters, 46, 364
OR, 74, 75
   logic table, 74
OUT, 73
outputting data, 50
parity, 46
PE option, 48, 366
PRINT, 50
PRINT#, 50
protocol, 46
protocol parameters, 46
quit routine, 70
RB option, 48, 366
reading a register, 73
receive buffer, 51
   emptying the buffer, 64
RESUME, 68
RIGHT$, 71
RS option, 47, 367
SEND subroutine, 63
setting a bit HIGH, 74
setting a bit LOW, 75
SGN, 79
SLEEP, 67
stop-bits, 46
STR$, 66
table of protocol parameters, 46
TB option, 48, 367
testing for a HIGH bit, 79
testing for a LOW bit, 78
TEX, 371
text-based utilities, 371
TIME$, 57
time delay, 67
TIMER, 66, 67
trapping keys, 70
TWOSCHECKSUM$ function, 72
WRITE#, 47
   problems with WRITE#, 51
writing to a register, 73
XON/XOFF not supported, 20
XOR, 77
   logic table, 77
quit routine, 70

RB option, 48, 366
RDR, *see* received data register
receive buffer
   emptying the buffer, 64
   RB option, 48, 366
received data register, 32
receiving data line, *see* RxD
reference clock, 28
   crystal frequencies, 29
   table of baud rate divisors, 28
references, 385
register-select lines, 27

registers, 26
   baud rate divisor latch register, 40
   bit-mapped registers, 31
   FIFO control register, 39
   interrupt enable register, 38
   interrupt identification register, 37
   line control register, 34
   line status register, 36
   modem control register, 33, 72
   modem status register, 35, 78
   numerical registers, 31
   offset, 31
   port address, 30
   reading a register, 73
   received data register, 32
   register addresses, 30
   setting a bit HIGH, 74
   setting a bit LOW, 75
   table giving offset, 31
   table of, 26, 30
   testing for a HIGH bit, 79
   testing for a LOW bit, 78
   transmitter holding register, 32
   writing to a register, 73
reinforced insulation, 91, 92
reply codes, 63
request to send, *see* RTS
resident clock, 17
RESUME, 68
RI, 8, 9
   and modem status register, 35
   monitoring RI status, 78
RIGHT$, 66, 71
ring indicator, *see* RI
RS option, 47, 367
RS control character, 347
RS-232 interface, *see* serial interface
RS-232 Standard, 3
RS-422, 10
RS-423, 10
RS-485, 10
RTS, 8, 41, 77
   and modem control register, 33, 72
   control line subroutine SETRTS, 77
   programming the RTS status, 72
   RS option, 47, 367
SETRTS subroutine, 77
RxD, 7, 8, 12

scan codes, 350
SEND subroutine, 63
serial interface, 3, 4
   base address, 30, 31
   circuits, 5, 8
   circuits renamed, 5
   compatibility with RS-423, 10
   connectors, 9

Index

control circuits, 7
data circuits, 7
diagram of circuits, 8
distance limitations, 11
DLAB, 31
ground circuits, 7, 11
input circuits, 8
number of serial ports, 25
opening the serial port, 45
output circuits, 8
problems with RS-232, 10
table for 9-pin connectors, 6, 349
table for 25/26-pin connectors, 6, 348
timing of line sampling, 16
voltages, 9
serial port, *see* serial interface
SETDTR subroutine, 77
SETRTS subroutine, 77
SGN, 79, 80
shield, 7
SHOW.COM, 65, 201, 284
SI control character, 345
SIA, 25
signal ground, 7, 8
simulator program, 358
SLEEP, 67
SO control character, 345
software handshaking, 19
 QBserial 2.0 program, 20
software tools, 100
SOH control character, 344
space/spacing, 9
spectral array plot, 102, 105, 106
spirometer
 Vitalograph Compact II, 272
spreadsheet packages, 100
Standards for electrical safety, 88
Standards for isolating transformers, 88
Standards for PCs, 88, 95
start-bit, 13, 15
statistical tests for oximetry data
 inferential procedures, 105
 table of, 107
statistics packages, 101
stop-bit, 13, 15, 34
 and line control register, 34
 and ON COM statement, 46
STR$, 66
STX control character, 20, 21, 344
SUB control character, 346
subroutine
 CHECKSUMHEX$, 71
 ELAPSEDTIME$, 66
 EMPTYBUFFER, 65
 FULLCODE, 57, 280
 GETREPLY, 63, 64
 SEND, 63

SETDTR, 77
SETRTS, 77
TWOSCHECKSUM$, 72
SYN control character, 346
syringe pump
 Graseby 3400, 211
 Ohmeda 9000, 241

Taylor oximetry program, 103
TB option, 48, 367
TC-checksum, *see* checksum
THR, *see* transmitter holding register
TIME$, 57
time
 ELAPSEDTIME$ function, 66
 resident clock, 17
 TIME$, 57
 TIMER, 66, 67
time delays, 67
time-out, 36, 46
 and line status register, 36
 CD option, 47, 366
 CS option, 47, 366
 CTS time-out, 42
 DS option, 47, 366
 DSR time-out, 42
 OP option, 47, 366
 using TIMER, 67
time plot, 102, 103
time series, 99
TIMER, 66, 67
tracking function, 99
trailing edge, 35
transmission control characters, 343
 table of, 20
transmit buffer
 remaining space using LOF, 50
 TB option, 48, 367
transmitter holding register, 32
transmitting data line, *see* TxD
trapping keys, 70
two's complement checksum, *see* checksum
TWOSCHECKSUM$ function, 72
TxD, 7, 8, 12
type B equipment, 93, 96
type BF equipment, 93
type CF equipment, 93

UART, 25
 8250, 25
 16450, 25
 16C1450, 33
 16550, 25
 16C1550, 33
 82510, 26
 bugs, 27
 DART, 25

DLAB, 27
FIFO buffers, 26
FIFO control register, 27
master clock, 28
port address, 30
protocol options, 29
reference clock, 28
register addresses, 30
register-select lines, 27
registers, 32
SIA, 25
table of baud rate divisors, 28
table of COM port addresses, 31
table of devices, 25
table of register addresses, 31
table of registers, 27
USART, 25
utilities for determining the UART, 29
UCASE$, 70
Ultima series of monitors (Datex), 176
US control character, 347

ventilator

Dräger Evita, 313
Ohmeda 7800, 295
VIEW.EXE, 65
viewing a data file, 65
Vitalograph Compact II spirometer, 272
voltage transition, 16
voltages, 9
VT control character, 345

WRITE#, 47
problems with WRITE#, 51

XMODEM, 21
XMODEM-1K, 21
XMODEM/CRC, 21
XOFF, 19, 20
and printers, 20
XON, 19, 20
and printers, 20
XOR, 77
logic table, 77

ZMODEM, 21